FINES PAYABLE
IF OVERDUE

This book is due for return on or before the last date shown below.

28 days
from 16/11.

Disorders of Thrombosis
and Hemostasis in Pregnancy

Hannah Cohen • Patrick O'Brien
Editors

Disorders of Thrombosis and Hemostasis in Pregnancy

A Guide to Management

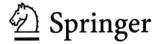 Springer

Editors

Hannah Cohen, MD, FRCP, FRCPath
Department of Haematology
University College London Hospitals
United Kingdom

Patrick O'Brien, FRCOG, FFSRH, FICOG
Department of Obstetrics and
Gynaecology
University College London Hospitals
United Kingdom

ISBN 978-1-4471-4410-6   ISBN 978-1-4471-4411-3   (eBook)
DOI 10.1007/978-1-4471-4411-3
Springer London Heidelberg New York Dordrecht

Library of Congress Control Number: 2012954610

Printed on acid-free paper

Springer is part of Springer Science+Business Media (www.springer.com)

Preface

This book provides a contemporary and comprehensive guide to all those involved in the management of hematological disorders in pregnancy. It covers a wide range of important clinical disorders that are associated with a potentially significant risk of morbidity and mortality in both the mother and the baby. The focus in each chapter is on authoritative, practical clinical advice, in the context of the available scientific evidence, on the management of women with both common and rare disorders of thrombosis and hemostasis in pregnancy. Included also are disorders where the management of thrombotic aspects are highly relevant such as cardiac disorders, hemoglobinopathies, and assisted conception. In addition, many chapters include case studies that highlight the pertinent clinical aspects of the topics covered. It is well recognized that in this population many recommendations are based on observational studies and extrapolation from other populations rather than on appropriately designed clinical trials, and this is reflected in some degree of variation in the opinions expressed in different chapters. The approach is multidisciplinary—the authorship brings together wide-ranging expertise in hematology, obstetrics and gynecology, obstetric medicine, cardiology, neonatology and assisted conception, resulting in a unique and clinically indispensable resource. This book will therefore be of interest and value to all those involved in the management of women with disorders of thrombosis and hemostasis in pregnancy and fertility treatment—hematologists, obstetricians and gynecologists, midwives and obstetric and general physicians, as well as neonatologists, at both consultant and trainee level.

Hannah Cohen, MD, FRCP, FRCPath
Patrick O'Brien, FRCOG, FFSRH, FICOG

Contents

Hemostatic Changes in Normal Pregnancy

Carolyn Millar and Mike Laffan

Abstract

Hemostasis represents a balance between pro- and anti-coagulant processes, with variations in this balance determining the net outcome. Significant physiological changes during pregnancy result in a hypercoagulable and hypofibrinolytic state that serves to protect the mother from bleeding complications at the time of placental separation. This chapter describes the effects of pregnancy on parameters of primary hemostasis, coagulation factors, anticoagulant pathways and the fibrinolytic system.

1.1 Introduction

Under normal conditions, blood flows within the vascular system, transporting oxygen, nutrients, and hormonal information around the body and removing metabolic waste. The confinement of circulating blood to the vascular bed and maintenance of blood fluidity are dependent upon a complex hemostatic system that involves interaction between the vasculature, platelets, coagulation factors, and the fibrinolytic system. Such interaction enables the stimulation of coagulation following injury, limits the extent of the response to the area of injury, and initiates the eventual breakdown of the clot as part of the process of healing. Thus, hemostasis may be viewed as a delicate balance between the pro- and anticoagulant processes, with variations in this balance determining the net outcome.

As well as a significant expansion in plasma volume, normal pregnancy is accompanied by major changes in the maternal hemostatic system, most likely mediated by hormonal influences, the net effect of which is to create a state of hypercoagulability and hypofibrinolysis. Together with the stemming of placental blood flow by myometrial contraction, these changes protect the mother from bleeding complications at the time of delivery. However, potentiation of the coagulation system also confers an increased risk of venous thromboembolism (VTE) and disseminated intravascular coagulation (DIC), leading causes of morbidity and mortality in pregnancy and the postpartum period.

In order to understand the physiological effects of pregnancy on the hemostatic system, an appreciation of hemostasis in the nonpregnant individual is required. Thus, while this chapter will focus on the hemostatic changes during pregnancy, each will

C. Millar, MD, MRCP, FRCPath (✉)
M. Laffan, DM, FRCP, FRCPath
Centre for Haematology,
Hammersmith Campus,
Imperial College London,
Du Cane Road,
London W12 0NN, UK
e-mail: c.millar@imperial.ac.uk; m.laffan@imperial.ac.uk

H. Cohen, P. O'Brien (eds.), *Disorders of Thrombosis and Hemostasis in Pregnancy*,
DOI 10.1007/978-1-4471-4411-3_1, © Springer-Verlag London 2012

be discussed in the context of normal hemostatic processes. It should be borne in mind that although these will be covered individually, they should not be considered to act in isolation. Furthermore, caution needs to be exercised when interpreting data obtained from studies in pregnancy. Data reported from these studies are often conflicting, and the study design and methods by which data are analyzed and reported require careful consideration. For example, it is generally preferable to obtain serial measurements from women throughout pregnancy rather than a set of cross-sectional data from different groups. This will allow the detection of subgroups and effects of starting (pre- or early pregnancy) values although it may be possible to derive reference ranges from cross-sectional studies providing the sample size is sufficiently large. Nonetheless, the reader should be aware that individual cases may deviate from the pooled data.

1.2 Primary Hemostasis

1.2.1 Platelets

Platelets are produced in the bone marrow by megakaryocytes and have a circulating life span of approximately 10 days. Following vascular injury, platelets adhere to the subendothelium, either directly to collagen via glycoprotein (GP) IaIIa and GPVI or indirectly via von Willebrand factor (VWF) and GPIb. Adhesion initiates platelet activation, with release of granular contents, notably ADP, and the synthesis of thromboxane A2. These factors have a positive feedback effect and activate more platelets, which are captured by VWF also released from platelet granules. Platelet activation is completed by a platelet shape change and a conformational change in the GPIIbIIIa receptor resulting in platelet aggregates held together by VWF and fibrinogen. These effects are normally counterbalanced by the active flow of blood and the endothelial production of prostacyclin, nitric oxide, and ADPase, which suppress platelet activation and prevent inappropriate platelet aggregation.

During pregnancy, there is a physiological decrease in the maternal platelet count of approximately 10 % [1–4]. While the resultant platelet count

at term is usually maintained within the normal range, the prevalence of gestational thrombocytopenia, as defined by a platelet count of less than $150 \times 10^9 \, L^{-1}$, has been shown to range between 5 and 12 % in population-based studies [4–6]. Subsequently, the platelet count has been shown to rise on days 2–5 postpartum [7]. The degree of thrombocytopenia is mild in most cases of gestational thrombocytopenia, with platelet counts of greater than $115 \times 10^9 \, L^{-1}$ reported in more than 80 % of cases, but a level down to $80 \times 10^9 \, L^{-1}$ is regarded as normal [4]. Factors such as hemodilution and accelerated platelet clearance that may contribute to the fall in platelet count have not been well defined. Earlier studies do not consistently show reduced platelet survival in pregnancy [8, 9], and means of directly assessing platelet lifespan are limited in pregnant women. It is possible that the increase in platelet volume reported in conjunction with falling platelet counts in the third trimester indicates a state of increased platelet destruction [10, 11]. Moreover, while enhanced platelet activation has been demonstrated in pregnancies complicated by hypertension or preeclampsia, it is less clear whether this occurs in normal pregnancy. Spontaneous platelet aggregation, increased platelet reactivity to arachidonic acid, and, more recently, increased platelet activation and adhesion have been variously demonstrated in normotensive pregnant women [12–14]. Increased numbers of circulating platelet aggregates and a rise in levels of β-thromboglobulin, platelet factor 4, and thromboxane B2 (the stable product of thromboxane A2) have also been reported, all suggestive of enhanced platelet reactivity [15–17]. Thus, there is some evidence of increased platelet activation in uncomplicated pregnancies, but it is not clear to what extent this contributes to the fall in platelet count. Some increased activation would be consistent with other evidence for coagulation activation that is exaggerated in preeclampsia. Platelet aggregation has been shown to return to normal by 6 weeks postpartum [12, 13].

1.2.2 Von Willebrand Factor

Von Willebrand factor is a multimeric glycoprotein synthesized by endothelial cells and megakaryocytes that mediates the adhesion of platelet to sites of injury and promotes platelet-platelet aggregation. In addition to its adhesive properties, VWF is a specific carrier for factor VIII (FVIII), and the VWF/FVIII complex usually circulates with a molar ratio of FVIII to VWF monomer of 1:50 (although this is defined as a ratio of 1 in units/dL). Levels of maternal VWF rise progressively with advancing gestational age, increasing early in the first trimester of pregnancy and continuing to increase thereafter [1, 18, 19]. By the time of delivery, levels of VWF may have reached double or more those of the nonpregnant state, falling rapidly following delivery and returning to baseline non-pregnant values within a few weeks [2, 18–21]. Factor VIII levels also increase progressively throughout pregnancy [2, 18, 19, 22], rising early in the first trimester and returning to near-normal values by around 8 weeks postpartum [22]. The increase in FVIII has been shown in some studies to parallel the rise in VWF levels, thus maintaining the VWF:Ag/FVIII ratio close to normal [18, 19, 23]. Other studies have demonstrated an increase in this ratio, in particular during the third trimester of pregnancy [2, 20, 21, 24, 25], reflecting a relatively greater rise in VWF levels with advancing gestation. This discrepancy may reflect variation in the degree of endothelial perturbation, as it is recognized that the rise in VWF levels is greater in conditions associated with endothelial cell damage such as preeclampsia [24, 25]. The functional activity of VWF is determined by its multimeric size, which is regulated by the protease ADAMTS13. Studies of ADAMTS13 during pregnancy have shown a mild progressive decrease in its activity from early in the second trimester until the first or second postpartum day [26, 27], and discrepancies between ADAMTS13 antigen and activity have been reported in pregnancy in older mothers [28]. A reduction in ADAMTS13 activity would be consistent with a reported disproportionate increase in large VWF multimers in the third trimester [24] and an increase in the specific functional activity of VWF, although this finding is not consistently reported [19, 21].

1.2.3 Hematocrit

Hematocrit also plays a role in primary hemostasis by influencing blood viscosity and platelet adhesion. However, as with the decreased platelet count, any decrease in platelet adhesion that may result from a reduction in hematocrit appears to be outweighed by the increase in VWF levels. This is discussed further when we consider global measures of primary hemostatic function.

1.3 Coagulation System

Blood coagulation pathways center on the generation of thrombin [29], which cleaves fibrinogen to generate fibrin, the structural scaffold that stabilizes platelet aggregates at sites of vascular injury [30].

1.3.1 Initiation of Coagulation

The extrinsic or tissue factor (TF)-dependent pathway of coagulation represents the major route by which thrombin generation is initiated in response to vessel damage. TF is an integral membrane protein and is the only procoagulant factor that does not require proteolytic activation. TF is primarily located at extravascular sites that are not usually exposed to the blood under normal physiological conditions [31]. As a result, the blood only encounters TF-presenting cells thus activating the extrinsic pathway, at sites of vascular injury. This dogma has been challenged by the identification of microparticle-associated TF and an alternatively transcribed, soluble TF molecule in blood, both of which have been implicated in the development of thrombosis [32, 33].

As well as being the principal initiator of coagulation, TF is essential for other cellular processes including implantation, embryogenesis, and angiogenesis [34]. The decidua and placenta are both rich sources of TF, with high levels of expression on syncytiotrophoblasts, while tissue factor pathway inhibitor (TFPI) is expressed in human umbilical vein endothelial cells [35]. Progesterone has been shown to upregulate TF gene expression by decidualized endometrial stromal cells, principally mediated by the promoter-specific transcription factor Sp1 [36]. This may be relevant in reducing postimplantation hemorrhage, although few studies have addressed the role of TF and TFPI in the pathogenesis of gestational complications [37].

1.3.2 Overview of Coagulation and Its Regulation

Following the exposure of TF-presenting cells to the blood, TF comes into contact with factor VII (FVII), a fraction (~1 %) of which circulates in its active form, FVIIa. TF binds both FVII and FVIIa with high affinity. The trace amount of TF-FVIIa that forms is enough to activate factor X (FX) both directly (extrinsic pathway) and indirectly via activation of factor IX (FIX) [38, 39]. However, FXa production by this route is rapidly terminated by the action of TFPI which binds FXa and VIIa forming an inactive TF-VIIa-Xa-TFPI complex. The limited quantities of FXa that are generated via this route facilitate the inefficient conversion of trace quantities of prothrombin to thrombin [40, 41]. The low concentrations of thrombin that arise mediate the feedback activation of the cofactors FVIII and factor V (FV). Binding of FIXa to FVIIIa forming the intrinsic tenase activates further FX thus bypassing the reliance upon TF-FVIIa as a source of FXa generation. The subsequent assembly of FXa and FVa on activated platelets (prothrombinase) leads to a rapid burst in thrombin generation at the site of vessel damage. Binding of the intrinsic tenase and prothrombinase complexes to the phospholipid surfaces expressed by platelets is mediated by calcium ions bound to the terminal gamma-carboxy residues on FXa and FIXa. Gamma-carboxylation of glutamic acid residues on FIX and FX as well as prothrombin and FVII requires vitamin K.

Fibrin is produced by proteolytic cleavage of fibrinogen by thrombin with the release of fibrinopeptides A and B and precipitation of insoluble fibrin monomer followed by polymerization and cross-linkage by factor XIII (FXIII). Thrombin has many functions that influence both coagulation and the vascular system; in addition to cleaving fibrinogen to produce fibrin and acti-

vating FVIII and FV as described above, other procoagulant functions of thrombin include the activation of platelets, factor XI (FXI), FXIII, and thrombin-activatable fibrinolysis inhibitor (TAFI).

1.3.3 Effect of Pregnancy on Coagulation Factors

As already discussed, normal pregnancy is accompanied by a rise in the plasma concentration of FVIII, which is likely to be secondary, at least in part, to increased VWF levels. Pregnancy also results in substantial progressive increases in the plasma concentrations of FVII [2, 42, 43] and fibrinogen [2, 3, 22, 42]. The increase in FVII levels appears to be greatest in the second trimester of pregnancy, with rises of around 50 % observed by the early third trimester [2, 42]. FVII levels fall sharply after delivery [2]. By term, levels of fibrinogen may reach double their prepregnancy values, and fall more slowly following delivery, returning to basal levels within 5 weeks postpartum [2, 3, 42]. A modest gradual increase in the plasma concentration of FX is apparent until around 30 weeks' gestation, following which there are reports of both a persistent elevation and a mild fall in levels through the remainder of pregnancy [2, 19, 20, 42]. Levels of prothrombin and FV remain unchanged throughout pregnancy [2, 19, 42, 44]. Data available regarding the effect of pregnancy on plasma concentrations of FIX and FXI are variable; several early studies reported a steady increase in FIX levels with advancing gestation [45–47], but no significant effect on FIX levels was shown in a subsequent cross-sectional study [19]. A longitudinal study has confirmed the earlier findings, demonstrating FIX levels at delivery to be above the nonpregnant upper reference value in approximately 50 % of women, with a further rise during the early puerperal period [42]. The finding of a prolonged activated partial thromboplastin time (APTT) at term not infrequently results in the incidental finding of reduced FXI levels, which subsequently normalize in the months following delivery. Indeed, a progressive decrease in FXI levels throughout pregnancy has been found in several studies, reaching a nadir at term [20, 48, 49]. There are also reports of unchanged FXI levels in pregnancy, although these studies report grouped data and may not detect individual trends [19, 42].

It has been shown that, following an initial early increase, FXIII levels have been shown to gradually fall throughout pregnancy, reaching levels around half nonpregnant values by term [50]. The significance of this is not clear because the minimum hemostatic level of FXIII is not established although some studies suggest that this might be low enough to increase the risk of bleeding.

There is considerable interindividual variation in the extent to which plasma levels of coagulation factors change with advancing gestational age. It is likely that some of the reduction is due to dilution caused by the progressive increase in plasma volume until around the 32nd week of gestation. However, as the plasma volume expands by approximately 50 %, increased synthesis is necessary to maintain clotting factor concentrations at equivalent nonpregnant values. This is most likely to be mediated by hormonal factors. Altered transcriptional activity in the presence of estrogenic factors has been demonstrated for some coagulation factors, with the identification of estrogen response elements in gene promoter regions [51]. Estrogen levels increase as pregnancy progresses; however, as with other placentally derived hormones, levels vary significantly between individuals [52].

1.4   Anticoagulant Pathways

The hemostatic response is confined to the site of injury by the action of inhibitory pathways preventing spontaneous activation of coagulation and generalized thrombosis. As already discussed, TFPI is the principal inhibitor of TF-mediated coagulation [53] and acts by binding and inhibiting FXa [54]. The resultant TFPI-FXa complex acts in a negative feedback loop through the binding and inactivation of TF-FVIIa [55] and in this way switches off the initiating procoagulant stimulus. This ensures that a small procoagulant stimulus does not elicit uncontrolled generation of thrombin. In addition to TFPI,

the normal hemostatic response is regulated by antithrombin and the protein C–protein S pathway. Together, these pathways modulate the generation and activity of thrombin and are critical for appropriate and controlled hemostatic plug formation.

1.4.1   Antithrombin

The half-life of thrombin in plasma is around 14 s. This is mainly due to the inhibitory action of antithrombin (previously designated antithrombin III), a plasma-borne serine protease inhibitor synthesized in the liver. Although antithrombin inactivates several protease substrates of the coagulation system, its main physiological targets are thrombin and FXa, and it is through the inhibition of these serine proteases that antithrombin exerts its anticoagulant function. These interactions are enhanced by the action of heparan sulfate proteoglycans, as well as exogenously administered heparins, on the surface of endothelial cells. The activity of antithrombin is reduced in liver disease and hypercoagulable states including DIC. However, there is little variation in the plasma concentration of antithrombin both during healthy pregnancy and following delivery [2, 3, 19, 20, 42, 56]. In contrast, modest effects on the thrombin inhibitors α_2-macroglobulin and heparin cofactor II (HCII) are found; the plasma concentration of α_2-macroglobulin is reduced and HCII activity increased in normal pregnancy [2, 57, 58], while HCII activity is reduced in pregnancies complicated by hypertension and preeclampsia [59].

1.4.2   Protein C and Protein S

Thrombin generation is also downregulated by the anticoagulant activities of protein C and its cofactor protein S, both vitamin K-dependent glycoproteins that are synthesized mainly in the liver. Protein C is activated by thrombin bound to thrombomodulin (TM), an integral membrane protein expressed on the surface of endothelial cells. This activation process is enhanced by a second endothelial cell surface protein, the endothelial cell protein C receptor (EPCR). Both the TM and

EPCR receptors are also expressed by placental trophoblasts. Aided by protein S, activated protein C (APC) catalyzes the inactivation of FVIIIa and FVa [60], thereby limiting further generation of thrombin. As the intact endothelium (i.e., adjacent to the site of vascular injury) normally expresses TM [61], thrombin diffusing away from the site of injury can bind to TM and its activity "switched" to impart an anticoagulant function [62]. Thus, the action of thrombin can be modulated depending on its location relative to the thrombus. In addition to its cofactor-mediated anticoagulant function, protein S has been shown to exhibit anticoagulant properties in the absence of APC, including cofactor activity for TFPI [63, 64].

Protein S circulates in plasma in two forms. Approximately 60 % is bound to complement 4b-binding protein (C4BP), a regulatory protein of the classical pathway of the complement system [65, 66], while the remaining 40 % is free. While it was previously thought that only protein S in its free form was active, APC cofactor activity for FVa and FVIIIa inactivation has now also been claimed for C4BP-bound protein S, albeit to a lesser degree than the activity of free protein S [67, 68]. Similarly, while TFPI cofactor activity has been suggested for bound protein S [63], recent data suggest that this is less potent than that of free protein S [69]. The implications of these recent findings for pregnancy-associated hemostasis remain to be clarified.

A decrease in the plasma concentration of protein S has been reported during both pregnancy and the puerperium, frequently to levels comparable to protein S-deficient heterozygotes. Two early cross-sectional studies showed plasma levels of both total and free protein S to be reduced in pregnancy, irrespective of whether the free protein S fraction was measured by an immunological or a functional method [70, 71]. The latter study showed more pronounced reductions in free protein S compared to total protein S that may be explained by the parallel increase in C4BP concentration; no change in C4BP was demonstrated in the former. Furthermore, concordant reductions in total and free protein S levels with no increase in C4BP have been found in women taking the combined oral contraceptive pill [71]. Together, these findings suggest that the reduction in protein S activity in pregnancy may not be wholly attributable to alterations in the free/bound protein S equilibrium. Similarly, progressive reductions throughout pregnancy in the plasma concentrations of both free and total protein S have subsequently been reported, with greater relative decreases in the free fraction [3, 19, 42]. The majority of studies report that the decrease in protein S levels begins early in the first trimester, with most reduction having occurred by the end of the second trimester [3, 19, 22, 42, 71]. A cross-sectional study demonstrated a significant decrease in the levels of free protein S from the 10th week of gestation, and total protein S levels from the 20th week, with no significant increase in C4BP at term compared to nonpregnant samples [72]. Total protein S has been shown to return to prepregnancy levels by the end of the first week postpartum [71], while levels of free protein S remain below the normal range in 15 % of women at 8 weeks postpartum [3, 22]; this should be considered when evaluating the results of thrombophilic tests.

It is possible that some of the discrepancies in findings are attributable to assay variability; however, the underlying mechanism for the decrease in protein S levels in pregnancy remains unclear. A dilution effect could account for some of the findings but would not explain the reduction in protein S levels associated with the combined oral contraceptive pill. Similarly, the reduction in free protein S levels may not be wholly attributable to increased C4BP levels, as has been the widely held view to date. Estrogen response elements have also been identified in the protein S gene promoter, which may alter the transcription activity of protein S, and this seems to offer the most likely explanation.

Unlike protein S, neither the concentration nor functional activity of protein C has been shown to be significantly affected by gestation [18, 19, 73]. Some minor variations in protein C activity have been demonstrated with a peak in levels in the second trimester; however, all values remained within the normal range [3, 18, 71]. Elevated protein C levels and activity have been reported in the early puerperal period with mean levels equivalent to nonpregnant upper reference values [19, 42, 74].

In addition to their anticoagulant activities, protein C and protein S appear to have other physiological effects including cellular protective, anti-inflammatory, and anti-apoptotic properties. Immunohistochemical analysis has recently demonstrated the deposition of protein S in damaged villi at the fetal-maternal interface, suggesting its involvement in the protection or restoration of damaged placental trophoblasts [72]. It is possible that protein S consumption at the fetal-maternal interface could contribute toward the observed reduction in its levels in pregnancy. Low levels of anti-protein S and anti-protein C antibodies have recently been shown in a cross-sectional study of healthy pregnant women, the significance of which is not known [75]. Plasma levels of anti-protein C antibodies were shown to decrease with advancing gestational age and were no longer detectable by the third trimester [75].

Measurable levels of soluble TM are found in plasma and are likely to derive from the proteolysis of endothelial cell TM. As well as being a potential marker of preeclampsia, TM levels have been shown to increase gradually during normal pregnancy and fall postpartum rapidly [76, 77].

1.5 Fibrinolytic System

The principal fibrinolytic enzyme is plasmin, which circulates in its inactive zymogen form, plasminogen. The activation of plasmin is mediated by two types of plasminogen activator: tissue type and urokinase type. Tissue plasminogen activator (tPA) is released into the blood by endothelium in its active form but does not activate plasminogen until they are brought together when they bind to fibrin. Plasmin is inhibited both directly by plasmin inhibitor (α_2-antiplasmin) and α_2-macroglobulin and indirectly by plasminogen activator inhibitor-1 (PAI-1) produced by endothelial cells and platelets. Plasmin activation is reduced by TAFI, which removes the terminal lysine residues from fibrin, to which tPA and plasminogen bind.

It has been a long-held view that maternal plasma fibrinolytic activity decreases in pregnancy, which has been attributed, at least in part, to the production of a plasminogen inhibitor by the placenta known as plasminogen activator inhibitor-2 (PAI-2) [2, 78, 79]. The decreased fibrinolytic activity reported by many of these studies is based on fibrin plate and clot lysis analyses of euglobulin fractions (which contain factors important in fibrinolysis: plasminogen, plasminogen activators (primarily tPA) and fibrinogen), although it is unclear how accurately these reflect the blood fibrinolytic capacity in pregnancy. In addition to PAI-2, the placenta and decidua are sources of PAI-1, levels of which have been shown to rise progressively throughout pregnancy, reaching at least fivefold basal values by term [1, 3, 22, 79]. The decidual expression of PAI-1 appears to be regulated by progesterone by similar mechanisms to those described for TF [80]. Circulating tPA antigen levels have been shown to remain constant or rise during pregnancy [76, 79, 81–83], and the increase in PAI-1 and PAI-2 leads to a decrease in the release of endothelial tPA [84] and its measurable activity [22, 79]. A rise in levels of urokinase-type plasminogen activator (uPA) antigen, which also appears to derive from the placenta, has also been demonstrated [83, 85]. Fibrinolytic activity may be further depressed in pregnancy by increased thrombin generation leading to an increase in TAFI activity [86–89]. A slight initial rise in α_2-macroglobulin levels followed by a steady fall throughout pregnancy and the postpartum period has been reported [2]. Levels of plasminogen and plasmin inhibitor appear to remain largely unchanged throughout pregnancy [83, 90]. A brisk fall in PAI-1 and rise in tPA activity immediately following delivery result in a rapid increase in fibrinolytic activity and a return to nonpregnant values within 3–5 days [2, 79, 83]. However, high levels of PAI-2 antigen persist for a further few days [83].

Despite the decrease in fibrinolytic activity, levels of fibrin degradation products including D-dimers have been shown to rise with advancing gestational age [3, 22, 42], but these reflect the enhanced coagulation activation in pregnancy. D-dimer concentrations rise above the level used for exclusion of VTE in over one quarter of women by the second trimester of pregnancy and in nearly all women by term [42], confounding their use in diagnosis. Levels peak at the first postpartum day and may take several weeks to return to normal [3, 22, 42]. Other measures that reflect increased in vivo thrombin generation or fibrin formation include the prothrombin fragment1.2 (PF1.2), thrombin-antithrombin complexes (TAT), and soluble fibrin polymer, all of which have been shown to increase during pregnancy [1, 3, 22, 91, 92].

1.6 Measures of Coagulation

1.6.1 Measures of Primary Hemostasis

The bleeding time is shortened in pregnant women [46], although its use in the evaluation of primary hemostasis has been largely abandoned or superseded by the platelet function analyzer (PFA-100™). The PFA-100 may be sensitive to quantitative and qualitative defects in platelets and VWF. The progressive shortening in PFA-100 closure times observed with advancing gestation mostly reflects the physiological rises in VWF levels.

1.6.2 Standard Coagulation Tests

The prothrombin time (PT), APTT and thrombin time (TT) may be normal or decreased in pregnancy with some variation in results according to the method and reagents used [3, 42, 46, 93]. While these findings may reflect some rises in procoagulant levels, standard coagulation tests are limited in their ability to reflect the overall coagulation potential of plasma.

1.6.3 Global Assays of Coagulation

The in vitro analysis of coagulation is facilitated by the use of global measures of hemostasis, which include thromboelastography (TEG) and rotational thromboelastometry (RoTEM). These assays take into consideration the activity of platelets and all plasma proteins relevant to coag-

ulation and therefore may provide a useful overall measure of thrombotic and hemorrhagic risk. TEG and RoTEM monitor hemostasis as a whole dynamic process, determining the kinetics of clot formation and growth as well as the strength and stability of the formed clot. These tests can be performed at the patient's bedside and are widely used in obstetric practice to provide an early and reliable assessment of coagulation problems associated with postpartum hemorrhage. The hypercoagulable state of pregnancy affects a number of the parameters recorded in the TEG and RoTEM profiles, resulting in shortening of the time for clot formation to reach a defined amplitude (k time and clot formation time [CFT], respectively), an increase in the clot amplitude early in clot formation, and an increase in maximum amplitude (MA) of the TEG tracing and its RoTEM equivalent, the maximum clot firmness (MCF) [46, 93, 94]. These findings are all consistent with increased concentrations of coagulation initiators (FVIIa-TF) and procoagulant factors, resulting in increased generation of thrombin. The shortened CFT and increased MCF are apparent in the first trimester, with the greatest changes occurring during the second trimester and persisting into the third trimester [93]. Shortening of the time from the start of measurement until the start of clot formation has been demonstrated by TEG (r time) [94]; however, surprisingly the equivalent measurement by RoTEM (clotting time, CT) has been shown not to be affected by pregnancy [93]. No effects on fibrinolytic parameters have been reported [93].

1.6.4 APC Resistance

The procoagulant state in pregnancy is also demonstrated in vitro as a poor anticoagulant response of plasma to APC, known as APC resistance (APCR) [95]. APCR is usually demonstrated by a reduction in the ratio of APTT in the presence and absence of added APC, known as the classic APC-sensitivity ratio (APC-SR). APCR mostly results from a mutation at an APC cleavage site in FV, R506Q, widely known as factor V Leiden [96], although it may be acquired in the presence of antiphospholipid antibodies [97] or other factors affecting the APTT such as high levels of FVIII or FIX [98, 99]. APCR is found to be increased in as many as 60 % of pregnancies, as well in users of oral contraceptives and hormone replacement therapy [22, 99–101]. While it is likely that increased FVIII and FIX levels contribute to the acquired APCR in pregnancy [19], correlation between these variables has not been consistently reported [19, 22, 102, 103].

The physiological significance of acquired APCR in pregnancy is not clear; APCR has been shown to be associated with an increased risk of preeclampsia; however, it is not routinely assessed in pregnant women [104].

1.7 Hemostasis in the Uteroplacental Circulation

The placenta is a highly vascularized organ functioning as the interface between fetal blood, which is confined to the villous blood vessels, and maternal blood, which flows in decidual arteries and washes the intervillous spaces in contact with syncytiotrophoblasts. Placental separation at birth presents a significant hemostatic challenge, and the interruption of blood flow to the placental site achieved by the combined effects of myometrial contraction and thrombotic occlusion of the sheared maternal vessels is balanced against maintaining the fluidity of maternal blood at the fetal-maternal interface. A detailed description of the physiological adaptation of the uteroplacental vasculature facilitating increased blood flow is beyond the scope of this book, and our understanding of hemostasis in the uteroplacental circulation is hampered by extremely limited available data. A transitory shortening of whole blood clotting time and pronounced increase in FVIII activity during placental separation have previously been demonstrated in blood samples obtained from the uterine vein [105]. Uterine venous samples have also demonstrated higher levels of fibrinolytic activity when compared to peripheral blood both during and immediately following placental separation [105]. Levels of TAT complexes, soluble fibrin polymer, D-dimers, and plasmin-

α2-antiplasmin complexes have all been shown to be higher in the uterine than peripheral maternal circulations [106].

1.8 Microparticles

Microparticles (MP) are formed by cytoskeleton structural rearrangements and are shed from cell membranes upon activation or apoptosis. MPs may be produced by all cell types; however, those derived from platelets, monocytes, and endothelial cells have been implicated in a number of prothrombotic disorders. MPs influence hemostasis by a variety of mechanisms, including increased TF and platelet activation, provision of a catalytic surface for assembly of intrinsic tenase and prothrombinase complexes, and endothelial activation resulting in increased VWF expression. Normal pregnancy is characterized by increased levels of platelet- and endothelial-derived MPs [107]; however, their relevance in gestational complications remains unclear. MPs are also produced during syncytiotrophoblast differentiation (often called STBMs) and are detectable in normal pregnancies by the second trimester, their numbers significantly increasing in the third trimester. STBMs interact with immune and endothelial cells and may contribute to the systemic maternal inflammatory reaction associated with pregnancy. This reaction is exaggerated in preeclampsia, in which higher levels of circulating STBMs have been demonstrated [108].

1.9 Summary

Hemorrhage remains a leading cause of maternal morbidity and mortality worldwide. The hypercoagulable state of pregnancy confers some degree of protection from hemorrhage during implantation and placental separation at delivery. However, this in turn predisposes women to VTE, which until recently was the most common direct cause of maternal mortality in the UK [109, 110]. Furthermore, the hypercoagulable state may contribute toward many complications of pregnancy including placental abruption and preeclampsia.

The change in the balance of hemostasis during pregnancy results from some major physiological changes which have been described here. It is important that these are not confused with similar changes outside pregnancy when their significance is quite different.

Learning Points

- Pregnancy is associated with a significant overall increase in the activity and potential of the hemostatic system.
- Pregnancy results in substantial rises in plasma levels of fibrinogen, VWF, FVII, and FVIII and modest rises in FIX and FX.
- Protein S and platelet levels fall during normal pregnancy.
- Levels of prothrombin, FV, antithrombin, and protein C do not vary significantly in pregnancy.
- The increase in coagulation activity may manifest in some standard laboratory tests such as D-dimer and APTT.
- Many of the coagulation changes take 6–8 weeks to return to normal after delivery.

References

1. Cadroy Y, Grandjean H, Pichon J, et al. Evaluation of six markers of haemostatic system in normal pregnancy and pregnancy complicated by hypertension or preeclampsia. Br J Obstet Gynaecol. 1993;100:416–20.
2. Stirling Y, Woolf L, North WR, Seghatchian MJ, Meade TW. Haemostasis in normal pregnancy. Thromb Haemost. 1984;52:176–82.
3. Bremme K, Ostlund E, Almqvist I, Heinonen K, Blomback M. Enhanced thrombin generation and fibrinolytic activity in normal pregnancy and the puerperium. Obstet Gynecol. 1992;80:132–7.
4. Boehlen F, Hohlfeld P, Extermann P, Perneger TV, de Moerloose P. Platelet count at term pregnancy: a reappraisal of the threshold. Obstet Gynecol. 2000;95:29–33.
5. Burrows RF, Kelton JG. Fetal thrombocytopenia and its relation to maternal thrombocytopenia. N Engl J Med. 1993;329:1463–6.
6. Sainio S, Kekomaki R, Riikonen S, Teramo K. Maternal thrombocytopenia at term: a population-based study. Acta Obstet Gynecol Scand. 2000;79:744–9.
7. Dahlstrom BL, Nesheim BI. Post partum platelet count in maternal blood. Acta Obstet Gynecol Scand. 1994;73:695–7.
8. Wallenburg HC, van Kessel PH. Platelet lifespan in normal pregnancy as determined by a nonradioisotopic technique. Br J Obstet Gynaecol. 1978;85:33–6.
9. Rakoczi I, Tallian F, Bagdany S, Gati I. Platelet lifespan in normal pregnancy and pre-eclampsia as determined by a non-radioisotope technique. Thromb Res. 1979;15:553–6.
10. Fay RA, Hughes AO, Farron NT. Platelets in pregnancy: hyperdestruction in pregnancy. Obstet Gynecol. 1983;61:238–40.
11. Sill PR, Lind T, Walker W. Platelet values during normal pregnancy. Br J Obstet Gynaecol. 1985;92:480–3.
12. Burgess-Wilson ME, Morrison R, Heptinstall S. Spontaneous platelet aggregation in heparinised blood during pregnancy. Thromb Res. 1986;41:385–93.
13. Morrison R, Crawford J, MacPherson M, Heptinstall S. Platelet behaviour in normal pregnancy, pregnancy complicated by essential hypertension and pregnancy-induced hypertension. Thromb Haemost. 1985;54:607–11.
14. Karalis I, Nadar SK, Al Yemeni E, Blann AD, Lip GY. Platelet activation in pregnancy-induced hypertension. Thromb Res. 2005;116:377–83.
15. O'Brien WF, Saba HI, Knuppel RA, Scerbo JC, Cohen GR. Alterations in platelet concentration and aggregation in normal pregnancy and preeclampsia. Am J Obstet Gynecol. 1986;155:486–90.
16. Fitzgerald DJ, Mayo G, Catella F, Entman SS, FitzGerald GA. Increased thromboxane biosynthesis in normal pregnancy is mainly derived from platelets. Am J Obstet Gynecol. 1987;157:325–30.
17. Douglas JT, Lowe GD, Forbes CD, Prentice CR. Beta-thromboglobulin and platelet counts – effect of malignancy, infection, age and obesity. Thromb Res. 1982;25:459–64.
18. Mahieu B, Jacobs N, Mahieu S, et al. Haemostatic changes and acquired activated protein C resistance in normal pregnancy. Blood Coagul Fibrinolysis. 2007;18:685–8.
19. Clark P, Brennand J, Conkie JA, McCall F, Greer IA, Walker ID. Activated protein C sensitivity, protein C, protein S and coagulation in normal pregnancy. Thromb Haemost. 1998;79:1166–70.
20. Hellgren M, Blomback M. Studies on blood coagulation and fibrinolysis in pregnancy, during delivery and in the puerperium. I. Normal condition. Gynecol Obstet Invest. 1981;12:141–54.
21. Sanchez-Luceros A, Meschengieser SS, Marchese C, et al. Factor VIII and von Willebrand factor changes during normal pregnancy and puerperium. Blood Coagul Fibrinolysis. 2003;14:647–51.
22. Kjellberg U, Andersson NE, Rosen S, Tengborn L, Hellgren M. APC resistance and other haemostatic variables during pregnancy and puerperium. Thromb Haemost. 1999;81:527–31.
23. Sie P, Caron C, Azam J, et al. Reassessment of von Willebrand factor (VWF), VWF propeptide, factor VIII:C and plasminogen activator inhibitors 1 and 2

during normal pregnancy. Br J Haematol. 2003;121: 897–903.

24. Brenner B, Zwang E, Bronshtein M, Seligsohn U. von Willebrand factor multimer patterns in pregnancy-induced hypertension. Thromb Haemost. 1989;62: 715–7.

25. Bergmann F, Rotmensch S, Rosenzweig B, How H, Chediak J. The role of von Willebrand factor in pre-eclampsia. Thromb Haemost. 1991;66:525–8.

26. Sanchez-Luceros A, Farias CE, Amaral MM, et al. von Willebrand factor-cleaving protease (ADAMTS13) activity in normal non-pregnant women, pregnant and post-delivery women. Thromb Haemost. 2004;92:1320–6.

27. Mannucci PM, Canciani MT, Forza I, Lussana F, Lattuada A, Rossi E. Changes in health and disease of the metalloprotease that cleaves von Willebrand factor. Blood. 2001;98:2730–5.

28. Feys HB, Deckmyn H, Vanhoorelbeke K. ADAMTS13 in health and disease. Acta Haematol. 2009;121:183–5.

29. Mann KG. Thrombin formation. Chest. 2003;124: 4S–10.

30. Savage B, Cattaneo M, Ruggeri ZM. Mechanisms of platelet aggregation. Curr Opin Hematol. 2001;8: 270–6.

31. Wilcox JN, Smith KM, Schwartz SM, Gordon D. Localization of tissue factor in the normal vessel wall and in the atherosclerotic plaque. Proc Natl Acad Sci USA. 1989;86:2839–43.

32. Bogdanov VY, Balasubramanian V, Hathcock J, Vele O, Lieb M, Nemerson Y. Alternatively spliced human tissue factor: a circulating, soluble, thrombogenic protein. Nat Med. 2003;9:458–62.

33. Falati S, Liu Q, Gross P, et al. Accumulation of tissue factor into developing thrombi in vivo is dependent upon microparticle P-selectin glycoprotein ligand 1 and platelet P-selectin. J Exp Med. 2003;197:1585–98.

34. Mackman N. Role of tissue factor in hemostasis, thrombosis, and vascular development. Arterioscler Thromb Vasc Biol. 2004;24:1015–22.

35. Aharon A, Brenner B, Katz T, Miyagi Y, Lanir N. Tissue factor and tissue factor pathway inhibitor levels in trophoblast cells: implications for placental hemostasis. Thromb Haemost. 2004;92:776–86.

36. Krikun G, Schatz F, Mackman N, Guller S, Demopoulos R, Lockwood CJ. Regulation of tissue factor gene expression in human endometrium by transcription factors Sp1 and Sp3. Mol Endocrinol. 2000;14:393–400.

37. Dusse LM, Carvalho MG, Cooper AJ, Lwaleed BA. Tissue factor and tissue factor pathway inhibitor: a potential role in pregnancy and obstetric vascular complications? Clin Chim Acta. 2006;372:43–6.

38. Morrison SA, Jesty J. Tissue factor-dependent activation of tritium-labeled factor IX and factor X in human plasma. Blood. 1984;63:1338–47.

39. Osterud B, Rapaport SI. Activation of factor IX by the reaction product of tissue factor and factor VII:

additional pathway for initiating blood coagulation. Proc Natl Acad Sci USA. 1977;74:5260–4.

40. Esmon CT, Owen WG, Jackson CM. The conversion of prothrombin to thrombin. V. The activation of prothrombin by factor Xa in the presence of phospholipid. J Biol Chem. 1974;249:7798–807.

41. Dahlback B, Stenflo J. The activation of prothrombin by platelet-bound factor Xa. Eur J Biochem. 1980;104: 549–57.

42. Szecsi PB, Jorgensen M, Klajnbard A, Andersen MR, Colov NP, Stender S. Haemostatic reference intervals in pregnancy. Thromb Haemost. 2010;103:718–27.

43. Dalaker K, Prydz H. The coagulation factor VII in pregnancy. Br J Haematol. 1984;56:233–41.

44. Nilsson IM, Kullander S. Coagulation and fibrinolytic studies during pregnancy. Acta Obstet Gynecol Scand. 1967;46:273–85.

45. Todd ME, Thompson Jr JH, Bowie EJ, Owen Jr CA. Changes in blood coagulation during pregnancy. Mayo Clin Proc. 1965;40:370–83.

46. Beller FK, Ebert C. The coagulation and fibrinolytic enzyme system in pregnancy and in the puerperium. Eur J Obstet Gynecol Reprod Biol. 1982;13:177–97.

47. Fresh JW, Ferguson JH, Lewis JH. Blood-clotting studies in parturient women and the newborn. Obstet Gynecol. 1956;7:117–27.

48. Phillips LL, Rosano L, Skrodelis V. Changes in factor XI (plasma thromboplastin antecedent) levels during pregnancy. Am J Obstet Gynecol. 1973;116:1114–6.

49. Nossel HL, Lanzkowsky P, Levy S, Mibashan RS, Hansen JD. A study of coagulation factor levels in women during labour and in their newborn infants. Thromb Diath Haemorrh. 1966;16:185–97.

50. Persson BL, Stenberg P, Holmberg L, Astedt B. Transamidating enzymes in maternal plasma and placenta in human pregnancies complicated by intrauterine growth retardation. J Dev Physiol. 1980;2:37–46.

51. Di Bitondo R, Hall AJ, Peake IR, Iacoviello L, Winship PR. Oestrogenic repression of human coagulation factor VII expression mediated through an oestrogen response element sequence motif in the promoter region. Hum Mol Genet. 2002;11:723–31.

52. Smith R, Smith JI, Shen X, et al. Patterns of plasma corticotropin-releasing hormone, progesterone, estradiol, and estriol change and the onset of human labor. J Clin Endocrinol Metab. 2009;94:2066–74.

53. Bajaj MS, Birktoft JJ, Steer SA, Bajaj SP. Structure and biology of tissue factor pathway inhibitor. Thromb Haemost. 2001;86:959–72.

54. Huang ZF, Wun TC, Broze Jr GJ. Kinetics of factor Xa inhibition by tissue factor pathway inhibitor. J Biol Chem. 1993;268:26950–5.

55. Broze Jr GJ, Warren LA, Novotny WF, Higuchi DA, Girard JJ, Miletich JP. The lipoprotein-associated coagulation inhibitor that inhibits the factor VII-tissue factor complex also inhibits factor Xa: insight into its possible mechanism of action. Blood. 1988;71: 335–43.

56. Weiner CP, Brandt J. Plasma antithrombin III activity in normal pregnancy. Obstet Gynecol. 1980;56:601–3.

57. Massouh M, Jatoi A, Gordon EM, Ratnoff OD. Heparin cofactor II activity in plasma during pregnancy and oral contraceptive use. J Lab Clin Med. 1989;114:697–9.

58. Uchikova EH, Ledjev II. Changes in haemostasis during normal pregnancy. Eur J Obstet Gynecol Reprod Biol. 2005;119:185–8.

59. Bellart J, Gilabert R, Cabero L, Fontcuberta J, Monasterio J, Miralles RM. Heparin cofactor II: a new marker for pre-eclampsia. Blood Coagul Fibrinolysis. 1998;9:205–8.

60. Esmon CT. The protein C pathway. Chest. 2003;124: 26S–32.

61. Maruyama I, Bell CE, Majerus PW. Thrombomodulin is found on endothelium of arteries, veins, capillaries, and lymphatics, and on syncytiotrophoblast of human placenta. J Cell Biol. 1985;101:363–71.

62. Esmon CT, Esmon NL, Harris KW. Complex formation between thrombin and thrombomodulin inhibits both thrombin-catalyzed fibrin formation and factor V activation. J Biol Chem. 1982;257:7944–7.

63. Hackeng TM, Sere KM, Tans G, Rosing J. Protein S stimulates inhibition of the tissue factor pathway by tissue factor pathway inhibitor. Proc Natl Acad Sci USA. 2006;103:3106–11.

64. Hackeng TM, van't Veer C, Meijers JC, Bouma BN. Human protein S inhibits prothrombinase complex activity on endothelial cells and platelets via direct interactions with factors Va and Xa. J Biol Chem. 1994;269:21051–8.

65. van de Poel RH, Meijers JC, Bouma BN. The interaction between anticoagulant protein S and complement regulatory C4b-binding protein (C4BP). Trends Cardiovasc Med. 2000;10:71–6.

66. Dahlback B. Inhibition of protein Ca cofactor function of human and bovine protein S by C4b-binding protein. J Biol Chem. 1986;261:12022–7.

67. Maurissen LF, Thomassen MC, Nicolaes GA, et al. Re-evaluation of the role of the protein S-C4b binding protein complex in activated protein C-catalyzed factor Va-inactivation. Blood. 2008;111:3034–41.

68. van de Poel RH, Meijers JC, Bouma BN. C4b-binding protein inhibits the factor V-dependent but not the factor V-independent cofactor activity of protein S in the activated protein C-mediated inactivation of factor VIIIa. Thromb Haemost. 2001;85:761–5.

69. Maurissen LFA, Castoldi E, Simioni P, Rosing J, Hackeng TM. Thrombin generation-based assays to measure the activity of the TFPI-protein S pathway in plasma from normal and protein S-deficient individuals. J Thromb Haemost. 2010;8:750–8.

70. Comp PC, Thurnau GR, Welsh J, Esmon CT. Functional and immunologic protein S levels are decreased during pregnancy. Blood. 1986;68:881–5.

71. Malm J, Laurell M, Dahlback B. Changes in the plasma levels of vitamin K-dependent proteins C and S and of C4b-binding protein during pregnancy and oral contraception. Br J Haematol. 1988;68:437–43.

72. Matsumoto M, Tachibana D, Nobeyama H, et al. Protein S deposition at placenta: a possible role of protein S other than anticoagulation. Blood Coagul Fibrinolysis. 2008;19:653–6.

73. Faught W, Garner P, Jones G, Ivey B. Changes in protein C and protein S levels in normal pregnancy. Am J Obstet Gynecol. 1995;172:147–50.

74. Mannucci PM, Vigano S, Bottasso B, et al. Protein C antigen during pregnancy, delivery and puerperium. Thromb Haemost. 1984;52:217.

75. Torricelli M, Sabatini L, Florio P, et al. Levels of antibodies against protein C and protein S in pregnancy and in preeclampsia. J Matern Fetal Neonatal Med. 2009;22:993–9.

76. de Moerloose P, Mermillod N, Amiral J, Reber G. Thrombomodulin levels during normal pregnancy, at delivery and in the postpartum: comparison with tissue-type plasminogen activator and plasminogen activator inhibitor-1. Thromb Haemost. 1998;79:554–6.

77. Boffa MC, Valsecchi L, Fausto A, et al. Predictive value of plasma thrombomodulin in preeclampsia and gestational hypertension. Thromb Haemost. 1998;79: 1092–5.

78. Astedt B, Hagerstrand I, Lecander I. Cellular localisation in placenta of placental type plasminogen activator inhibitor. Thromb Haemost. 1986;56:63–5.

79. Wright JG, Cooper P, Astedt B, et al. Fibrinolysis during normal human pregnancy: complex interrelationships between plasma levels of tissue plasminogen activator and inhibitors and the euglobulin clot lysis time. Br J Haematol. 1988;69:253–8.

80. Lockwood CJ. Regulation of plasminogen activator inhibitor 1 expression by interaction of epidermal growth factor with progestin during decidualization of human endometrial stromal cells. Am J Obstet Gynecol. 2001;184:798–804. discussion –5.

81. Halligan A, Bonnar J, Sheppard B, Darling M, Walshe J. Haemostatic, fibrinolytic and endothelial variables in normal pregnancies and pre-eclampsia. Br J Obstet Gynaecol. 1994;101:488–92.

82. Cerneca F, Ricci G, Simeone R, Malisano M, Alberico S, Guaschino S. Coagulation and fibrinolysis changes in normal pregnancy. Increased levels of procoagulants and reduced levels of inhibitors during pregnancy induce a hypercoagulable state, combined with a reactive fibrinolysis. Eur J Obstet Gynecol Reprod Biol. 1997;73:31–6.

83. Kruithof EK, Tran-Thang C, Gudinchet A, et al. Fibrinolysis in pregnancy: a study of plasminogen activator inhibitors. Blood. 1987;69:460–6.

84. Robb AO, Mills NL, Din JN, et al. Acute endothelial tissue plasminogen activator release in pregnancy. J Thromb Haemost. 2009;7:138–42.

85. Shimada H, Takashima E, Soma M, et al. Source of increased plasminogen activators during pregnancy and puerperium. Thromb Res. 1989;54:91–8.

86. Mousa HA, Downey C, Alfirevic Z, Toh CH. Thrombin activatable fibrinolysis inhibitor and its fibrinolytic effect in normal pregnancy. Thromb Haemost. 2004; 92:1025–31.

87. Ku DH, Arkel YS, Paidas MP, Lockwood CJ. Circulating levels of inflammatory cytokines (IL-1 beta and TNF-alpha), resistance to activated protein C, thrombin and fibrin generation in uncomplicated pregnancies. Thromb Haemost. 2003;90:1074–9.

88. Chabloz P, Reber G, Boehlen F, Hohlfeld P, de Moerloose P. TAFI antigen and D-dimer levels during normal pregnancy and at delivery. Br J Haematol. 2001;115:150–2.

89. Watanabe T, Minakami H, Sakata Y, Matsubara S, Sato I, Suzuki M. Changes in activity of plasma thrombin activatable fibrinolysis inhibitor in pregnancy. Gynecol Obstet Invest. 2004;58:19–21.

90. Chen J, Fu X, Wang Y, et al. Oxidative modification of von Willebrand factor by neutrophil oxidants inhibits its cleavage by ADAMTS13. Blood. 2010;115:706–12.

91. Rosen T, Kuczynski E, O'Neill LM, Funai EF, Lockwood CJ. Plasma levels of thrombin-antithrombin complexes predict preterm premature rupture of the fetal membranes. J Matern Fetal Med. 2001;10:297–300.

92. Comeglio P, Fedi S, Liotta AA, et al. Blood clotting activation during normal pregnancy. Thromb Res. 1996;84:199–202.

93. Huissoud C, Carrabin N, Benchaib M, et al. Coagulation assessment by rotation thrombelastometry in normal pregnancy. Thromb Haemost. 2009;101:755–61.

94. Steer PL, Krantz HB. Thromboelastography and Sonoclot analysis in the healthy parturient. J Clin Anesth. 1993;5:419–24.

95. Dahlback B, Carlsson M, Svensson PJ. Familial thrombophilia due to a previously unrecognized mechanism characterized by poor anticoagulant response to activated protein C: prediction of a cofactor to activated protein C. Proc Natl Acad Sci USA. 1993;90:1004–8.

96. Bertina RM, Koeleman BP, Koster T, et al. Mutation in blood coagulation factor V associated with resistance to activated protein C. Nature. 1994;369:64–7.

97. Bokarewa MI, Bremme K, Falk G, Sten-Linder M, Egberg N, Blomback M. Studies on phospholipid antibodies, APC-resistance and associated mutation in the coagulation factor V gene. Thromb Res. 1995;78:193–200.

98. Laffan MA, Manning R. The influence of factor VIII on measurement of activated protein C resistance. Blood Coagul Fibrinolysis. 1996;7:761–5.

99. Lowe GD, Rumley A, Woodward M, Reid E, Rumley J. Activated protein C resistance and the FV:R506Q mutation in a random population sample–associations with cardiovascular risk factors and coagulation variables. Thromb Haemost. 1999;81:918–24.

100. Kemmeren JM, Algra A, Meijers JC, et al. Effect of second- and third-generation oral contraceptives on the protein C system in the absence or presence of the factor VLeiden mutation: a randomized trial. Blood. 2004;103:927–33.

101. Mathonnet F, de Mazancourt P, Bastenaire B, et al. Activated protein C sensitivity ratio in pregnant women at delivery. Br J Haematol. 1996;92:244–6.

102. Cumming AM, Tait RC, Fildes S, Yoong A, Keeney S, Hay CR. Development of resistance to activated protein C during pregnancy. Br J Haematol. 1995;90:725–7.

103. Bokarewa MI, Wramsby M, Bremme K, Blomback M. Variability of the response to activated protein C during normal pregnancy. Blood Coagul Fibrinolysis. 1997;8:239–44.

104. Clark P, Sattar N, Walker ID, Greer IA. The Glasgow outcome, APCR and lipid (GOAL) pregnancy study: significance of pregnancy associated activated protein C resistance. Thromb Haemost. 2001;85:30–5.

105. Bonnar J, Prentice CR, McNicol GP, Douglas AS. Haemostatic mechanism in the uterine circulation during placental separation. Br Med J. 1970;2:564–7.

106. Higgins JR, Walshe JJ, Darling MR, Norris L, Bonnar J. Hemostasis in the uteroplacental and peripheral circulations in normotensive and preeclamptic pregnancies. Am J Obstet Gynecol. 1998;179:520–6.

107. Bretelle F, Sabatier F, Desprez D, et al. Circulating microparticles: a marker of procoagulant state in normal pregnancy and pregnancy complicated by preeclampsia or intrauterine growth restriction. Thromb Haemost. 2003;89:486–92.

108. Germain SJ, Sacks GP, Sooranna SR, Sargent IL, Redman CW. Systemic inflammatory priming in normal pregnancy and preeclampsia: the role of circulating syncytiotrophoblast microparticles. J Immunol. 2007;178:5949–56.

109. Liston W. Haemorrhage. In: Lewis G, editor. The confidential enquiry into maternal and child health (CEMACH). Saving mothers' lives: reviewing maternal deaths to make motherhood safer – 2003–2005. The seventh report on confidential enquiries into maternal deaths in the United Kingdom. London: CEMACH; 2007.

110. Drife J. Centre for Maternal and Child Enquiries (CMACE). Saving Mothers' Lives: reviewing maternal deaths to make motherhood safer: 2006–08. The Eighth Report on Confidential Enquiries into Maternal Deaths in the United Kingdom. G. Lewis (ed.). BJOG 2011;118(Suppl. 1):57–65 and 71–6.

Systemic Thromboembolism in Pregnancy: Heritable and Acquired Thrombophilias

2

Trevor Baglin

Abstract

Normal pregnancy is a hypercoagulable state. The predisposition to thrombosis may be exacerbated in women with heritable or acquired predisposition to thrombosis, known as thrombophilia. For a variety of reasons, the precise contribution of these thrombophilias to pregnancy morbidity is uncertain. However, there is evidence of an association between heritable thrombophilia and pregnancy morbidity including early and late pregnancy loss, preeclampsia, and intrauterine growth restriction. There also appears to be a weak association with placental abruption. Management of pregnant women with a thrombophilia relies on an accurate assessment of individual risk based on her personal and family history.

2.1 Introduction

Pregnancy results in an acquired hypercoagulable state due to pregnancy-associated changes in the hemostatic system (see Chap. 1). At delivery the placental bed spiral arteries, which lack a muscular layer, must quickly thrombose to limit and stop maternal hemorrhage. While contraction of the uterus is essential for prevention of major blood loss, it is likely that the evolutionary development of the hemostatic response to pregnancy (reviewed in Chap. 1) has provided a material survival advantage to both mother and fetus.

However, the progressive hypercoagulability increases the risk of venous thrombosis during pregnancy (and the postpartum period) and in some women may contribute to pregnancy complications.

Venous thrombosis (deep vein thrombosis and pulmonary embolus, also referred to collectively as venous thromboembolism), pregnancy loss, preeclampsia, and intrauterine growth restriction are common pregnancy complications. These risks may be amplified in women with a heritable or acquired predisposition to thrombosis, so-called thrombophilia. Testing for heritable thrombophilias in women with previous pregnancy morbidity is now common in clinical practice. Consequently, hematologists and obstetricians are frequently asked for advice on intervention with antithrombotic therapy for subsequent pregnancies in women found to have laboratory evidence of heritable thrombophilia. However, the

T. Baglin, PhD, FRCP, FRCPath
Department of Haematology, Addenbrooke's Hospital,
Cambridge University Hospitals NHS Trust,
Cambridge CB2 0QQ, UK
e-mail: trevor.baglin@addenbrookes.nhs.uk

H. Cohen, P. O'Brien (eds.), *Disorders of Thrombosis and Hemostasis in Pregnancy*,
DOI 10.1007/978-1-4471-4411-3_2, © Springer-Verlag London 2012

Table 2.1 Heritable and acquired conditions that predispose to venous thrombosis and hence which increase the risk of pregnancy-associated venous thrombosis

Heritable thrombophilia	Possible heritable component	Acquired risk factors for venous thrombosis
Antithrombin deficiency	High factor VIII/VWF	Increasing age (over 35 in pregnancy)
Protein C deficiency	High factor IX	Pregnancy
Protein S deficiency	High factor XI	COC/HRT
F5G1691A (factor V Leiden)	High fibrinogen	Obesity
F2G20210A (Sickle and thalassaemia disorders)	Factor XIII (qualitative)	Smoking
	High homocysteine	Immobility
	Hypofibrinolysis	Dehydration (hyperemesis)
		Hospitalization
		Antiphospholipid syndrome (APS)
		Heart failure
		Inflammatory disease
		Chronic respiratory disease
		Nephrotic syndrome
		Cancer
		Myeloproliferative disorders (PV, ET, PMF)
		Paroxysmal nocturnal hemoglobinuria (PNH)

VWF Von Willebrand Factor, *COC* combined oral contraceptive, estrogen containing, *HRT* hormone replacement therapy, *PV* polycythemia vera, *ET* essential thrombocythemia, *PMF* primary myelofibrosis

material contribution of heritable thrombophilia to pregnancy morbidity and hence the value of testing and using the results to inform clinical management decisions are still uncertain.

- The association between a diagnosis of heritable thrombophilia and pregnancy morbidity is weak as (1) the laboratory tests are imprecise, (2) the tests performed do not comprehensively assess the genetic framework of thrombophilia, and (3) both laboratory abnormalities and pregnancy morbidity are common and so it is inevitable that abnormalities are frequently found in women who are investigated.

- If there is a true association, then causation might be expected to be related to a common underlying pathology in which the likelihood of venous thrombosis and pregnancy morbidity is increased. However, while limited, studies reported so far do not support a common underlying pathology, at least for venous thromboembolism and pregnancy loss. Furthermore, based on biological plausibility, there is reason to believe that there may be different mechanistic pathology.

- Finally, if there is a causative link between an underlying predisposition to thrombosis and pregnancy morbidity, then testing for a limited

number of thrombophilias using imprecise laboratory methodology may have little theoretical or practical clinical utility as the test results do not discriminate between women with and without an underlying predisposition to pregnancy morbidity.

The management of pregnancy-associated venous thromboembolism is detailed in Chap. 4 with specific treatment in relation to heritable thrombophilia addressed in Section 2.4.1 below. The association of pregnancy morbidity and late pregnancy complications with hereditary and acquired thrombophilias is reviewed in detail in Chap. 3. In this chapter, generic aspects of thrombophilia are considered, and a summary is presented of:

- The spectrum of established heritable thrombophilias associated with an increased risk of venous thrombosis

- The limitations of laboratory measurement and the implications for establishing a causal relationship and developing testing strategies that might have clinical utility

- An overview of heritable thrombophilia as it relates to pregnancy-associated venous thrombosis

- An overview of heritable thrombophilia as it relates to pregnancy morbidity

Acquired conditions that predispose to venous thrombosis, which therefore increase the risk of pregnancy-associated venous thrombosis, are included for the sake of completeness alongside the definite and possible heritable thrombophilias listed in Table 2.1.

2.2 Heritable Thrombophilias Associated with an Increased Risk of Venous Thrombosis

The heritable thrombophilias shown to be associated with at least a twofold increased risk of venous thrombosis are deficiencies of the natural anticoagulants antithrombin, protein C, and protein S, due to mutations in the corresponding genes *SERPINC1*, *PROC*, and *PROS*, and the two common mutations in genes encoding procoagulant factor: *F5G1691A* (FVR506Q, factor V Leiden) and *F2G20210A* (commonly referred to as the prothrombin gene mutation) (Table 2.1). The causal association between these heritable thrombophilias and venous thrombosis has been confirmed by comparing the prevalence of defects in patients with venous thrombosis and controls. The expression of heritable thrombophilia as a disease (venous thrombosis) is dependent on a strong gene-environment interaction and, in this respect, there is a strong interaction with pregnancy [29].

Numerous acquired medical conditions and environmental factors increase the risk of venous thrombosis (Table 2.1). Risk factors for venous thrombosis generally interact synergistically. This means that risk factors are not additive, rather that they multiply. For example, if two risk factors A and B each increase the risk of venous thrombosis threefold, then the combination of factors increases the risk nine times (3 x 3), not six times (3 + 3). Pregnancy is an independent risk factor for venous thrombosis, so the presence of additional heritable and acquired thrombophilias and environmental factors act synergistically to increase the risk of venous thrombosis in pregnancy. The baseline risk of venous thrombosis in women of reproductive age is low at approximately 1 per 10,000.

Consequently, the relative increased risk of venous thrombosis associated with pregnancy translates into an absolute risk of only 1 per 1,000 live births overall. However, in an individual woman, a relative increase in risk due to multiple interacting factors may translate into a high absolute risk. This is the basis for assessing the risk of venous thrombosis and offering thromboprophylaxis in high-risk pregnancies (see Chap. 4).

2.2.1 Antithrombin Deficiency

Antithrombin is a protease inhibitor. Based on kinetic rates of inhibition, its primary targets are thrombin and factor Xa, and hence antithrombin both regulates generation of thrombin and inhibits thrombin that has been generated. Inhibition of target proteases is increased approximately 1,000-fold by glycosaminoglycan activation of antithrombin, which is the mechanism by which heparin acts as a pharmacological anticoagulant. The activation process involves an induced conformational change in the structure of antithrombin which enables formation of an irreversible covalent complex with the target protease [15]. The complex undergoes a further dramatic conformational change involving both the inhibitor and the inhibited protein which alters the properties of each, resulting in rapid clearance from the circulation.

Two laboratory (intermediate) phenotypes of heritable antithrombin deficiency are recognized. Type I is characterized by a quantitative reduction of antithrombin with a parallel reduction in function (measured as inhibitory activity against factor Xa or thrombin) and the level of protein in the plasma (measured immunologically as the antigenic level). Type 2 deficiency is due to the production of a qualitatively abnormal antithrombin protein characterized by disturbance of the complex inhibitory mechanism of protease inhibition as a result of a mutation in the *SERPINC1* gene. The functional activity is discrepantly low compared to the antigenic level. Type 2 deficiency is subclassified according to the nature of the functional deficit:

- Type 2 reactive site (RS) in which mutations alter the sequence of the mobile reactive center loop, thus reducing the ability to inhibit thrombin or factor Xa either in the presence or absence of heparin in a laboratory assay
- Type 2 heparin binding site (HBS) in which mutations affect the ability of antithrombin to bind and be activated by glycosaminoglycans, resulting in reduced ability to inhibit thrombin or factor Xa only in the presence of heparin in a laboratory assay
- Type 2 pleiotropic (PE) in which a single mutation produces multiple effects on the structure-function relationship of the molecule which is often associated with low plasma levels due to effects on either secretion or stability

Approximately 100 point mutations (missense, nonsense, or insertions or deletions causing frameshifts) and several whole or partial gene deletions have been identified as causes of type 1 deficiency. Numerous point mutations causing qualitative type 2 deficiency have been identified. Homozygous type 1 deficiency and type 2RS mutations are incompatible with life. Type 2 HBS and some PE mutations are associated with a lower risk of thrombosis; homozygosity, and compound heterozygosity, involving these mutations is compatible with life.

Functional activity assays typically use a chromogenic substrate and factor Xa as the target protease. The total amount of antithrombin protein can be measured immunologically with antibodies, for example, by enzyme-linked immunosorbent assay (ELISA). As antithrombin antigen levels may be normal or near normal in type 2 deficiency, immunological assays may fail to identify patients with these variants and so a functional assay should be used as the initial assay.

Although there is little reported variation in the plasma concentration of antithrombin both during healthy pregnancy and following delivery (as stated in Chap. 1), antithrombin levels may be slightly reduced in pregnancy and are reduced in women taking estrogen preparations, as well as in other situations. Consequently, the clinical significance of a low antithrombin level must be interpreted by an experienced clinician who is aware of all the relevant factors that may have influenced the test result in a specific patient.

2.2.2 Protein C Deficiency

Protein C is the zymogen precursor of activated protein C (APC). Protein C is activated to APC by thrombin bound to thrombomodulin on the endothelial surface. APC inactivates the activated cofactors (VIIIa and Va) and so inhibits thrombin generation. Factors VIII and V are activated by small amounts of thrombin during initiation of coagulation to nonenzymatic cofactors required for assembly of macromolecular complexes that are required for the full thrombin explosion. The enzymatic components of these complexes are factors IXa and Xa, and so inactivation of VIIIa and Va by APC leads to disassembly of the enzymatic complexes, thus attenuating thrombin generation.

Protein C deficiency is classified into type 1 and 2 defects on the basis of functional and antigenic assays. The relative risk of thrombosis in relation to type 1 and the various type 2 defects has not been characterized. Most heritable protein C deficiency is due to type 1 abnormalities. The majority of type 1 defects are due to point mutations. Multiple type 2 defects due to mutations in the *PROC* gene have been reported affecting the catalytic active site, the phospholipid-binding Gla domain, the propeptide cleavage activation site, and the sites of interaction with substrates or cofactors. In this case, there is discordance between the functional and antigenic levels.

The laboratory diagnosis of protein C deficiency is based on a functional assay. As protein C antigen levels may be normal or near normal in type 2 deficiency, immunological assays may fail to identify patients with these variants, so a functional assay should be used as the initial assay. Most commercially available functional assays use a snake venom to activate protein C and a chromogenic substrate to quantify APC activity. A chromogenic assay will detect type 1 and most type 2 defects. The diagnosis of type 1 protein C deficiency is problematic because of the wide overlap in protein C activity between heterozygous carriers and unaffected individuals. The diagnosis of type 2 defects is problematic because a chromogenic assay will only detect defects affecting the enzymatic site.

Protein C levels are not affected by pregnancy or estrogen exposure. Acquired low levels of protein C occur during anticoagulant therapy with oral vitamin K antagonists, vitamin K deficiency, disseminated intravascular coagulation (DIC), and liver disease. Consequently, the clinical significance of a low protein C level must be interpreted by an experienced clinician who is aware of all the relevant factors that may have influenced the test result in a specific patient.

2.2.3   Protein S Deficiency

Protein S is a vitamin K-dependent glycoprotein produced in the liver, endothelial cells, and megakaryocytes. Protein S is a nonenzymatic cofactor for APC-mediated inactivation of factors VIIIa and Va and additionally is involved with tissue factor pathway inhibitor-dependent natural anticoagulation. Approximately 60 % of protein S circulates bound to C4b-binding protein and is inactive. The remaining 40 %, designated free protein S, is uncomplexed and is the active form. Free protein S increases the affinity of activated protein C for negatively charged phospholipid surfaces on platelets or the endothelium and increases complex formation of APC with the activated forms of factors VIII and V (VIIIa & Va). However, the degree of C4b binding has not yet been shown to be a determinant of thrombosis risk. In addition to APC cofactor activity, protein S has an independent anticoagulant activity as a cofactor for TFPI (tissue factor pathway inhibitor).

Protein S is usually quantified immunologically rather than measured functionally. Nowadays, monoclonal antibodies that detect only free protein are used to quantify free protein S. Functional protein S assays are imprecise and are not used in the majority of coagulation laboratories.

Protein S levels are significantly lower in females, so much so that different normal reference ranges are required for males and females.

There is a significant risk of a false-positive diagnosis of protein S deficiency in women. Protein S levels are reduced by estrogens and fall progressively during normal pregnancy. Acquired low levels of protein S occur during anticoagulant therapy with oral vitamin K antagonists, vitamin K deficiency, DIC, and liver disease.

Protein S defects are divided into three types:
- In type I deficiency, both total and free protein S levels are low (and functional activity, if measured, is found to be low).
- Type II defects are characterized by reduced activity in the presence of normal total and free levels of protein S. Type II deficiency is difficult to diagnose because functional protein S assays are imprecise.
- In type III deficiency, the total protein S level is normal but the free protein S level is low. Some type III deficiency is thought to be a phenotypic variation of type 1 resulting from the same genetic mutations. However, it is now apparent that many patients with an apparent type III phenotype do not have heritable protein S deficiency. This may be related to an increase in C4b levels.

This complicated classification reflects the complexity of the biology of protein S but has no mechanistic reference to disturbance of natural anticoagulant activity. Given these limitations and the imprecision of laboratory methodology, the diagnosis of heritable protein S deficiency is less precise and the clinical implication of a low protein S level in an individual is more uncertain than it is for antithrombin or protein C.

2.2.4   *F5G1691A* (FVR506Q, Factor V Leiden)

Factor V is a cofactor required for thrombin generation. Factor V has no cofactor activity until cleaved by thrombin or factor Xa. Activated factor V (Va) is inactivated by APC (see protein C above). Resistance to activated protein C (APC resistance) is a laboratory phenomenon in which there is a suboptimal anticoagulant response to addition of APC to a patient's plasma. In 95 % of cases of familial APC resistance, this is due to the same point mutation in the gene for FV, a guanine to adenine transition at nucleotide position 1691 in exon 10 (*F5G1691A*), resulting in a mutant protein FVR506Q. The mutation is known as the factor V Leiden mutation and the mutant factor Va has normal procoagulant activity, but substitution of glutamine for arginine at position 506 (which is an APC cleavage site) results in slower inactivation by APC. Nowadays, the mutation is frequently detected by direct DNA analysis (rather than by a clotting assay) to detect the presence of the mutant protein.

The mutation is present in around 4 % of the Caucasian population and around 15 % of unselected consecutive Caucasian patients with a first venous thrombosis. The prevalence is highest in Northern Europeans. The mutation is infrequent in other populations. The high prevalence and founder effect suggest positive selection, and this may relate to a favorable effect on embryo implantation and hence reproduction [7] rather than a lower risk of fatal hemorrhage in females during childbirth, as originally thought.

Acquired APC resistance is common, in part often due to increased FVIII levels, and is observed in pregnancy and in association with estrogen exposure.

2.2.5   *F2G20210A*

A single nucleotide change of guanine to adenine at position 20210 in the 3′ untranslated region of the prothrombin gene is a mild risk factor for venous thrombosis. The prevalence of the *F2G20210A* mutation is around 2 % in Caucasians with a higher prevalence in Southern compared to Northern Europeans. The mutation increases the plasma level of prothrombin by around 30 %, but the mechanism responsible for this has not been identified. No specific clotting test for the presence of the mutation has been described, and diagnosis depends on detection of the genetic mutation by DNA analysis.

2.2.6   Other Candidate Heritable Thrombophilias

A number of other anticoagulant proteins have been investigated as potential factors causing thrombophilia, but a relationship between venous thrombosis and low protein levels or associated gene mutations has not been established.

Increased levels of factors VIII, IX, and XI are associated with an increased risk of venous thrombosis, but a heritable basis for high levels associated with venous thrombosis is not established. There is equivocal evidence for a causal relationship between fibrinogen levels and venous thrombosis. Polymorphisms in the prothrombin gene have been described that may further increase the risk of venous thrombosis associated with the *F2G20210A* mutation, but the effect is mild. It was previously thought that deficiency of factor XII was a risk factor for venous thromboembolism, but subsequent investigation strongly indicates that this is unlikely. A protective effect against venous thrombosis has been reported for a polymorphism in the factor XIII gene (FXIIIV341L).

A causal relationship between levels of specific individual proteins involved in regulating fibrinolysis and venous thrombosis has not been established. However, in a case–control study using a global measure of fibrinolytic potential, there was an approximately doubled risk of venous thrombosis in patients with clot lysis times above the 90th percentile of controls [16]. Further analysis of a larger study confirmed this finding and demonstrated that hypofibrinolysis in combination with established acquired and genetic risk factors, such as F5G1691A, had a synergistic effect on venous thrombosis risk [18]. The genetic basis for hypofibrinolysis in these patients was not investigated.

Hyperhomocysteinemia may be caused by genetic abnormalities but only the severe inherited abnormalities of homocysteine metabolism (homozygous cystathionine beta-synthase deficiency and homozygous deficiency of methylenetetrahydrofolate reductase) result in congenital homocystinuria associated with an increased risk of both arterial and venous thrombosis, as well as premature atherosclerosis and mental retardation, epilepsy, and skeletal and eye problems. Fifty percent of patients present with venous or arterial thrombosis before the age of 30 years. The thermolabile variant of methylenetetrahydrofolate reductase (MTHFR), due to a common genetic polymorphism (C677T), is not a risk factor for venous thrombosis [3, 5].

2.2.7 Antiphospholipid Syndrome (APS)

The antiphospholipid syndrome (APS) is the most common acquired form of thrombophilia. APS is diagnosed when a patient with arterial or venous thrombosis (or pregnancy morbidity in women) is found to have antiphospholipid antibodies (anticardiolipin, aCL; and/or lupus anticoagulant, LA; and/or anti-beta-2-glycoprotein I, aβ2-GPI). The updated international consensus (revised Sapporo) classification criteria for definite antiphospholipid syndrome [20] require the presence of a LA and/or IgG or IgM aCL present in medium or high titer (i.e., >40 GPL or MPL or > the 99th percentile) and/or aβ$_2$GPI (IgG and/or IgM) >99th percentile. These aPL should be persistent, defined as being present on two or more consecutive occasions at least 12 weeks apart. The international consensus criteria were originally designed for scientific clinical studies, and there remains a need for firm diagnostic criteria for routine clinical use which may differ from these. APS has conventionally been divided into primary and secondary forms, the latter being associated with systemic lupus erythematosus (SLE) or a related rheumatological condition. However, this distinction was abandoned in the revised Sapporo classification [20] on the basis that it is unknown whether APS and SLE are two diseases coinciding in an individual, underlying SLE offers a setting for the development of APS, or APS and SLE represent two elements of the same process.

Laboratory test results are subject to considerable pre-analytical variation. In addition, transiently abnormal results may be found in normal healthy individuals. For these reasons, for a patient to be considered to have antiphospholipid activity (aCL, LA, or aβ2-GPI), test results must be positive on two separate occasions. The probability of misdiagnosing APS has been reduced by stricter criteria for antibody titers (>40 GPL or MPL for aCL or >90th percentile for aCL or aβ2-GPI) and demonstration of persistence of antibodies (present on at least 2 consecutive occasions at least 12 weeks apart) [25]. Positivity in all 3 assays (aCL, LA, aβ2-GPI) is associated most strongly with thrombosis and pregnancy complications. Recent evidence suggests that the antibodies most strongly associated with thrombosis and pregnancy morbidity are against domain I of β2-GPI; these antibodies are responsible for lupus anticoagulant activity specifically associated with clinical events and are responsible for positive aCL results. While the criteria for diagnosis of APS are unlikely to change again soon, it is possible that the laboratory identification of clinically relevant antibodies to domain I β2-GPI will eventually simplify the diagnosis and improve the clinical utility of laboratory tests.

2.3 Limitations of Laboratory Measurement and the Implications for Establishing a Causal Relationship and Developing Testing Strategies with Clinical Utility

The laboratory diagnosis of heritable thrombophilias is difficult as the tests are subject to considerable pre-analytical variables. Low levels of antithrombin, protein C, and protein S occur in a variety of circumstances and test results, and the clinical implications of both positive and negative results, are frequently misinterpreted. If testing is performed during pregnancy, results must be interpreted with reference to the effect of the pregnancy.

Functional assays should be used for which accuracy and imprecision are acceptable. However, no single method will detect all defects. Even in families with characterized defects, a phenotypic assay may fail to accurately discriminate affected and non-affected individuals. True heritable deficiencies may not be detected and false positive diagnoses are common.

Low levels of antithrombin, protein C, or protein S may relate to age, sex, acquired illness, or drug therapy, so interpretation requires knowledge of the patient's condition at the time of blood sampling. Low levels of antithrombin, protein C, or protein S suspected to be the result of heritable mutations should be confirmed on one or more separate samples. Demonstrating a low level in other family members supports a diagnosis of heritable deficiency, and characterization of the genetic mutation can be confirmatory.

As well as specific limitations relating to individual factors, there are a number of common generic issues which limit accuracy and precision of laboratory diagnosis and consequently contribute to limiting the clinical utility of thrombophilia testing. These can be summarized as follows:

• The laboratory diagnosis of heritable thrombophilias is difficult as the tests are subject to numerous biological and pre-analytical variables.
• The fact that venous thrombosis has a multiple genetic basis with incomplete penetrance and a strong gene-environment interaction makes counseling in relation to thrombophilia testing uncertain.
• In families with known heritable thrombophilias, the risk of venous thrombosis can be increased in unaffected members as well as affected, so a negative thrombophilia result does not exclude an increased risk of venous thrombosis.
• Even in families with characterized defects, a phenotypic assay may fail to accurately discriminate affected and non-affected individuals.
• True heritable deficiencies may not be detected and false positive diagnoses are common.
• Low levels of antithrombin, protein C, and protein S occur in a variety of circumstances, and test results and the clinical implications of both positive and negative results are frequently misinterpreted.

• Testing for heritable thrombophilias in selected patients, such as those with a strong family history of unprovoked recurrent thrombosis, may influence decisions regarding duration of anticoagulation. Unfortunately, in this regard, identifying patients for testing is not straightforward as criteria for defining thrombosis-prone families have not been validated and the association between family history of thrombosis and detection of inherited thrombophilia is weak.

In order to limit inaccuracy and imprecision, the British Society for Haematology has published clinical guidelines for testing for heritable thrombophilia [2] which include the following generic recommendations:

• Testing at the time of acute venous thrombosis is not indicated as the utility and implications of testing need to be considered and the patient needs to be counseled before testing. As treatment of acute venous thrombosis is not influenced by test results, testing can be performed later.
• The prothrombin time (PT) should be measured to detect the effect of oral vitamin K antagonists which will cause a reduction in protein C and S levels.
• Functional assays should be used to determine antithrombin and protein C levels.
• Chromogenic assays of protein C activity are less subject to interference than clotting assays and are therefore preferable.
• Immunoreactive assays of free protein S antigen are preferable to functional assays. If a protein S activity assay is used in the initial screen, low results should be further investigated with an immunoreactive assay of free protein S.
• Repeat testing for identification of deficiency of antithrombin, protein C, and protein S is indicated, and a low level should be confirmed on one or more separate samples. Deficiency should not be diagnosed on the basis of a single abnormal result.

In addition to factors that limit the accuracy and precision of laboratory testing, there is potentially a fundamental flaw in attempting to quantify the degree of thrombophilia in an individual patient by using a dichotomous testing strategy in which a limited number of factors are designated normal or abnormal. The "thrombophilic condition" is dependent on a large complex genetic framework subject to strong environmental influence [1, 29, 30].

2.4 Overview of Heritable Thrombophilia as It Relates to Pregnancy-Associated Venous Thrombosis

2.4.1 Treatment of Pregnancy-Associated Venous Thrombosis

There are limited data in relation to treatment specifically of pregnancy-associated venous thrombosis in women with heritable thrombophilia. However, there is no evidence that issues that have been clarified in nonpregnant patients are different in pregnant women:

- There is no evidence that heritable thrombophilia should influence the initial intensity of anticoagulation with heparin.
- When warfarin is introduced following delivery, there is no evidence that heritable thrombophilia should influence the intensity of anticoagulation.
- Warfarin-induced skin necrosis is extremely rare, even in patients with protein C or S deficiency, such that most individuals with protein C or S deficiency do not develop skin necrosis.
- There is no evidence that recurrent venous thrombosis while on anticoagulant treatment is more likely in patients with heritable thrombophilia.

In nonpregnant patients with antithrombin deficiency, heparin resistance is infrequent and recurrence or extension of thrombosis while on treatment is no more frequent than that observed in individuals without antithrombin deficiency. However, there are anecdotes of pregnant women with heritable antithrombin deficiency who have low anti-Xa levels despite therapeutic doses of low-molecular-weight heparin. It is advisable for pregnant women with venous thrombosis and antithrombin deficiency to be referred urgently to a hematologist with appropriate expertise for supervision of treatment.

The most important clinical factor predicting likelihood of recurrent venous thrombosis is whether or not a first episode of venous thrombosis was unprovoked or provoked. Pregnancy is a relatively strong provocation for venous thrombosis and the risk of spontaneous recurrent venous thrombosis after pregnancy-associated venous thrombosis in women with heritable thrombophilia is low, and long-term anticoagulation is not indicated. Long-term prospective cohort outcome studies have shown that finding a heritable thrombophilia does not reliably predict recurrence in unselected patients even after an episode of unprovoked venous thrombosis. However, studies were not powered to exclude an increased risk of recurrence specifically in relation to rare thrombophilias, such as antithrombin or protein C deficiency. Therefore, it remains uncertain if mutations affecting the *SERPINC1*, *PROC*, and *PROS* genes causing deficiency of the corresponding protein might predict a sufficiently high risk of thrombosis to justify long-term (lifelong) anticoagulation after a single episode of venous thrombosis. Following an episode of pregnancy-associated venous thrombosis, women with heritable thrombophilia should be referred to a thrombophilia specialist for consideration of future management, including duration of anticoagulation and need for thromboprophylaxis in subsequent pregnancies.

2.4.2 Prevention of Pregnancy-Associated Venous Thrombosis

Pregnancy is associated with a 5- to 10-fold increased risk of venous thrombosis compared to nonpregnant women of comparable age and has an absolute risk of 1 per 1,000 deliveries. There is an increased relative risk of pregnancy-associated venous thrombosis in women with thrombophilia (Table 2.2), but this translates into a low absolute risk. For example, the relative risks of 34 and 8 associated with homozygosity and heterozygosity for the factor V Leiden mutation, respectively

Table 2.2 Results of systematic review of thrombophilia in pregnancy

	Pregnancy-associated VTE	Recurrent pregnancy loss in first trimester	Non-recurrent second trimester loss	Late pregnancy loss	Preeclampsia	Intrauterine growth restriction
Antithrombin deficiency	(8/11)/(242/815) 4.7 (1.3–17.0)	–	–	(1/1)/(17/61) 7.6 (0.3–196)	(1/1)/(57/131) 3.9 (0.2–97)	–
Protein C deficiency	(23/32)/(232/715) **4.8** (2.1–10.6)	–	–	(3/234)/(18/524) 3.0 (0.2–38.5)	(3/3)/(60/104) 5.1 (0.3–102)	–
Protein S deficiency	(16/28)/(250/911) **3.2** (1.5–6.9)	–	–	(14/15)/(258/801) 20.1 (3.7–109)	(14/20)/(158/402) 2.8 (0.8–10.6)	–
Homozygous *F5G1691A*	(29/91)/(145/1,248) **34.4** (9.9–120)	Heterozygous and homozygous	–	(7/212)/(2/118) 2.0 (0.4–9.7)	(4/5)/(608/1,143) 1.9 (0.4–7.9)	(1/1)/(60/153) 4.6 (0.2–115)
Heterozygous *F5G1691A*	(96/226)/(263/1,595) **8.3** (5.4–12.7)	(173/287)/(1,390/2,285) **1.9** (1.01–3.6)	(34/58)/(98/432) **4.12** (1.9–8.8)	(27/382)/(124/1,121) **2.1** (1.1–3.9)	(161/249)/(1790/3,673) **2.2** (1.5–3.3)	(25/49)/(512/1,147) 2.7 (0.6–12.1)
Homozygous *F2G20210A*	(2/2)/(40/253) 26.4 (1.2–559)	–	–	–	–	–
Heterozygous *F2G20210A*	(42/61)/(277/1,005) **6.8** (2.5–18.8)	(54/78)/(627/1,428) **2.7** (1.4–5.3)	(4/11)/(22/271) 8.6 (2.2–34)	(15/36)/(348/1,134) **2.7** (1.3–5.5)	(42/71)/(937/2,028) **2.5** (1.5–4.2)	(25/44)/(583/1,375) 2.9 (0.6–13.7)
Homozygous MTHFR (C677T)	(20/128)/(89/543) 0.7 (0.2–2.5)	(22/39)/(21/368) 0.9 (0.4–1.7)	–	(69/323)/(198/1,059) 1.3 (0.9–1.9)	(221/482)/(1234/3,205) **1.4** (1.1–1.8)	(62/121)/(460/961) 1.2 (0.8–1.8)
Hyperhomocysteinemia	(33/37)/(128/235) **6.2** (1.4–28.4)	(12/16)/(47/113) 4.3 (1.3–13.9)	–	(2/7)/(16/55) 1.0 (0.2–5.6)	(37/41)/(257/364) **3.5** (1.2–10.1)	–

Lupus anticoagulant	(59/107)/(581/1,728) **3.0** (1.03–8.6)	–	(9/17)/(13/178) 14.3 (4.7–43)	(15/242)/(124/730) 2.4 (0.8–7.0)	(63/89)/(426/981) 1.5 (0.8–4.6)	–
Anticardiolipin antibodies	(127/149)/(869/1,956) **3.4** (1.3–8.7)	(116/120)/(551/647) **5.0** (1.8–14.0)	–	(52/242)/(124/730) **3.3** (1.6–6.7)	(130/217)/(803/2,428) **2.7** (1.7–4.5)	(7/60)/(15/800) **6.9** (2.7–17.7)

From Robertson et al. [28]

Each box indicates in brackets number of women in total (women with thrombophilia/women with event)/(women with no thrombophilia/women with event), odds ratios calculated on the random effects model (not the fixed effect model) to provide a more conservative result, indicated to 1 decimal place with 95 % confidence intervals in brackets. Statistically significant results are indicated in bold if $n > 20$ for thrombophilia group equate to absolute risks of 3.4 and 0.8 %, based on an overall absolute risk of 0.1 % (1 per 1,000 deliveries). Based on the calculated odds ratios in Table 2.2, absolute risks of pregnancy-associated venous thrombosis would only be expected to exceed 1 % for homozygosity for the factor V Leiden mutation. However, where a statistically significant increase in risk is demonstrated, the possibility of rates greater than 1 % cannot be excluded (based on the upper 95 % confidence intervals) for deficiencies of antithrombin, protein C, and protein S; heterozygosity for the $F5$G1691A (factor V Leiden); and homozygous and heterozygous $F2$G20210A mutations. Homozygosity for the thermolabile variant of MTHFR (C677T) is not associated with an increased risk of pregnancy-associated venous thrombosis (Table 2.2).

The risk of thrombosis, compared to the general age-matched female population, is increased 100-fold in pregnancy in women with a previous thrombosis. Thrombosis in pregnancy rarely occurs in women whose initial venous thrombosis was provoked, unless the provocation was use of an estrogen-containing contraceptive. In general, the absolute risk of pregnancy-associated venous thrombosis in women with heritable thrombophilia with no previous history is small, but the risk is considered greatest in women with antithrombin deficiency, those homozygous for the FVR506Q or the $F2$G20210A mutations or those who are double heterozygotes for FVR506Q and $F2$G20210A. The number of women with these defects is very small. The most appropriate management of these women is uncertain and recommendations are based on low-level evidence. Retrospective studies in women with laboratory evidence of thrombophilia and previous venous thrombosis for whom detailed information of the type of thrombophilia was available indicate that the rate of recurrence is similar in women with and without thrombophilia. However, a limitation of studies published to date is that women with high-risk thrombophilias were excluded (deficiency of antithrombin, protein C, and protein S, and combined defects).

In women with a previous history of venous thrombosis, the major factor in determining whether prophylaxis should be given is whether or not the prior venous thrombosis was provoked. If the episode was unprovoked, prophylaxis should be considered and thrombophilia testing is not required if prophylaxis is given. In women with a first provoked event, the decision to test or not should be influenced by the strength of the provocation, for example, thrombosis associated with major trauma and subsequent immobility would not be an indication for prophylaxis or testing. In women with a first-degree relative with thrombosis, the decision to test should be influenced by whether or not the event in the relative was unprovoked or provoked and the strength of the provocation. If the event in the first-degree relative was pregnancy or COC-associated, then testing and finding thrombophilia should prompt consideration of prophylaxis, particularly if the symptomatic relative was known to have the same defect, especially deficiency of antithrombin or protein C. When testing in pregnancy is performed, it is necessary to interpret the results with reference to the effect of pregnancy on the test results.

In summary:

- Women should be assessed for risk of pregnancy-associated venous thrombosis primarily in relation to clinical risk factors; this assessment should be performed when first seen in pregnancy and again if circumstances change during pregnancy, for example, the woman develops preeclampsia or is admitted to hospital.
- Most women with a previous unprovoked venous thrombosis or pregnancy or COC-related thrombosis will qualify for thromboprophylaxis on the basis of clinical risk alone, so testing for heritable thrombophilia may not be contributory.
- Women with a previous event due to a major provoking factor, for example, surgery or major trauma, would not usually require prophylaxis or testing.
- Women with a previous event due to a minor provoking factor, for example, travel, should be tested and considered for prophylaxis if a thrombophilia is found.
- In asymptomatic women with a family history of venous thrombosis, testing is not required if the clinical risks alone are sufficient to result in thromboprophylaxis during pregnancy.
- Asymptomatic women with a family history of venous thrombosis should be tested if an

event in a first-degree relative was unprovoked or provoked by pregnancy, COC exposure, or a minor risk factor. The result will be more informative if the first-degree relative has a known thrombophilia, so the interpretation of the result in the asymptomatic woman is with reference to the defect in the symptomatic affected relative.

2.5 Overview of Heritable Thrombophilia as It Relates to Pregnancy Morbidity

There is evidence of an association between heritable thrombophilia and pregnancy morbidity including early and late pregnancy loss, preeclampsia, and intrauterine growth restriction. There also appears to be a weak association with placental abruption [28]. A simple hypothesis is that thrombophilia may increase the risk of placental insufficiency due to placental vascular thrombosis. If thrombophilia results in pathology which mechanistically results from thrombosis, it might be expected that women with a predisposition to venous thrombosis would have a higher incidence of pregnancy morbidity thought to be due to placental vascular thrombosis. However, in a case–control study, pregnancy loss was no more frequent in women with a history of venous thrombosis than in controls, although pregnancy-induced hypertension and preeclampsia were more common. The stillbirth rate was not significantly higher [23]. The placental vasculature is not formed until 10–12 weeks of gestation so a thrombotic pathology does not explain why the majority of women with thrombophilia have early pregnancy loss before 12 weeks. An alternative "non-thrombotic" hypothesis is that trophoblast apoptosis is the underlying mechanism. In vitro studies have demonstrated that antiphospholipid antibodies inhibit trophoblast differentiation and placentation [4, 32]. Experimental studies in mice with genetic disruption of the protein C pathway indicate that the fetal loss that occurs before 10 weeks is similarly due to inhibition of trophoblast growth by coagulation proteases [11].

Meta-analysis indicates an increased prevalence of thrombophilias in case–control studies comparing women with pregnancy complications to those without. However, the point estimates of odds ratios calculated from case–control studies are low, indicating that any causal association is weak. Importantly, the predictive value of a positive thrombophilia test result for recurrence of a particular pregnancy complication has not yet been determined. Randomized trials demonstrating that the presence of a thrombophilia should modify management of subsequent pregnancies have yet to be reported. Nevertheless, many clinicians have instituted a policy of offering anticoagulant drugs to women with a history of pregnancy morbidity, particularly recurrent miscarriage or stillbirth, on the basis of finding laboratory evidence of a thrombophilic defect. Thromboprophylactic dose of low-molecular-weight heparin (LMWH) is usually the preferred option and, while the risk of treatment is low, it is not zero. Allergic skin reactions occur in 1–2 % [8] although heparin-induced thrombocytopenia with thrombosis that often manifests with skin necrosis at injection sites rarely if ever occurs in pregnancy. Regional analgesia is considered to be contraindicated if within 12 h of subcutaneous prophylactic dose heparin [31]. There seems to be little if any risk of osteoporosis with the use of low-dose LMWH for the duration of a pregnancy. A review of almost 3,000 women prescribed low-dose LMWH in pregnancy revealed a very low incidence of complications including bleeding [8].

Systematic reviews of the results of studies reported up to 2005 investigating the association between heritable thrombophilia and pregnancy loss have been published [10, 13, 27, 28]. The summary of results of the most recent is shown in Table 2.2.

2.5.1 Pregnancy Loss

The largest study of pregnancy loss and thrombophilia investigated an association with the factor V Leiden mutation in over 1,000 consecutive Caucasian women [26]. No association was demonstrated with congenital APC resistance (due to the factor V Leiden mutation), but acquired APC resistance was more common in women with a history of miscarriage. Acquired APC resistance reflects the physiological hypercoagulable state of pregnancy, and there may be an association between pregnancy loss and other pregnancy morbidity; however, in this study, the women were tested in the nonpregnant state. A retrospective analysis of 64 women homozygous for the factor V Leiden mutation compared pregnancy outcomes to those in 54 age-matched control women [24]. The stillbirth rate in the affected women was 3.3 % compared to 1.7 % in the controls and rates of miscarriage were 12 and 10 % respectively, results that were not significantly different. While the statistically insignificant results may have resulted from the low power of the study, a major difference in outcome between heterozygous and homozygous women is unlikely, a finding suggested also by systematic review (Table 2.2). The only prospective controlled study investigating the association between heritable thrombophilia and pregnancy loss showed no increased risk in 48 affected women compared to 60 controls [35].

The systematic review published by Robertson and colleagues [28] showed that recurrent first trimester pregnancy loss in association with anticardiolipin antibodies was higher than for any heritable thrombophilia, and second trimester pregnancy loss was strongly associated with lupus anticoagulant activity (Table 2.2). Late pregnancy loss appeared to be most strongly associated with protein S deficiency, but the number of women with protein S deficiency was only 15 and, as indicated in Section 2.3, the diagnosis of heritable protein S deficiency is often inaccurate.

Individual studies have produced conflicting findings on the association between MTHFR homozygosity and recurrent pregnancy loss: some found an association [22, 33] but others did not [6, 9, 17], and a meta-analysis suggested that there is no association (Table 2.2). Adequate folic acid supplementation silences the phenotypic expression of this polymorphism.

2.5.2 Preeclampsia and Intrauterine Growth Restriction

The association between heritable thrombophilia and preeclampsia and intrauterine growth restriction appears to be similar to other pregnancy morbidity, but fewer data are available. Anticardiolipin antibodies appear to be relatively strongly associated with growth restriction (Table 2.2).

A meta-analysis suggested that MTHFR homozygosity was associated with an increased risk only for preeclampsia (Table 2.2). However, this polymorphism may be associated with an increased risk of other pregnancy complications, including placental abruption or infarction [34], preeclampsia [14, 21], and pregnancy-induced hypertension [12]. As mentioned above, adequate folic acid supplementation silences the phenotypic expression of this polymorphism.

2.5.3 Recommendations

Randomized controlled trials, with a no treatment or a placebo arm, in women with a history of pregnancy complications are in progress. The British Society for Haematology has recommended that results from these trials should be awaited before recommending that anticoagulant drugs are given to pregnant women based on testing for heritable thrombophilia, but the issue remains contentious [2]. Provisional studies suggest a benefit of intervention in women with thrombophilia but the benefit, if true, may not be restricted to women with thrombophilia. In small studies, live birth rates of around 70 % were reported compared to live birth rates of around 30 % in previous pregnancies. However, these studies involved small cohorts and there were no control groups. If hypercoagulability, and a related mechanism such as protease-induced trophoblastic apoptosis, is a material contributory factor in many cases of pregnancy morbidity, then administration of low-dose LMWH may be beneficial regardless of whether or not there is laboratory evidence of thrombophilia. If there is an increased relative risk in women with a laboratory "marker," then a beneficial effect will be more readily demonstrated in women with thrombophilia, even though the magnitude of benefit may be the same in women with the same underlying pathology but no identifiable thrombophilia "marker." Therefore, until the results of trials in women at high risk of pregnancy complications and the results of trials specifically in women with thrombophilia are known, many experts suggest that decisions to use low-dose heparin for prevention of pregnancy morbidity should not be made in relation to the results of thrombophilia tests.

In all future studies, criteria for both diagnosis of heritable thrombophilia and pregnancy morbidity must be clearly defined a priori [19]. Many studies to date have not defined criteria for the diagnosis of thrombophilia, they have often relied on results of single laboratory measurements in individuals, and they have not used strict criteria for pregnancy morbidity, for example, the use of ultrasound for accurate clinical assessment.

2.6   Purpura Fulminans in the Newborn

Purpura fulminans is a rare syndrome characterized by progressive hemorrhagic skin necrosis that occurs in neonates with congenital severe protein C or S deficiency at birth or in the first few days of life (an alternative form of the condition occurs in association with infection in children and adults, and this condition is typically associated with acquired severe protein S deficiency). If a neonate develops purpura fulminans, levels of protein C and S should be measured urgently. Levels are normally low at birth, but the condition is associated with undetectable levels. Measurement of levels in the parents may help to interpret the neonate's results. Neonatal purpura fulminans due to deficiency of protein C or S requires urgent replacement therapy with factor concentrate or fresh frozen plasma when concentrate is not immediately available.

In cases of pregnancy where one partner is known to have protein C deficiency, some experts would consider testing the other partner to determine if there is the possibility of the child having severe protein C deficiency at birth, with a view to antenatal detection of a homozygous infant. However, this approach is extremely problematic and counseling and interpretation of test results must be undertaken by an expert. Given the unreliability of phenotypic diagnosis, genetic analysis is mandatory if antenatal diagnosis is going to be considered with a view to termination. Some experts would consider this approach only if there was a previously affected infant.

References

1. Baglin T. Unravelling the thrombophilia paradox: from hypercoagulability to the prothrombotic state. J Thromb Haemost. 2010;8:228–33.
2. Baglin T, Gray E, Greaves M, Hunt B, Keeling D, Machin S, Mackie I, Makris M, Nokes T, Perry D, Tait R, Walker I, Watson H. Clinical guidelines for testing for heritable thrombophilia. Br J Haematol. 2010 [Epub ahead of print]. http://www.ncbi.nlm.nih.gov/pubmed/20128794?itool=EntrezSystem20128792.PEntrez.Pubmed.Pubmed_ResultsPanel.Pubmed_RVDocSum&ordinalpos=20128791.
3. Bezemer ID, Doggen CJ, Vos HL, Rosendaal FR. No association between the common MTHFR 677C->T polymorphism and venous thrombosis: results from the MEGA study. Arch Intern Med. 2007;167:497–501.
4. Bose P, Black S, Kadyrov M, Weissenborn U, Neulen J, Regan L, Huppertz B. Heparin and aspirin attenuate placental apoptosis in vitro: implications for early pregnancy failure. Am J Obstet Gynecol. 2005;192:23–30.
5. Brown K, Luddington R, Baglin T. Effect of the MTHFRC677T variant on risk of venous thromboembolism: interaction with factor V Leiden and prothrombin (F2G20210A) mutations. Br J Haematol. 1998;103:42–4.
6. Foka ZJ, Lambropoulos AF, Saravelos H, Karas GB, Karavida A, Agorastos T, Zournatzi V, Makris PE, Bontis J, Kotsis A. Factor V Leiden and prothrombin G20210A mutations, but not methylenetetrahydrofolate reductase C677T, are associated with recurrent miscarriages. Hum Reprod. 2000;15:458–62.
7. Gopel W, Ludwig M, Junge AK, Kohlmann T, Diedrich K, Moller J. Selection pressure for the factor-V-Leiden mutation and embryo implantation. Lancet. 2001;358:1238–9.
8. Greer IA, Nelson-Piercy C. Low-molecular-weight heparins for thromboprophylaxis and treatment of venous thromboembolism in pregnancy: a systematic review of safety and efficacy. Blood. 2005;106:401–7.
9. Holmes ZR, Regan L, Chilcott I, Cohen H. The C677T MTHFR gene mutation is not predictive of risk for recurrent fetal loss. Br J Haemost. 1999;105:98–101.

10. Howley HE, Walker M, Rodger MA. A systematic review of the association between factor V Leiden or prothrombin gene variant and intrauterine growth restriction. Am J Obstet Gynecol. 2005;192:694–708.

11. Isermann B, Sood R, Pawlinski R, Zogg M, Kalloway S, Degen JL, Mackman N, Weiler H. The thrombomodulin-protein C system is essential for the maintenance of pregnancy. Nat Med. 2003;9:331–7.

12. Kosmas IP, Tatsioni A, Ioannidis JP. Association of C677T polymorphism in the methylenetetrahydrofolate reductase gene with hypertension in pregnancy and pre-eclampsia: a meta-analysis. J Hypertens. 2004;22:1655–62.

13. Kovalevsky G, Gracia CR, Berlin JA, Sammel MD, Barnhart KT. Evaluation of the association between hereditary thrombophilias and recurrent pregnancy loss: a meta-analysis. Arch Intern Med. 2004;164: 558–63.

14. Lachmeijer AM, Arngrimsson R, Bastiaans EJ, Pals G, ten Kate LP, de Vries JI, Kostense PJ, Aarnoudse JG, Dekker GA. Mutations in the gene for methylenetetrahydrofolate reductase, homocysteine levels, and vitamin status in women with a history of preeclampsia. Am J Obstet Gynecol. 2001;184:394–402.

15. Langdown J, Johnson DJ, Baglin TP, Huntington JA. Allosteric activation of antithrombin critically depends upon hinge region extension. J Biol Chem. 2004;279:47288–97.

16. Lisman T, de Groot PG, Meijers JC, Rosendaal FR. Reduced plasma fibrinolytic potential is a risk factor for venous thrombosis. Blood. 2005;105:1102–5.

17. Makino A, Nakanishi T, Sugiura-Ogasawara M, Ozaki Y, Suzumori N, Suzumori K. No association of C677T methylenetetrahydrofolate reductase and an endothelial nitric oxide synthase polymorphism with recurrent pregnancy loss. Am J Reprod Immunol. 2004;52:60–6.

18. Meltzer ME, Lisman T, Doggen CJ, de Groot PG, Rosendaal FR. Synergistic effects of hypofibrinolysis and genetic and acquired risk factors on the risk of a first venous thrombosis. PLoS Med. 2008;5:e97.

19. Middeldorp S. Thrombophilia and pregnancy complications: cause or association? J Thromb Haemost. 2007;5 Suppl 1:276–82.

20. Miyakis S, Lockshin MD, Atsumi T, Branch DW, Brey RL, Cervera R, Derksen RHWM, de Groot PG, Koike T, Meroni PL, Reber G, Shoenfeld Y, Tincani A, Vlachoyiannopoulos PG, Krilis SA. International consensus statement on an update of the classification criteria for definite antiphospholipid syndrome (APS). J Thromb Haemost. 2006;4:295–306.

21. Murakami S, Matsubara N, Saitoh M, Miyakaw S, Shoji M, Kubo T. The relation between plasma homocysteine concentration and methylenetetrahydrofolate reductase gene polymorphism in pregnant women. J Obstet Gynaecol Res. 2001;27:349–52.

22. Nelen WL, Blom HJ, Steegers EA, den Heijer M, Eskes TK. Hyperhomocysteinemia and recurrent early pregnancy loss: a meta-analysis. Fertil Steril. 2000;74:1196–9.

23. Pabinger I, Grafenhofer H, Kaider A, Ilic A, Eichinger S, Quehenberger P, Husslein P, Mannhalter C, Lechner K. Preeclampsia and fetal loss in women with a history of venous thromboembolism. Arterioscler Thromb Vasc Biol. 2001;21:874–9.

24. Pabinger I, Nemes L, Rintelen C, Koder S, Lechler E, Loreth RM, Kyrle PA, Scharrer I, Sas G, Lechner K, Mannhalter C, Ehrenforth S. Pregnancy-associated risk for venous thromboembolism and pregnancy outcome in women homozygous for factor V Leiden. Hematol J. 2000;1:37–41.

25. Pengo V, Tripodi A, Reber G, Rand JH, Ortel TL, Galli M, De Groot PG. Update of the guidelines for lupus anticoagulant detection. J Thromb Haemost. 2009;7:1737–40.

26. Rai R, Shlebak A, Cohen H, Backos M, Holmes Z, Marriott K, Regan L. Factor V Leiden and acquired activated protein C resistance among 1000 women with recurrent miscarriage. Hum Reprod. 2001;16: 961–5.

27. Rey E, Kahn SR, David M, Shrier I. Thrombophilic disorders and fetal loss: a meta-analysis. Lancet. 2003;361:901–8.

28. Robertson L, Wu O, Langhorne P, Twaddle S, Clark P, Lowe GD, Walker ID, Greaves M, Brenkel I, Regan L, Greer IA. Thrombophilia in pregnancy: a systematic review. Br J Haematol. 2006;132:171–96.

29. Rosendaal FR. Venous thrombosis: a multicausal disease. Lancet. 1999;353:1167–73.

30. Rosendaal FR, Bovill EG. Heritability of clotting factors and the revival of the prothrombotic state. Lancet. 2002;359:638–9.

31. Royal College of Obstetricians & Gynaecologists. Green-top guideline no. 37. Thrombosis and embolism during pregnancy and the puerperium, reducing the risk. 2009.

32. Sebire NJ, Regan L, Rai R. Biology and pathology of the placenta in relation to antiphospholipid antibody-associated pregnancy failure. Lupus. 2002;11: 641–3.

33. Unfried G, Griesmacher A, Weismuller W, Nagele F, Huber JC, Tempfer CB. The C677T polymorphism of the methylenetetrahydrofolate reductase gene and idiopathic recurrent miscarriage. Obstet Gynecol. 2002;99:614–9.

34. Van der Molen EF, Arends GE, Nelen WL, Van der Put NJ, Heil SG, Eskes TK, Blom HJ. A common mutation in the 5,10-methylenetetrahydrofolate reductase gene as a new risk factor for placental vasculopathy. Am J Obstet Gynecol. 2000;182:1258–63.

35. Vossen CY, Preston FE, Conard J, Fontcuberta J, Makris M, van der Meer FJ, Pabinger I, Palareti G, Scharrer I, Souto JC, Svensson P, Walker ID, Rosendaal FR. Hereditary thrombophilia and fetal loss: a prospective follow-up study. J Thromb Haemost. 2004;2: 592–6.

Systemic Thromboembolism in Pregnancy: Thromboprophylaxis

3

Charlotte J. Frise, Peter K. MacCallum,
Lucy H. Mackillop, and Catherine Nelson-Piercy

Abstract

Venous thromboembolism is a significant cause of maternal death in the UK, despite being a preventable condition for which clear risk factors have been identified. The introduction of routine antenatal and postnatal thromboprophylaxis for women identified by risk assessment tools has been linked to a steady reduction in the number of deaths. This chapter discusses the risk factors for the development of thromboembolism as well as the options for prophylactic intervention, and the specific clinical situations which can alter the treatment advice.

C.J. Frise, MA, MRCP
Department of Acute General Medicine, John Radcliffe
Hospital, Oxford University Hospitals NHS Trust,
Headley Way, Headington, Oxford OX3 9DU, UK
e-mail: cjfrise@doctors.org.uk

P.K. MacCallum, MD, FRCP, FRCPath
Barts and The London School of Medicine and Dentistry,
Queen Mary University of London,
and Barts Health NHS Trust,
Charterhouse Square, EC1M 6BQ, London, UK
e-mail: p.k.maccallum@qmul.ac.uk

L.H. Mackillop, MA, MRCP
John Radcliffe Hospital, Oxford University Hospitals
NHS Trust, Headley Way, Headington,
Oxford OX3 9DU, UK
e-mail: lucymackillop@hotmail.com

C. Nelson-Piercy, MA, FRCP, FRCOG (✉)
Guy's and St Thomas' Foundation Trust and Imperial
College Healthcare Trust, Westminster Bridge Road,
London SE1 7EH, UK
e-mail: catherine.nelson-piercy@gstt.nhs.uk

3.1 Introduction

Venous thromboembolism (VTE) is a preventable condition, yet pulmonary embolus remains a leading direct cause of maternal death in the UK [17]. In recent years, attention has been drawn to the assessment of every person admitted to hospital to attempt to risk stratify individuals and institute appropriate preventive measures to reduce the rate of venous thromboembolic events [83]. Pregnancy is a prothrombotic state, meaning that women are at increased risk of venous thromboembolic disease from the first trimester, and in particular in the puerperium.

Regular assessment of a pregnant woman, repeated every time there is a change in her clinical condition (whether inpatient or outpatient), is the cornerstone of successful prevention of VTE. Low-molecular-weight heparins (LMWHs) are the most commonly used agents for thromboprophylaxis

H. Cohen, P. O'Brien (eds.), *Disorders of Thrombosis and Hemostasis in Pregnancy*,
DOI 10.1007/978-1-4471-4411-3_3, © Springer-Verlag London 2012

as they are safe, effective, and well tolerated in pregnancy and the postnatal period.

This chapter aims to summarize the risk factors for venous thromboembolic disease in pregnancy and the rationale for different treatment approaches depending on the risk factors present in each individual. It is based on the VTE prophylaxis guidelines of the Royal College of Obstetricians and Gynaecologists [83].

3.2 Assessment of Thromboembolic Risk

Physiological changes in the hemostatic system produce a hypercoagulable state and make pregnancy an independent risk factor for VTE. VTE is still a rare event, however, in pregnant women without other risk factors. Therefore, a search for other risk factors and stratification of those risks is critical to enable decisions about thromboprophylaxis. Known risk factors may be characterized as preexisting, those directly relating to the pregnancy, and transient risk factors that might be present for part of the pregnancy only.

The assessment and reassessment of thrombotic risk are of utmost importance. Assessment of risk should take place at the initial consultation whether that is in primary or secondary care, if clinical parameters change, on any admission to hospital and immediately postnatally. Risk factors for VTE, which are shown in Table 3.1, must be reviewed and documented. The latest evidence for risk factor assessment is presented below.

3.2.1 Thrombophilia: Heritable

A heritable thrombophilia is found in 20–50 % of women with pregnancy-related VTE [48]. However, different thrombophilias have different levels of risk. In a retrospective study of 72,000 pregnancies in which women with VTE were investigated for a thrombophilic tendency and the background prevalence of these defects was known, the risk of VTE in pregnancy was estimated to be 1:2.8 in type I antithrombin deficiency (with reduced activity and antigen), 1:42 for type

II antithrombin deficiency (with reduced activity and normal antigen level), 1:113 for protein C deficiency, and 1:437 for factor V Leiden [61].

3.2.1.1 Factor V Leiden and Prothrombin G20210A

The most common heritable thrombophilic tendencies in the UK are factor V Leiden and prothrombin F2G20210A, present in around 4 % and 2 % of the population, respectively. Case–control studies show that individuals heterozygous for these genes are at roughly fivefold increased risk of VTE in both the general population and pregnancy [31, 71, 80]. However, the absolute risk appears to be small (<1 %). Cohort studies undertaken in the general population and a further study in women heterozygous for factor V Leiden recorded three episodes of VTE in 752 pregnancies [11, 23, 36, 51]. Therefore, the benefit of thromboprophylaxis at this level of risk would be limited.

The absolute risk may be higher, however, in women with a family history of VTE and a thrombophilic genotype. In a meta-analysis [10, 11], 2 % of factor V Leiden carriers had a pregnancy-related VTE. In the cohort studies where the cases were selected because of family screening, that is, two or more first-degree relatives with VTE but exclusion of the proband from analysis, 3 % of factor V Leiden carriers had a pregnancy-related VTE compared to 0.6 % in family members who were not carriers. This absolute risk is similar in magnitude to that seen in retrospective analyses in women with pregnancy-related thrombosis and with the F2G20210A prothrombin gene variant, selected because of a family history of VTE, and to those observed in a retrospective family study in carriers of factor V Leiden and F2G20210A [5, 56, 84]. A review of heterozygous factor V Leiden carriers with at least one symptomatic first-degree relative estimated the incidence of the first episode of VTE occurring in association with pregnancy at 2.1 %. The risk *during* pregnancy, however, was only 0.4 % compared to 1.7 % in the postpartum period. Very similar incidences were estimated for the prothrombin variant – 0.5 % in pregnancy and 1.9 % postpartum [62].

Table 3.1 Risk factors for VTE

Preexisting	
Previous VTE	Single
	Estrogen or pregnancy related
	Thrombophilia related
	Unprovoked
	Related to temporary risk factor
	Recurrent events
Thrombophilia	Heritable
	Antithrombin deficiency
	Protein C deficiency
	Protein S deficiency
	Factor V Leiden
	Prothrombin gene G20210A
	Acquired
	Antiphospholipid syndrome – persistent lupus anticoagulant or persistent moderate/high-titre anticardiolipin or β2-glycoprotein 1 antibodies
Medical comorbidities including	SLE
	Nephrotic syndrome
	Heart disease
	Sickle cell disease
	Cancer
	Inflammatory conditions, e.g. inflammatory bowel disease
Others	Age >35 years
	Obesity BMI > 30 kg/m^2 either prior to pregnancy or in early pregnancy
	Parity $\geq$ 3
	Smoking
	Varicose veins: gross, symptomatic, above knee, or with phlebitis or skin changes
	Paraplegia
	Family history of VTE
Obstetric	
Antenatal	Multiple pregnancy, assisted reproduction therapy (ART)
	Preeclampsia
Delivery	Caesarean section
	Prolonged labor, midcavity rotational operative delivery
Postnatal	Postpartum hemorrhage (>1 L)
	Blood transfusion
New onset/transient	
Early pregnancy	Hyperemesis gravidarum
	Ovarian hyperstimulation syndrome
Any time in pregnancy	Surgical procedure, e.g. ERPC, appendicectomy, postpartum sterilization
	Admission or immobility, e.g. symphysis pubis dysfunction
	Dehydration
	Systemic infection, e.g. pneumonia, pyelonephritis, wound infection
	Travel of duration >4 h

Adapted from RCOG guideline no. [35]

The risk of pregnancy-related VTE also appears to increase with compound (combined defects) or homozygous states. In previously asymptomatic women, the risk is higher in compound heterozygotes for factor V Leiden and F2G20210A, with an absolute risk of approximately 4 %, although a retrospective family cohort study did not confirm this increased risk [19, 56, 57]. A systematic review suggests that women who are homozygous for factor V Leiden or F2G20210A are also at much higher risk of pregnancy-related VTE, and absolute risks of 9–16 % have been reported for homozygous factor V Leiden [51, 76].

3.2.1.2 Antithrombin, Protein C, and Protein S Deficiencies

Outside pregnancy, the risk of the first VTE appears to be higher in individuals with deficiencies of antithrombin, protein C, or protein S compared to V Leiden and the F2G20210A [47]. Asymptomatic women with protein C or protein S deficiency probably have a moderately increased risk of VTE associated with pregnancy, again with most events occurring postpartum. The risk associated with antithrombin deficiency appears to vary according to the subtype but may be associated with a very high absolute risk of 15–50 % [15].

In a more recent retrospective cohort study of women from families with hereditary antithrombin, protein C, or protein S deficiency, 12 pregnancy-related VTE episodes were objectively diagnosed in 162 pregnancies (7 %), two-thirds of which occurred in the postpartum period [26]. In a recent review, in women with a deficiency of antithrombin, protein C, or protein S and at least one symptomatic first-degree relative, the incidence of the first episode of VTE occurring in association with pregnancy was estimated at 4.1 % (1.7–8.3 %). Again, the incidence appeared to be higher during the postpartum period than during pregnancy, 3 % and 1.2 %, respectively [62].

3.2.1.3 MTHFR

Homozygosity for a thermolabile variant of the gene for methylenetetrahydrofolate reductase (C677T MTHFR) is sometimes included in thrombophilia testing, but there is no evidence of an association with a clinically relevant increase in the risk of VTE in pregnancy [76].

3.2.2 Thrombophilia: Antiphospholipid Syndrome

Antiphospholipid syndrome (APS) is defined as the presence of persistently positive antiphospholipid antibodies (aPL) – lupus anticoagulant (LA) and/or anticardiolipin (aCL) and/or β2-glycoprotein 1 (β2 GP1) antibodies of medium or high titre on two consecutive occasions at least 12 weeks apart ("persistently positive") in association with a history of arterial or venous thrombosis or adverse pregnancy outcome. An adverse pregnancy outcome is defined as either a fetal death after 10 weeks' gestation, a preterm birth at less than 34 weeks' gestation due to severe preeclampsia or intrauterine growth restriction, or the occurrence of three or more unexplained miscarriages before 10 weeks' gestation [63].

Antiphospholipid antibodies, in particular persistent LA or moderate/high-titre aCL antibodies or β2 GP1 antibodies, are associated with an increased risk of recurrent thrombosis, and it is common for such women to be on long-term warfarin after a first event [18, 25, 27].

Optimal management for the prevention of recurrent thrombosis in pregnancy is unclear. There is a lack of randomized trials and very few prospective studies of women with APS and prior thrombosis. In one study, 98 of 565 women tested were found to have positive aPL and were divided into low, high, or very high risk based on their clinical history, that is, asymptomatic, three or more pregnancy losses, or prior venous or arterial thrombosis, respectively [8]. Women who were low risk received 2 weeks of postpartum LMWH and antenatal LMWH if there were additional risk factors. Women in the latter two groups received prophylactic or high-prophylactic-dose LMWH (dalteparin 50–100 IU/kg/day and 100–200 IU/kg/day, respectively) from enrollment until 6 weeks postpartum (or until oral anticoagulation was recommenced). They also received low-dose aspirin from weeks 12 to 36. There were no VTE events in the low- or high-risk groups, but there were two events in the 28 patients in the very-high-risk group, suggesting a significant risk of thrombosis. In a further series of 33 women with primary APS, women who had no previous history of thrombosis and no other risk factors were given 3–5 days of thromboprophylaxis postpartum only, and there were no thrombotic events in this subgroup [88].

3.2.3 Previous Venous Thromboembolism

Women with previous VTE have an increased risk of recurrence in pregnancy and postpartum, with reported recurrence rates of 1.4–11.1 %, and this risk appears to be constant over the whole duration of pregnancy [40, 67]. A retrospective comparison of the recurrence rate of VTE during pregnancy and the nonpregnant period revealed recurrence rates of 10.9 % during and 3.7 % outside pregnancy, giving a relative risk during pregnancy of 3.5 (95 % CI 1.6–7.8) [66].

In order to aid risk assessment, women with previous VTE can be stratified into those with recurrent or single previous VTE. The latter group may be further subdivided into those with:

- A temporary risk factor associated with the VTE, for example, major trauma or surgery
- Estrogen-provoked, that is, pregnancy or estrogen-containing contraception
- Unprovoked
- Thrombophilia, either heritable or acquired or associated with a family history of VTE

3.2.3.1 Recurrent VTE
Individuals with recurrent VTE are at increased risk of further recurrence [42]. Many will therefore be on long-term therapeutic dose warfarin. Although data are lacking, these women would be expected to have a high risk of recurrence in pregnancy.

3.2.3.2 Temporary Risk Factor-Associated VTE
Outside pregnancy, there is a low risk of recurrence of VTE which resulted from a transient major risk factor. This is also likely to be the case in pregnancy, as both a prospective and a retrospective study suggested that the risk of antenatal recurrence is very low if the prior VTE was provoked by a transient major risk factor that is no longer present [13, 20]. Examples of this include a DVT post surgery or trauma or in an intravenous drug user who is no longer injecting.

3.2.3.3 Single Previous Estrogen Related
Although prior estrogen-provoked VTE was not found to be a risk factor for VTE in subsequent pregnancy in the study by Brill-Edwards and colleagues [13], other retrospective studies suggest the contrary [20, 66, 67]. For example, in women whose previous VTE was associated with the use of estrogen-containing contraception, the recurrence rate was 9.5 % in subsequent pregnancies where thromboprophylaxis was withheld [20]. The risk was very similar (9.8 %, 95 % CI 4.2–20.9 %) if the prior VTE had occurred during a previous pregnancy. In another study comparing pregnant women whose prior episode was provoked by estrogen-containing contraception and those women without a history of contraceptive use at the time of VTE, the recurrence rates were 10 % and 2.7 %, respectively [67].

A retrospective study using Californian hospital discharge data analyzed recurrence rates in women with a previous single pregnancy-related VTE and in women with a previous unprovoked thromboembolic event [92]. The overall recurrence rates over the following 6–60 months were lower in the group with pregnancy-related VTE initially (5.8 % compared to 10.4 %), but the rate of recurrence in subsequent pregnancies was higher (4.5 % compared to 2.7 %). Of the recurrent events in the women who had previously had a pregnancy-related VTE, 35 % occurred in a subsequent pregnancy, compared to 8.7 % in the group with previous unprovoked VTE. Furthermore, 71 % of the recurrences were antenatal in the former group compared to 54 % in the latter. This adds further support to the stratification of women with previous estrogen-related VTE as being at high risk of VTE in subsequent pregnancy and the puerperium.

3.2.3.4 Single Previous Unprovoked

In non-pregnant populations, unprovoked VTE has been shown to be associated with an increased risk of recurrence compared to those provoked by a temporary risk factor that is no longer present [42]. A prospective study of 125 pregnant women with a single prior episode of VTE showed that 5.9 % of women with VTE that was unprovoked or associated with a thrombophilia had a recurrence, in contrast to women with a previous VTE that was associated with a temporary risk factor and no thrombophilia, in whom no recurrences were seen [13]. In this study, estrogen-provoked VTE was included as a temporary risk factor. A retrospective study of 155 pregnancies in 88 women with a previous VTE compared the recurrence rate in women with a previous unprovoked VTE who were not given thromboprophylaxis to that in women where the prior VTE was associated with a transient risk factor. The recurrence rate was 4.2 % in the former group and none in the latter [20].

In contrast, Pabinger and colleagues [66] found that the presence or absence of a temporary risk factor did not affect the risk of recurrence in a subsequent pregnancy, although again estrogen-provoked VTE was included as a temporary risk factor, which may have influenced the results.

3.2.3.5 Thrombophilia Related

Outside pregnancy, the most common heritable thrombophilias do not substantially increase the risk of recurrence after a single event. This was shown in a systematic review of prospective studies [55] where being a heterozygote carrier of factor V Leiden increased the relative risk of recurrence with an OR of 1.39 (95 % CI 1.15–1.67). Data regarding the effect of heritable thrombophilia on the risk of recurrent VTE in pregnancy are extremely sparse.

3.2.4 Obesity

Obesity is common in the non-pregnant population, and a body mass index (BMI) above 30 kg/m² was seen in 19 % of women aged 25–34 and 25 % of women aged 35–44 years [35]. Any increase in weight above a normal BMI appears to be associated with an increased risk of VTE in pregnancy. Being overweight (BMI 25–30 kg/m²) is very common in pregnancy, with a prevalence of approximately 50 %, and this is a risk factor for pregnancy-related VTE. The risk of VTE appears to increase further with increasing obesity, although the data are limited [77]. In one study, obesity was more strongly associated with pulmonary embolism than with deep vein thrombosis, with odds ratios of 14.9 (95 % CI 3.0– 74.8) and 4.4 (95 % CI 1.6–11.9), respectively [46].

Obesity has been identified as a particular concern in two reports from the UK's Centre for Maternal and Child Enquiries (CMACE). For the triennium 2003–2005, there were 33 deaths from pulmonary embolus [16]. In the 21 cases where BMI was recorded, 12 women were obese, that is, BMI > 30 kg/m². In the report from 2006–2008, 30 % of mothers who died from direct causes and for whom the BMI was known were obese, as were 24 % of women who died from indirect causes (27 % overall) [17].

3.2.5 Age

Age greater than 35 years increases the risk of antenatal and postnatal VTE, with an odds ratio of 1.3 (95 % CI 1.0–1.7) compared to that of women aged 20–34 years [50]. Simpson and colleagues [86] also showed that postnatal events were significantly associated with maternal age greater than 35 years (OR 1.4, 95 % CI 1.0–2.0).

3.2.6 First-Trimester Events

The risk of VTE may increase further in the first trimester due to other complications such as hyperemesis gravidarum (OR 2.5, 95 % CI 2.0–3.2) or ovarian hyperstimulation (OR 4.3, 95 % CI 2.0–9.4) [39, 40]. Women with ovarian hyperstimulation are at particular risk of internal jugular vein VTE [3]. There is also an increased risk of VTE associated with surgery during pregnancy, including termination of pregnancy and ectopic pregnancy. Postsurgical thromboprophylaxis is therefore advised if indicated in these circumstances, as it is after delivery.

3.2.7 Mode of Delivery

Compared with vaginal birth, Caesarean section increases the risk of postpartum VTE. In a Canadian retrospective population-based cohort study of 46,766 women who underwent a planned Caesarean section for breech presentation and 2,292,420 women who planned to deliver vaginally, an increased risk of postpartum VTE with Caesarean section was demonstrated, with an odds ratio of 2.2 (95 % CI 1.5–3.2) [52].

Compared to elective Caesarean section, emergency Caesarean further increases the risk of VTE. A Swedish study included both elective and emergency Caesarean sections and showed a relative risk of VTE of 6.7 compared to vaginal delivery [79]. A Scottish study also compared emergency with elective Caesarean section and showed that the risk of VTE was doubled following emergency [54].

RCOG guidelines were published in 1995 that recommended thromboprophylaxis after emergency Caesarean section [81]. The CEMACE reports for the subsequent four triennia show that during this period (1997–2008), there were 26 deaths from VTE following Caesarean section compared to 27 following vaginal delivery [17]. As the latter make up 70–80 % of all deliveries, this suggests that Caesarean section remains a risk factor for fatal PE despite the published guidelines on thromboprophylaxis.

3.2.8 Immobility

Immobility is known to be a risk factor for the development of VTE in non-pregnant patients, but the information available for pregnant patients is limited. One case–control study looked at antepartum immobilization, defined as strict bed rest for 1 week or more prior to delivery, in patients with a BMI of greater than 25 kg/m². The results showed a multiplicative effect on the risk

of antepartum and postpartum VTE with odds ratios of 62.3 and 40.1, respectively [39]

The UK's National Institute for Health and Clinical Excellence (NICE) guideline on antenatal care [64] and the UK's Royal College of Obstetricians and Gynaecologists (RCOG) Scientific Advisory Committee Opinion Paper on air travel in pregnancy [82] state that long-haul air travel increases the risk of VTE, but the current RCOG guideline considers all long-distance travel longer than 4 h duration, and not just by air, to be a risk factor for VTE in pregnancy [83].

3.2.9 Hospital Admission

In non-pregnant medical and surgical patients, hospitalization is now recognized as a major risk factor for VTE, and it is believed that at least 25,000 deaths per year in England resulting from PE complicating hospital admission may be preventable. An independent expert working group set up by the UK Chief Medical Officer recommended that it be mandatory for all patients to be risk assessed for VTE on admission to hospital, and this report has been accepted by the Department of Health [22]. NICE guidelines on prevention of VTE in patients admitted to hospital recommend consideration of VTE prophylaxis with LMWH for women who are pregnant or have given birth within 6 weeks who are admitted to hospital and have one or more risk factors [65].

3.3 Thromboprophylaxis

3.3.1 Efficacy

Thromboprophylaxis has been shown to reduce the incidence of VTE in pregnancy. In a study of 284 pregnancies in women with a prior event, there were no recurrent events in the 87 in which thromboprophylaxis was administered compared with eight in the 197 pregnancies where it was not [67]. In a prospective cohort study in families with antithrombin, protein C, or protein S deficiency or factor V Leiden, two VTEs occurred in 28 pregnancies (7 %) in women who did not receive thromboprophylaxis, whereas there were no episodes in 43 women who did receive thromboprophylaxis [90]. Another study compared the incidence of postpartum VTE before and after the introduction of thromboprophylaxis across Scottish maternity hospitals in 1995. There were approximately 1.55 million maternities between 1980 and 2005, and there was a significant reduction in the incidence of VTE between 1996 and 2004 compared to 1980–1995 [34].

3.3.2 Pharmacological Agents

3.3.2.1 Low Molecular Weight Heparins (LMWHs)

LMWHs have been shown to be as effective as, and safer than, unfractionated heparin (UFH) when used to prevent VTE in pregnancy [33, 85]. UFH can cause heparin-induced thrombocytopenia (HIT), but the risk of this is much lower when LMWHs are used. Current guidelines support monitoring the platelet count in patients on LMWH only when there has been previous exposure to UFH. Prolonged use of UFH during pregnancy can result in osteoporosis and fractures, but this risk is very low with LMWH [69]. In a systematic review of prophylactic and treatment dose LMWH use in 2,777 pregnancies, there were no cases of HIT; the incidence of osteoporotic fractures was 0.04 % and of allergic skin reactions was 1.8 % [33]. Significant bleeding was seen in 1.98 % and was usually related primarily to obstetric causes.

Table 3.3 gives suggested prophylactic and therapeutic subcutaneous doses of LMWH in pregnancy and postpartum. Doses of LMWH are based on booking weight rather than BMI or weight later in pregnancy (although some authorities calculate the dose according to current weight). Data from the UK Obstetric Surveillance Study (UKOSS) show that overweight and obese women develop VTE while on prophylactic LMWH at doses appropriate for those of lower weight [43]. There is no consensus on the appropriate prophylactic dosing of obese women, so some units may prescribe the usual prophylactic dose twice daily for women over 90 kg.

It may be appropriate to use higher doses of LMWH as prophylaxis in women who are usually on long-term oral anticoagulation because of previous recurrent VTE or thrombophilia. Anti-Xa level monitoring may also be helpful in guiding therapy in women at very high risk because of antithrombin deficiency, but this should be done in association with an expert in hemostasis.

3.3.2.2 Unfractionated Heparin

UFH has a shorter half-life than LMWH, and there is more complete reversal of its activity by protamine sulfate. UFH has several disadvantages compared to LMWH. In addition to the association with HIT and osteoporosis, when used for thromboprophylaxis, more frequent administration is required due to its shorter half-life [89].

In some women, for example those at very high risk of thrombosis or increased risk of hemorrhage, UFH may be preferred around the time of delivery so that use of regional anesthesia or analgesia is not prevented. For example, if no LMWH has been given for 24 h but the woman has not yet delivered and there is concern about delaying further doses of LMWH, a prophylactic dose of 5,000 units subcutaneously of UFH could be used and repeated every 12 h until LMWH can be safely resumed after delivery. The required interval between a prophylactic dose of UFH and regional analgesia or anesthesia is less than with LMWH (4 and 12 h, respectively), and there is less concern regarding neuraxial hematoma with UFH [37].

3.3.2.3 Danaparoid

Danaparoid, a heparinoid with a half-life of approximately 24 h, is used mostly in patients intolerant of heparin. A recent review of the use of prophylactic and treatment doses of danaparoid in pregnant women with (current or a history of) HIT or skin allergy to heparin (32 and 19 cases, respectively) showed four maternal bleeding events, two of which were fatal due to placental problems (previa and abruption) [49]. In three lactating women with measurable plasma levels, no anti-Xa activity was detected in the cord blood of five infants tested, and no anti-Xa activity was found in breast milk. There were no adverse fetal outcomes attributed to danaparoid. Use of this agent should be managed in conjunction with a consultant hematologist with expertise in this area.

3.3.2.4 Fondaparinux

Fondaparinux is a synthetic indirect factor Xa inhibitor, licensed in the UK for the prevention and treatment of VTE outside pregnancy, and is similar in efficacy to LMWH [59]. No placental transfer of fondaparinux was found in a human cotyledon model [44], but anti-Xa activity of approximately 10 % of that in maternal plasma was found in the umbilical cord plasma in newborns of five mothers being treated with fondaparinux [21]. There is limited experience of its use in pregnancy, where it may be useful in women with a history of HIT. Although no adverse effects were observed in the newborns, it is premature to conclude that it is safe, and its use should be reserved for women intolerant of heparin compounds. The regular prophylactic dose is 2.5 mg subcutaneously daily, and it does not seem necessary to alter this dose in pregnancy [30].

It is unknown whether fondaparinux is excreted in breast milk and, although oral absorption seems unlikely, its use in the postpartum setting is not currently advised.

3.3.2.5 Low Dose Aspirin

There are no controlled trials on the use of aspirin for thromboprophylaxis in pregnancy, so conclusions about its efficacy have been extrapolated from other trials in the non-pregnant population. A meta-analysis of trials of short-term antiplatelet therapy in surgical and medical patients showed a significant reduction in both DVT and PE with antiplatelet prophylaxis [1]. Another meta-analysis, focusing on patients at high risk for occlusive vascular events, found a statistically significant 25 % reduction in the odds of pulmonary embolism associated with antiplatelet therapy [2].

Another trial, much criticized, suggested that, compared to placebo, low dose aspirin reduces by 36 % the risk of VTE after orthopedic surgery, even in some patients taking concomitant heparin therapy [72]. The Women's Health Study, however, found aspirin to be no better than placebo for long-term primary prevention of VTE in older women in a secondary end-point analysis [32]. The American College of Chest Physicians' guidelines recommend against the use of aspirin for VTE prophylaxis in any patient group [7, 28].

No adverse fetal outcomes were reported in the meta-analyses of large randomized controlled trials of low dose aspirin in pregnancy for the prevention of preeclampsia [24]. Use of low dose aspirin is appropriate for women with APS to improve fetal outcome [75] and as conjunctive therapy when LMWH is used in pregnant women with mechanical heart valves.

3.3.2.6 Warfarin

Warfarin use in pregnancy is restricted to a few situations where heparin is considered unsuitable, that is, in some patients with mechanical heart valves. It is therefore generally not used for thromboprophylaxis antenatally.

Warfarin can be safely used following delivery and in breastfeeding mothers, although it requires close monitoring and visits to an anticoagulant clinic and, compared with LMWH, carries an increased risk of postpartum hemorrhage and perineal hematoma. It is appropriate for those on maintenance warfarin outside pregnancy to restart postnatally, but this should be delayed for at least 5–7 days after delivery to minimize the risk of hemorrhage during the period of overlap of LMWH and warfarin. It is not appropriate for those women who require short-term postpartum prophylaxis, for example, 7 days.

3.3.2.7 Dextran

Dextran should be avoided antenatally and intrapartum, primarily because of the risk of anaphylactoid reaction, which has been associated with uterine hypertonus, fetal distress, fetal neurological abnormalities, and death [6, 9]. As there are now many alternatives, dextran is of little value in modern obstetric practice.

3.3.2.8 Oral Thrombin and Xa Inhibitors

Dabigatran and rivaroxaban are licensed for the prevention of VTE after major orthopedic surgery and the latter is now licensed for treatment of acute DVT. They are not licensed for use in pregnancy where there is no experience in their use and thus should be avoided.

3.3.3 Contraindications to Pharmacological Thromboprophylaxis

LMWH should be avoided, discontinued, or postponed in women who are at risk of bleeding, after careful consideration of the balance of risks of bleeding and thrombosis. Nonpregnancy-related risk factors for bleeding in pregnancy are extrapolated from data obtained from non-pregnant populations.

Women with major antepartum hemorrhage, progressive wound hematoma, suspected intra-abdominal bleeding, and postpartum hemorrhage are therefore at high risk of further hemorrhage and may be more appropriately managed with UFH or anti-embolism stockings. If a woman develops a hemorrhagic problem while on LMWH, the treatment should be stopped and expert hema-

---

Risk Factors for Bleeding

- Active antenatal or postpartum bleeding
- Increased risk of major hemorrhage (e.g. placenta previa)
- Bleeding diathesis, for example, von Willebrand's disease, some types of hemophilia, acquired coagulopathy
- Thrombocytopenia (platelet count $<75 \times 10^9$ per liter)
- Acute stroke in the last 4 weeks (ischemic or hemorrhagic)
- Uncontrolled hypertension (BP >200 mmHg systolic or >120 mmHg diastolic)
- Severe liver disease (prothrombin time above normal range or known varices)
- Severe renal disease (GFR <30 mL/min/1.73m²)

---

tological advice sought. Excessive blood loss and blood transfusion are also risk factors for VTE, so thromboprophylaxis should be begun or reinstituted as soon as the immediate risk of hemorrhage is reduced, again emphasizing the need for repeated review of the individual patient [38, 39].

Renal impairment is not an absolute contraindication to LMWH use, but a dose reduction is required in severe renal impairment (because of the risk of accumulation of LMWH and the association of platelet dysfunction with uremia). The dose reduction depends on the specific LMWH. For example, the dose of enoxaparin and dalteparin should be reduced in patients with creatinine clearance less than 30 mL/min, but the dose of tinzaparin should be reduced if the creatinine clearance is less than 20 mL/min.

3.3.4 Graduated Compression Stockings

Previous British Committee for Standards in Haematology (BCSH) guidelines advised that all women with a history of VTE should be encouraged to wear graduated compression stockings (GCSs) throughout their pregnancy and for 6–12 weeks after delivery [91]. This guidance was based on evidence extrapolated from studies using GCS in hospitalized, nonpregnant populations as there are no trials specifically looking at pregnant women. Small studies have shown that GCSs significantly improve venous emptying in pregnant women and increase the blood flow while decreasing the lumen diameter of the superficial femoral and common femoral veins in late pregnancy and early postpartum [14, 41].

The advantages and limitations of GCS and other mechanical methods of VTE prevention in the nonpregnancy setting were reviewed by the ACCP [28]. The conclusion was that such methods should be used primarily in patients at high risk of bleeding and thus unable to receive pharmacological thromboprophylaxis and as an adjunct to anticoagulant thromboprophylaxis where this had been shown to improve efficacy, for example, in surgical patients. Attention should be given to their proper application. In hospitalized medical patients, their recommended use was limited to those who had a contraindication to anticoagulant thromboprophylaxis.

In the 2008 ACCP guidelines on thromboprophylaxis in pregnancy [7], the use of GCS was recommended for women considered to be at high risk of VTE after Caesarean section, and antenatally and postpartum for all women with a previous DVT. However, this latter indication was not included in the 2012 ACCP guidelines [93]. In patients with a symptomatic DVT, a tighter-fitted GCS should be worn during the day, that is, with an ankle pressure gradient of 30–40 mmHg. This should be worn for 2 years to reduce the risk of post-thrombotic syndrome and longer if there are post-thrombotic sequelae [42]. This recommendation should apply in pregnancy where possible.

GCSs of an appropriate size are therefore suggested in pregnancy for those who are hospitalized in whom LMWH is contraindicated, those who are at particularly high risk of VTE (previous VTE or more than three risk factors) and hospitalized post-Caesarean section, outpatients with prior VTE, and women traveling for more than 4 h.

There are few data regarding the most efficacious length of GCS to use in pregnancy. Calf vein DVTs are more common in the nonpregnant population in comparison to pregnant populations in whom most DVTs are iliofemoral. Reviews outside pregnancy suggest equivalent efficacy of knee- and thigh-length GCS but better compliance with the former [12, 70]. Studies in pregnancy have assessed only thigh-length stockings [41]. Hydrostatic pressures on standing tend to counteract venous compression from GCS, so GCS may be of less benefit in the ambulant population compared with those confined to bed [53, 68]. On balance, therefore, properly applied thigh-length GCSs are advocated for pregnant women, but knee-length GCS should be considered if thigh-length GCSs are ill-fitting or compliance is poor.

3.3.5 Monitoring

Anti-Xa levels can be used to monitor the effect of LMWH. Anti-Xa levels are only an indication of the concentration of LMWH present, and levels provide little or no evidence on the efficacy in relation to prevention of thrombosis. Experience indicates that monitoring of anti-Xa levels is not required when LMWH is used for thromboprophylaxis, provided that the woman has normal renal function [4]. In women at extremes of body weight, it may be reasonable to check anti-Xa levels. Due to the relatively short half-life of LMWH, it is important to check with the local laboratory as to when to check the levels. Many laboratories have a reference range for 4 h post dose, whereas some use a trough level.

3.3.6 Timing

Many studies have shown that the VTE risk in the first trimester is significant. A meta-analysis shows that most VTEs occur antenatally with an equal distribution throughout gestation [74]. CMACE found that two-thirds of antenatal fatal pulmonary VTE in 2003–2005 occurred in the first trimester [16] and half in the 2006–2008 report [17]. Women at high risk of VTE either because of a previous event, thrombophilia, or multiple risk factors should therefore be offered pre-pregnancy counseling to ensure that treatment is started as soon as pregnancy is confirmed. It is advisable that an assessment of risk factors should occur at first contact with a healthcare professional and be repeated at every hospital admission or intercurrent illness. The period of greatest risk per day is postpartum [7, 38]. Therefore, many women who did not meet the threshold for significant risk antenatally should be reconsidered for thromboprophylaxis postnatally. Any woman taking antenatal thromboprophylaxis should continue it postnatally unless contraindications have developed, and all women with prior VTE should receive postpartum prophylaxis. Given this increased risk postnatally, further assessment of the risk of VTE is required following delivery, taking into consideration mode of delivery, bleeding risk, and any complications or comorbidities that may have developed.

3.3.7 Duration

As detailed in Chap. 1, the prothrombotic changes associated with pregnancy can take several weeks to normalize. A study of thromboelastography (TEG) data from 71 women after normal delivery showed that all parameters remain abnormal at 1 week postpartum but normalize over the subsequent 3 weeks [58], although prothrombotic coagulation factor and naturally occurring anticoagulant abnormalities may persist for longer (see Chap. 1). The clinical data from several observational studies, however, show that the risk persists for up to 6 weeks postpartum, although to a lesser degree in weeks 5 and 6 [36, 38, 71, 81].

In view of this persistent increased risk, it is advisable for high-risk women, that is, those on antenatal thromboprophylaxis, to continue for 6 weeks postpartum. There has been much debate as to the optimal duration of thromboprophylaxis in women at intermediate risk of VTE (see Fig. 3.1 and Table 3.2). There is little evidence to support recommendations regarding

duration of thromboprophylaxis in such women, and research in this area is needed. In view of the data regarding postpartum prothrombotic changes, a minimum of 7 days' thromboprophylaxis is suggested. In addition, women with ongoing additional risk factors should be considered potentially high risk, and it may be necessary to extend the 7-day period of prophylaxis for up to 6 weeks, for example, if hospital discharge is delayed due to sepsis.

3.4 Management in Specific Situations

The management of pregnant women with respect to their risk of VTE starts with accurate assessment of risk factors at their first presentation in pregnancy or ideally before, together with regular reassessment throughout the pregnancy and puerperium.

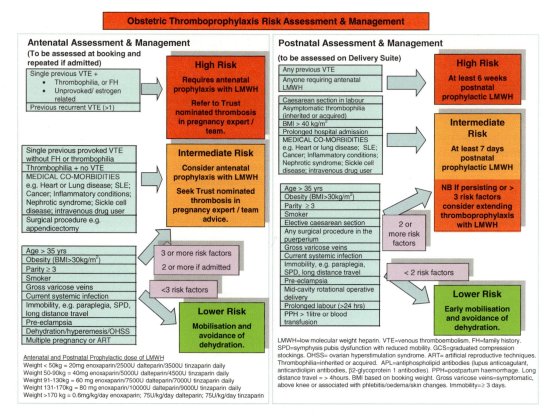

Fig. 3.1 An example of a risk assessment tool

Table 3.2 Stratification of VTE risk by type of thrombophilia and history

Very high risk	*Treatment recommendation*
Previous VTE on long-term warfarin	Antenatal high-dose LMWH and at least 6 weeks' postnatal LMWH or warfarin
Antithrombin deficiency	
Antiphospholipid syndrome + previous VTE	
High risk	*Treatment recommendation*
Previous recurrent or unprovoked VTE	Antenatal and 6 weeks' postnatal LMWH
Previous estrogen-related VTE	
Previous VTE + thrombophilia	
Previous VTE + family history of VTE	
Asymptomatic thrombophilia – combined defects, homozygous FVL	
Intermediate risk	*Treatment recommendation*
Single previous VTE associated with transient risk factor, no family history, or thrombophilia	7 days postnatal prophylactic LMWH 6 weeks if other risk factors present
Asymptomatic thrombophilia (other than those above)	

Management also requires accurate and sensitive counseling of women and their families so that they understand the risks of VTE, the signs and symptoms of VTE, and the requirement for thromboprophylaxis. Women should be taught how to give the subcutaneous injections and require support from primary and secondary care to facilitate continued compliance. They should be counseled about delivery and management of their LMWH and require sensitive discussion around how this might influence their birth plan. Women receiving thromboprophylaxis require referral to an obstetric anesthetist, preferably antenatally, for discussion of pain management during labor.

The decision about the threshold for thromboprophylaxis in a woman with risk factors is discussed under each risk factor below. This is summarized in Fig. 3.1, an algorithm to aid thromboprophylaxis decision making, based on that in the recent RCOG guidelines [83].

3.4.1 Thrombophilia

Current evidence supports antenatal thromboprophylaxis and postnatal thromboprophylaxis for 6 weeks in women with an identified thrombophilia and previous VTE. For very-high-risk individuals (those with a compound thrombophilia or antithrombin deficiency or previous recurrent VTE on long-term anticoagulation), discussion with a clinician with expertise in

hemostasis and pregnancy is imperative to determine the appropriate level of anticoagulation for pregnancy, as high prophylactic (twice daily) dose or therapeutic anticoagulation may be indicated.

Management of asymptomatic women (without prior VTE) with a known heritable thrombophilia is not straightforward because there are limited reliable data on the benefits of thromboprophylaxis in this setting. It is desirable to discuss the options as fully as possible with the woman, ideally in conjunction with a clinician with expertise in this area. It is important that laboratory thrombophilia results are not viewed in isolation but considered along with the family history and other risk factors before a conclusion is reached about the risk of VTE, and therefore the benefit of thromboprophylaxis, in the individual. In the family history, factors considered should include the number of affected relatives, the age at which thrombosis developed, and the presence or absence of additional risk factors in the affected relatives [91].

Since the risk of VTE is lower in asymptomatic women, antenatal thromboprophylaxis is usually necessary only in those with antithrombin deficiency or with combined or homozygous defects [29, 60, 91]. However, since asymptomatic thrombophilia is a risk factor, if combined with other risk factors such as increased age, obesity, or immobility, it may be justified to use antenatal thromboprophylaxis.

Similarly, for asymptomatic women with thrombophilia without either a personal or family history of VTE, 6 weeks of postpartum thromboprophylaxis may be unnecessary. Again, decisions regarding whether to recommend postnatal thromboprophylaxis should be based on a risk assessment for that individual immediately after delivery.

The validity of this approach was reported in a prospective study in which women classified as low risk were managed by clinical surveillance alone unless there were additional risk factors [8]. This group included those with heritable thrombophilia (excluding antithrombin deficiency) and no prior VTE. Of the 225 women in this group, 70 % had either a heritable laboratory-detected thrombophilia or a positive family history in a first-degree relative, and none developed a pregnancy-related episode of VTE. However, in practice, 85 % of the women in this group received antenatal thromboprophylaxis because of additional risk factors, and the median time of treatment initiation was at 24 weeks' gestation (range 4–41 weeks). The duration of postpartum thromboprophylaxis the women received was intended to be 2 weeks, but other studies suggest that the risk of VTE remains elevated for up to 6 weeks postpartum, and therefore, if thromboprophylaxis is given antenatally for a persisting risk factor, it should be continued postpartum for 6 weeks [36, 38].

3.4.1.1 Antithrombin Deficiency

Women with antithrombin deficiency, particularly type 1, have a very high risk of first and recurrent thrombosis and probably require higher doses of LMWH in pregnancy. They are likely to be on long-term anticoagulation with warfarin, and therefore an intermediate or treatment dose of LMWH may be indicated throughout pregnancy and continued postpartum for a minimum of 6 weeks or until converted back to long-term warfarin. Heparins may not be as effective in antithrombin deficiency as their mode of action is antithrombin dependent, and it is reasonable to monitor anti-Xa levels in this setting, aiming for a level 4 h post injection of 0.35–0.5 u/mL [91]. Such women should be managed in collaboration with a hematologist with expertise in thrombosis in pregnancy.

3.4.1.2 Antiphospholipid Syndrome

On the basis of the perceived high risk of recurrent thrombosis, it is recommended in the most recent ACCP guidelines that pregnant women with APS and previous VTE should receive antenatal thromboprophylaxis with LMWH [7]. It is suggested that women on warfarin convert to LMWH before the sixth week of pregnancy and that those not on warfarin commence LMWH in the first trimester as soon as possible after diagnosis of the pregnancy. For women with a single previous VTE event, a high prophylactic (i.e. twice daily) dose of LMWH is often used [88]. For women with a history of recurrent VTE, particularly where this has entailed an increase in the usual target INR from 2.0 to 3.0, a high prophylactic, that is, 75 % of treatment dose, or full treatment dose can be used. Low dose aspirin is recommended for all women with APS [75]. A survey by the European Antiphospholipid Forum of clinicians who regularly manage patients with APS concluded that in women with APS associated with a previous VTE event, the majority would advise therapeutic dose LMWH during pregnancy, aiming for a 4-h anti-Xa level of 0.5–1.0 (personal communication, MC Boffa, 2009). The presence of antiphospholipid antibodies alone, even if persistent, without previous APS-classifiable pregnancy loss or thrombosis, does not equate to APS, and such women do not require antenatal LMWH [87].

After delivery, women on antenatal LMWH should continue at the same dose until reestablished on long-term oral anticoagulation or for a minimum of 6 weeks if not on long-term therapy. In women with APS featuring recurrent miscarriage or fetal loss without thrombosis, the risk of postpartum VTE is unclear, but data from randomized trials suggest the risk is likely to be low. Antenatal antithrombotic therapy administered to improve pregnancy outcome in these trials was typically stopped between 34 weeks and delivery, and no maternal VTE events were reported [45, 73], However, many clinicians advocate postpartum thromboprophylaxis for 6 weeks in a similar way to those with asymptomatic inherited thrombophilia [7]. In women with persistent lupus anticoagulant or high-titre antiphospholipid antibodies but without APS, that is, no prior thrombosis, recurrent miscarriage, or fetal loss, the risk of VTE is small. It is, however, reasonable to administer LMWH postnatally at a prophylactic dose for 7 days, even in the absence of additional risk factors.

3.4.2 Previous VTE

It is recommended that women with previous VTE are stratified into intermediate-risk, high-risk, and very high risk groups (Table 3.2) [7].

Women in the high and very high risk groups will therefore benefit from referral for pre-pregnancy counseling to construct a prospective management plan for thromboprophylaxis in pregnancy. Those who become pregnant before receiving such counseling require early referral for specialist management by an expert in hemostasis and pregnancy.

Women with recurrent VTE or a previous unprovoked or estrogen-related VTE or a previous VTE along with a family history of VTE are at higher risk than the normal population and should be offered thromboprophylaxis both antenatally and for 6 weeks postpartum. All women with a previous history of confirmed VTE should have postpartum prophylaxis.

Women on warfarin for recurrent VTE should be counseled about the risks to the fetus and advised to stop warfarin and change to LMWH as soon as pregnancy is confirmed, ideally within 2 weeks of the missed period, i.e., before 6 weeks' gestation. Women with recurrent VTE but not on warfarin should be advised to start LMWH as soon as they have a positive pregnancy test. For some women in this category, higher doses of LMWH may be appropriate. Advice should be sought from a clinician with expertise in hemostasis and pregnancy.

Where objective documentation is not available, the previous diagnosis of VTE can be assumed in cases where the woman gives a good history and received prolonged (>6 weeks)

therapeutic anticoagulation. Any woman with objective documentation of previous VTE should have a careful history documented and undergo testing for both heritable and acquired thrombophilias if appropriate, preferably before pregnancy (see below).

3.4.2.1 Thrombophilia Testing

Testing for an underlying heritable thrombophilia is indicated only in certain circumstances in pregnancy and should be performed only when the outcome of the test will influence subsequent management. Pregnancy can also affect circulating coagulation factors; for example, protein S levels are reduced by pregnancy, deficiency cannot be diagnosed in pregnancy. If testing is planned, counseling is required to ensure that the woman and her family are aware of the potential implications of a positive diagnosis.

In women with a previous VTE, if this was unprovoked or estrogen related, then thrombophilia testing is not required as thromboprophylaxis is already indicated.

Testing is therefore useful in two main settings. In women with a previous VTE related to a minor temporary risk factor, if a thrombophilia was detected, then they would be offered antenatal prophylaxis. If antiphospholipid or antithrombin deficiency was detected, then the dose of LMWH would be increased during pregnancy.

3.4.3 Obesity

All women with class 3 obesity (BMI > 40 kg/m^2) should be considered for thromboprophylaxis for 7 days after delivery (whether vaginal or Caesarean section), even if young and no other risk factors are present. The weight-related doses for different types of LMWH are provided in Table 3.3.

3.4.4 Mode of Delivery

The increased risk of VTE following Caesarean section, particularly as an emergency procedure, supports the routine prescription of postpartum prophylactic LMWH in all women undergoing an

Table 3.3 Suggested doses for antenatal and postnatal LMWH thromboprophylaxis

Weight	Enoxaparin	Dalteparin	Tinzaparin
<50 kg	20 mg daily	2,500 units daily	3,500 units daily
50–90 kg	40 mg daily	5,000 units daily	4,500 units daily
91–130 kg	60 mg daily[a]	7,500 units daily[a]	7,000 units daily[a]
131–170 kg	80 mg daily[a]	10,000 units daily[a]	9,000 units daily[a]
>170 kg	0.6 mg/kg/day[a]	75 u/kg/day[a]	75 u/kg/day[a]
50–90 kg, high prophylactic	40 mg twice daily	5,000 units twice daily	4,500 units twice daily
Treatment dose (antenatal)	1 mg/kg/twice daily	100 u/kg/twice daily	175 u/kg/day
Treatment dose (postnatal)	1.5 mg/kg/day	200 u/kg/day	175 u/kg/day

[a]Can be given in two divided doses

emergency Caesarean section and any woman with additional risk factors that undergoes elective Caesarean section. The duration of this should be at least 7 days, but extension of this period is recommended if additional risk factors are present or persisting, as the numbers of VTE after elective and emergency Caesarean sections are similar in weeks 1, 2, and 3 post delivery [39].

3.4.5 Thromboprophylaxis at Delivery

Pregnancy-associated prothrombotic changes are maximal soon after delivery. However, continuing thromboprophylaxis during labor to cover this time risks significant bleeding at the time of delivery and conflicts with techniques for administering regional anesthesia. The main concern with respect to regional anesthetic techniques is the potential for increasing the risk of epidural hematoma formation, either at the time of epidural or spinal injection or at removal of the epidural catheter. There is also an increased risk of wound hematoma following Caesarean section with both UFH and LMWH of around 2 % [33]. Women on LMWH should therefore be advised to discontinue it at the onset of labor or in the event of any vaginal bleeding and restart only after medical review and reassessment of risks of VTE and bleeding.

Regional techniques are not advised until at least 12 h after the previous prophylactic dose of LMWH or 24 h after a therapeutic dose (i.e. given on a 12-hourly basis). If an epidural has been sited, the catheter should not be removed within 12 h of the most recent prophylactic LMWH injection. A further 4 h should pass before the next dose of prophylactic LMWH is given. Prophylactic LMWH can be safely given 4 h after spinal anesthesia [37].

If women have been receiving antenatal prophylactic LMWH and an elective Caesarean section is planned, the normal dose can be given on the day prior to delivery. On the day of delivery, any morning dose can be omitted and the operation performed that morning. The same prophylactic dose of LMWH should be given 4 h postoperatively or 4 h post epidural catheter removal. For example, if the woman normally takes her dose of LMWH at 6 p.m., she can take this the evening prior to delivery and then have the elective Caesarean section the following morning. If the epidural catheter is removed before 2 p.m., the next prophylactic dose of LMWH can be given as normal at 6 p.m.

If regional techniques cannot be used for a patient presenting in spontaneous labor as a result of insufficient time since the last dose, alternative analgesia such as opiate-based intravenous patient-controlled analgesia should be offered. This restriction of anesthetic options means that planned induction of labor can be an attractive option for patients on high-prophylactic-dose or treatment dose LMWH therapy so that treatment can be planned around delivery. For example, a multiparous woman could take the morning dose on the day prior to induction and then omit the evening dose. An elective epidural could then be sited the following day (24 h after the last dose) prior to induction. Alternatively, the dose could be reduced to the standard prophylactic dose on the day prior to induction of labor and continued at this dose during labor if appropriate, if plans had been made to use alternative methods of analgesia. This group of women would therefore benefit from antenatal anesthetic review.

Learning Points
- Assessment of risk factors for VTE is required at booking and postpartum and should be reassessed at every hospital admission or development of intercurrent illness.
- The increased risk of VTE is present from early pregnancy. Therefore, if thromboprophylaxis is indicated antenatally, it should be instituted at the earliest opportunity.
- Low-molecular-weight heparin is the agent of choice for thromboprophylaxis in pregnancy, and the dose depends on maternal weight and any risk factors present.
- Anti-embolism stockings can be useful if pharmacological thromboprophylaxis is contraindicated, and these should be thigh length and properly fitted.
- All women with a previous history of confirmed VTE should be offered thromboprophylaxis for 6 weeks postpartum.

References

1. Antiplatelet Trialists' Collaboration. Collaborative overview of randomised trials of antiplatelet therapy – III: reduction in venous thrombosis and pulmonary embolism by antiplatelet prophylaxis among surgical and medical patients. BMJ. 1994;308:235–46.
2. Antithrombotic Trialists' Collaboration. Collaborative meta-analysis of randomised trials of antiplatelet therapy for prevention of death, myocardial infarction, and stroke in high risk patients. BMJ. 2002;324: 71–86.
3. Arya R, Shehata HA, Patel RK, Sahu S, Rajasingam D, Harrington K, Nelson-Piercy C, Parsons J. Internal jugular vein thrombosis following assisted conception therapy. Br J Haematol. 2001;115:153–6.
4. Baglin T, Barrowcliffe TW, Cohen A, Greaves M, for the British Committee for Standards in Haematology. Guidelines on the use and monitoring of heparin. Br J Haematol. 2006;133:19–34.
5. Bank I, Libourel EJ, Middeldorp S, van Pampus ECM, Koopman MMW, Hamulyak K, Prins MH, van der Meer J, Buller HR. Prothrombin 20210A mutation: a mild risk factor for venous thromboembolism but not

for arterial thrombotic disease and pregnancy-related complications in a family study. Arch Intern Med. 2004;164(17):1932–7.
6. Barbier P, Jongville AP, Autre TE, Coureau C. Fetal risks with dextran during delivery. Drug Saf. 1992; 7:71–3.
7. Bates SM, Greer IA, Pabinger I, Sofaer S, Hirsh J. Venous thromboembolism, thrombophilia, antithrombotic therapy, and pregnancy: American College of Chest Physicians Evidence-Based Clinical Practice Guidelines (8th Edition). Chest. 2008;133(6 Suppl): 844S–86.
8. Bauersachs RM, Dudenhausen J, Faridi A, Fischer T, Fung S, Geisen U, et al. Risk stratification and heparin prophylaxis to prevent venous thromboembolism in pregnant women. Thromb Haemost. 2007;98(6): 1237–45.
9. Berg EM, Fasting S, Sellevold OF. Serious complications with dextran-70 despite hapten prophylaxis. Is it best avoided prior to delivery? Anaesthesia. 1991;46: 1033–5.
10. Bezemer ID, van der Meer FJ, Eikenboom JC, Rosendaal FR, Doggen CJ. The value of family history as a risk indicator for venous thrombosis. Arch Intern Med. 2009;169(6):610–5.
11. Biron-Andreani C, Schved J-F, Daures J-P. Factor V Leiden mutation and pregnancy-related venous thromboembolism. Thromb Haemost. 2006;96:14–8.
12. Brady D, Raingruber B, Peterson J, Varnau W, Denman J, Resuello R, De Contreaus R, Mahnke J. The use of knee-length versus thigh-length compression stockings and sequential compression devices. Crit Care Nurs Q. 2007;30(3):255–62.
13. Brill-Edwards P, Ginsberg JS, for the Recurrence Of Clot In This Pregnancy (ROCIT) Study Group. Safety of withholding antepartum heparin in women with a previous episode of venous thromboembolism. N Engl J Med. 2000;343:1439–44.
14. Buchtemann AS, Steins A, Volkert B, Hahn M, Klyscz T, Junger M. The effect of compression therapy on venous haemodynamics in pregnant women. Br J Obstet Gynaecol. 1999;106:563–9.
15. Conard J, Horellou MH, van Dreden P, Le Compte T, Samama M. Thrombosis in pregnancy and congenital deficiencies in AT III, protein C or protein S: study of 78 women. Thromb Haemost. 1990;63:319–20.
16. Confidential Enquiry into Maternal and Child Health (CEMACH). Saving mothers' lives: reviewing maternal deaths to make motherhood safer, 2003–05. In: Lewis G, editors. The seventh report of the confidential enquiries into maternal deaths in the United Kingdom. London: CEMACH; 2007.
17. Centre for Maternal and Child Enquiries (CMACE). Saving mothers' Lives: reviewing maternal deaths to make motherhood safer: 2006–08. The eighth report on confidential enquiries into maternal deaths in the United Kingdom. BJOG. 2011;118(Suppl 1):1-203.
18. Crowther MA, Ginsberg JS, Julian J, Denburg J, Hirsh J, Douketis J, Laskin C, Fortin P, Anderson D, Kearon C, Clarke A, Geerts W, Forgie M, Green D,

Costantini L, Yacura W, Wilson S, Gent M, Kovacs MJ. A comparison of two intensities of warfarin for the prevention of recurrent thrombosis in patients with the antiphospholipid antibody syndrome. N Engl J Med. 2003;349:1133–8.

19. Danilenko-Dixon DR, Heit JA, Silverstein MD, Yawn BP, Petterson TM, Lohse CM, Melton 3rd LJ. Risk factors for deep vein thrombosis and pulmonary embolism during pregnancy or post partum: a population-based, case–control study. Am J Obstet Gynecol. 2001;184(2):104–10.

20. De Stefano V, Martinelli I, Rossi E, Battaglioli T, Za T, Mannuccio Mannucci P, Leone G. The risk of recurrent venous thromboembolism in pregnancy and puerperium without antithrombotic prophylaxis. Br J Haematol. 2006;135(3):386–91.

21. Dempfle CH. Minor transplacental passage of fondaparinux in vivo. N Engl J Med. 2004;350:1914–5.

22. Department of Health. Report of the independent expert working group on the prevention of venous thromboembolism in hospitalised patients. http://www.dh.gov.uk/dr_consum_dh/groups/dh_digitalassets/documents/digitalasset/dh_073953.pdf. Accessed Jan 2010.

23. Dizon-Townson D, Miller C, Sibai B, Spong CY, Thom E, Wendel Jr G, Wenstrom K, Samuels P, Cotroneo MA, Moawad A, Sorokin Y, Meis P, Miodovnik M, O'Sullivan MJ, Conway D, Wapner RJ, Gabbe SG, for the National Institute of Child Health and Human Development Maternal-F et al Medicine Units Network. The relationship of the factor V Leiden mutation and pregnancy outcomes for mother and fetus. Obstet Gynecol. 2005;106(3):517–24.

24. Duley L, Henderson-Smart DJ, Meher S, King JF. Antiplatelet agents for preventing pre-eclampsia and its complications. Cochrane Database Syst Rev. 2007;(2): CD004659. DOI: 10.1002/14651858.CD004659.pub2.

25. Finazzi G, Marchioli R, Brancaccio V, Schinco P, Wisloff F, Musial J, Baudo F, Berrettini M, Testa S, D'Angelo A, Tognoni G, Barbui T. A randomized clinical trial of high-intensity warfarin vs. conventional antithrombotic therapy for the prevention of recurrent thrombosis in patients with the antiphospholipid syndrome (WAPS). J Thromb Haemost. 2005;3: 848–53.

26. Folkeringa N, Brouwer JLP, Korteweg FJ, Veeger JGM, Erwich JJHM, van der Meer J. High risk of pregnancy-related venous thromboembolism in women with multiple thrombophilic defects. Br J Haematol. 2007;138:110–6.

27. Galli M, Luciani D, Bertolini G, Barbui T. Anti-beta 2-glycoprotein I, antiprothrombin antibodies, and the risk of thrombosis in the antiphospholipid syndrome. Blood. 2003;102(8):2717–23.

28. Geerts WH, Bergqvist D, et al. Prevention of venous thromboembolism. American College of Chest Physicians Evidence-Based Clinical Practice Guidelines (8th Edition). Chest. 2008;133:381–453.

29. Gerhardt A, Scharf RE, Zotz RB. Effect of hemostatic risk factors on the individual probability of thrombosis during pregnancy and the puerperium. Thromb Haemost. 2003;90:77–85.

30. Gerhardt A, Zotz RB, Stockschlaeder M, Scharf RE. Fondaparinux is an effective alternative anticoagulant in pregnant women with high risk of venous thromboembolism and intolerance to low-molecular-weight heparins and heparinoids. Thromb Haemost. 2007;97: 496–7.

31. Gerhardt A, Scharf RE, Beckman MW, et al. Prothrombin and factor V mutations in women with thrombosis during pregnancy and the puerperium. N Engl J Med. 2000;342:374–80.

32. Glynn RJ, Ridker PM, Goldhaber SZ, Buring JE. Effect of low-dose aspirin on the occurrence of venous thromboembolism: a randomized trial. Ann Intern Med. 2007;147(8):525–33.

33. Greer IA, Nelson-Piercy C. Low-molecular-weight heparins for thromboprophylaxis and treatment of venous thromboembolism in pregnancy: a systematic review of safety and efficacy. Blood. 2005;106:401–7.

34. Greer IA. Reduction in incidence of postpartum VTE following the introduction of thromboprophylaxis. Abstract presented at the International Society of Obstetric Medicine, Washington, 2008.

35. Health Survey for England – 2008 trend tables. Department of Health, http://www.ic.nhs.uk/statistics-and-data-collections/health-and-lifestyles-related-surveys/health-survey-for-england. Accessed 26 Jan 2010.

36. Heit JA, Kobbervig CE, James AH, Petterson TM, Bailey KR, Melton 3rd LJ. Trends in the incidence of venous thromboembolism during pregnancy or postpartum: a 30-year population-based study. Ann Intern Med. 2005;143:697–706.

37. Horlocker TT, et al. Regional anesthesia in the anticoagulated patient: defining the risks (the second ASRA Consensus Conference on Neuraxial Anesthesia and Anticoagulation). Reg Anesth Pain Med. 2003;28: 172–97.

38. Jacobsen AF, Skjeldestad FE, Sandet PM. Incidence and risk patterns of venous thromboembolism in pregnancy and puerperium – a register-based case–control study. Am J Obstet Gynecol. 2008;198:223–34.

39. Jacobsen AF, Skjeldestad FE, Sandset PM. Ante- and postnatal risk factors of venous thrombosis: a hospital-based case – control study. J Thromb Haemost. 2008;6(6):905–12.

40. James AH, Jamison MG, Brancazio LR, Myers ER. Venous thromboembolism during pregnancy and the postpartum period: incidence, risk factors, and mortality. Am J Obstet Gynecol. 2006;194(5):1311–5.

41. Jamieson R, Calderwood CJ, Greer IA. The effect of graduated compression stockings on blood velocity in the deep venous system of the lower limb in the postnatal period. BJOG. 2007;114:1292–4.

42. Kearon C, Kahn SR, Agnelli G, Goldhaber S, Raskob GE, Comerota AJ. Antithrombotic therapy for venous thromboembolic disease: American College of Chest Physicians Evidence-Based Clinical Practice Guidelines (8th Edition). Chest. 2008;133:454–545.

43. Knight M, on behalf of UKOSS. Antenatal pulmonary embolism: risk factors, management and outcomes. BJOG. 2008;115(4):453–61.
44. Lagrange F, Vergnes C, Brun JL, Paolucci F, Nadal T, Leng JJ, Saux MC, Banwarth B. Absence of placental transfer of pentasaccharide (fondaparinux, Arixtra®) in the dually perfused human cotyledon in vitro. Thromb Haemost. 2002;87:831–5.
45. Laskin CA, Spitzer CA, Clark C, et al. Low molecular weight heparin and aspirin for recurrent pregnancy loss: results from the randomized, controlled Hep ASA trial. J Rheumatol. 2009;36:279–87.
46. Larsen TB, Sorensen HT, et al. Maternal smoking, obesity, and risk of venous thromboembolism during pregnancy and the puerperium: a population-based nested case–control study. Thromb Res. 2007;120(4):505–9.
47. Lijfering WM, Brouwer JLP, Veeger NJGM, Coppens M, Middeldorp S, Hamulyak K, Prins M, Buller HR, van der Meer J. Selective testing for thrombophilia in patients with first venous thrombosis: results from a retrospective family cohort study on absolute thrombotic risk for currently known thrombophilic defects in 2479 relatives. Blood. 2009;113(21):5314–22.
48. Lim W, Eikelboom JW, Ginsberg JS. Inherited thrombophilia and pregnancy associated venous thromboembolism. BMJ. 2007;334:1318–21.
49. Lindhoff-Last E, Kreutzenbeck H-J, Magnani HN. Treatment of 51 pregnancies with danaparoid because of heparin intolerance. Thromb Haemost. 2005;93:63–9.
50. Lindqvist P, Dahlbäck B, Maršál K. Thrombotic risk during pregnancy: a population study. Obstet Gynecol. 1999;94:595–9.
51. Lindqvist PG, Svensson PJ, Marsal K, Grennert L, Luterkort M, Dahlback B. Activated protein C resistance (FV:Q506) and pregnancy. Thromb Haemost. 1999;81(4):532–7.
52. Liu S, Liston RM, Joseph KS, Heaman M, Sauve R, Kramer MS, et al. Maternal mortality and severe morbidity associated with low-risk planned cesarean delivery versus planned vaginal delivery at term. CMAJ. 2007;176(4):455–60.
53. Lord RA, Hamilton D. Graduated compression stockings (20–30 mmHg) do not compress leg veins in the standing position. ANZ J Surg. 2004;74:581–5.
54. Macklon NS, Greer IA. Venous thromboembolic disease in obstetrics and gynaecology: the Scottish experience. Scott Med J. 1996;41(3):83–6.
55. Marchiori A, Mosena L, Prins MH, Prandoni P. The risk of recurrent venous thromboembolism among heterozygous carriers of factor V Leiden or prothrombin G20210A mutation. A systematic review of prospective studies. Haematologica. 2007;92:1107–14.
56. Martinelli I, Battaglioli T, De Stefano V, Tormene D, Valdre L, Grandone E, Tosetto A, Mannucci PM, on behalf of the GIT (Gruppos Italiano Trombofilia). The risk of first venous thromboembolism during pregnancy and puerperium in double heterozygotes for factor V Leiden and prothrombin G20210A. J Thromb Haemost. 2008;6:494–8.
57. Martinelli I, Legnani C, Bucciarelli P, Grandone E, De Stefano V, Mannucci PM. Risk of pregnancy-related venous thrombosis in carriers of severe inherited thrombophilia. Thromb Haemost. 2001;86:800–3.
58. Maybury H, Waugh JJ, Gornall AS, Pavord S. There is a return to non-pregnant coagulation parameters after four not six weeks postpartum following spontaneous vaginal delivery. Obstet Med. 2008;1:92–4.
59. Mazzolai L, Hohlfeld P, Spertini F, Hayoz D, Schapira M, Duchosal MA. Fondaparinux is a safe alternative in case of heparin intolerance during pregnancy. Blood. 2006;108:1569–70.
60. McColl MD, Ellison J, Reid F, et al. Prothrombin 20210GA, MTHFR C677T mutations in women with venous thromboembolism associated with pregnancy. Br J Obstet Gynaecol. 2000;107:565–9.
61. McColl MD, Ramsay JE, Tait RC, Walker ID, McCall F, Conkie JA, Carty MJ, Greer IA. Risk factors for pregnancy associated venous thromboembolism. Thromb Haemost. 1997;78(4):1183–8.
62. Middeldorp S, van Hylckama Vlieg A. Does thrombophilia testing help in the clinical management of patients? Br J Haematol. 2008;143:321–35.
63. Miyakis S, Lockshin MD, Atsumi T, Branch DW, Brey RL, Cervera R, Derksen RHWM, De Groot PG, Koike T, Meroni PL, Reber G, Shoenfeld Y, Tincani A, Vlachoyannopoulos PG, Krilis SA. International consensus statement on an update of the classification criteria for definite antiphospholipid syndrome. J Thromb Haemost. 2006;4:295–306.
64. National Institute for Health and Clinical Excellence. Clinical Guideline no. 62. Antenatal Care. Routine care for the healthy pregnant woman. March 2008.
65. National Institute for Health and Clinical Excellence. Clinical Guideline no. 92. Venous thromboembolism: Reducing the risk of venous thromboembolism (deep vein thrombosis and pulmonary embolism) in patients admitted to hospital. January 2010.
66. Pabinger I, Grafenhofer H, Kyrle PA, Quehenberger P, Mannhalter C, Lechner K, Kaider A. Temporary increase in the risk for recurrence during pregnancy in women with a history of venous thromboembolism. Blood. 2002;100:1060–2.
67. Pabinger I, Grafenhofer H, Kaider A, Kyrle PA, Quehenberger P, Mannhalter C, Lechner K. Risk of pregnancy-associated recurrent venous thromboembolism in women with a history of venous thrombosis. J Thromb Haemost. 2005;3(5):949–54.
68. Partsch B, Partsch H. Calf compression pressure required to achieve venous closure from supine to standing positions. J Vasc Surg. 2005;42:734–8.
69. Pettila V, Leinonen P, Markkola A, Hiilesmaa V, Kaaja R. Postpartum bone mineral density in women treated for thromboprophylaxis with unfractionated heparin or LMW heparin. Thromb Haemost. 2002;87:182–6.

70. Phillips S, Gallagher M, Buchan H. Use graduated compression stockings postoperatively to prevent deep vein thrombosis. BMJ. 2008;336:943–4.

71. Pomp ER, Lenselink AM, Rosendaal FR, Doggen CJ. Pregnancy, the postpartum period and prothrombotic defects: risk of venous thrombosis in the MEGA study. J Thromb Haemost. 2008;6(4):632–7.

72. Pulmonary embolism prevention (PEP) Trial Collaborative Group. Prevention of pulmonary embolism and deep venous thrombosis with low dose aspirin: Pulmonary Embolism Prevention (PEP) trial. Lancet. 2000;355:1295–302.

73. Rai R, Cohen H, Dave M, Regan L. Randomised controlled trial of aspirin and aspirin plus heparin in pregnant women with recurrent miscarriage associated with phospholipid antibodies (or antiphospholipid antibodies). BMJ. 1997;314:253–7.

74. Ray JG, Chan WA. Deep vein thrombosis during pregnancy and the puerperium: a meta-analysis of the period of risk and the leg of presentation. Obstet Gynecol Surv. 1999;54(4):265–71.

75. Robertson B, Greaves M. Antiphospholipid syndrome: an evolving story. Blood Rev. 2006;20(4):201–12.

76. Robertson L, Wu O, Langhorne P, Twaddle S, Clark P, Lowe GDO, Walker ID, Greaves M, Brenkel I, Regan L, Greer IA, for The Thrombosis: Risk and Economic Assessment of Thrombophilia Screening (TREATS) Study. Br J Haematol. 2005;132(2):171–96.

77. Robinson HE, O'Connell CM, Joseph KS, McLeod NL. Maternal outcomes in pregnancies complicated by obesity. Obstet Gynecol. 2005;106(6):1357–64.

78. Ros HS, Lichtenstein P, Bellocco R, Petersson G, Cnattingius S. Increased risks of circulatory diseases in late pregnancy and puerperium. Epidemiology. 2001;12(4):456–60.

79. Ros HS, Lichtenstein P, Bellocco R, Petersson G, Cnattingius S. Pulmonary embolism and stroke in relation to pregnancy: how can high-risk women be identified? Am J Obstet Gynecol. 2002;186(2):198–203.

80. Rosendaal FR, Koster T, Vandenbroucke JP, Reitsma PH. High risk of thrombosis in patients homozygous for factor V Leiden (activated protein C resistance). Blood. 1995;85(5):1504–8.

81. Royal College of Obstetricians and Gynaecologists. Report of the RCOG Working Party on prophylaxis against thromboembolism in gynaecology and obstetrics. London: RCOG Press;1995.

82. Royal College of Obstetricians and Gynaecologists. Air travel and pregnancy. Scientific Advisory Committee Opinion Paper 1. London: RCOG Press; 2008.

83. Royal College of Obstetricians and Gynaecologists. Green-top guideline no. 37. Thrombosis and embolism during pregnancy and the puerperium, Reducing the risk. 2009

84. Samama MM, Rached RA, Horellou M-H, Aquilanti S, Mathieux VG, Plu-Bureau G, Elalamy I, Conard J. Pregnancy-associated venous thromboembolism (VTE) in combined heterozygous factor V Leiden (FVL) and prothrombin (FII) 20210 A mutation and in heterozygous FII single gene mutation alone. Br J Haematol. 2003;123:327–34.

85. Sanson BJ, Lensing AWA, Prins MH, et al. Safety of low-molecular-weight heparin in pregnancy: a systematic review. Thromb Haemost. 1999;81:668–72.

86. Simpson EL, Lawrenson RA, Nightingale AL, Farmer RDT. Venous thromboembolism in pregnancy and the puerperium: incidence and additional risk factors from a London perinatal database. BJOG. 2001;108:56–60.

87. Stone S, Langford K, Nelson-Piercy C, Khamashta M, Bewley S, Hunt BJ. Antiphospholipid antibodies do not a syndrome make. Lupus. 2002;11:130–3.

88. Stone S, Hunt BJ, Khamashta MA, Bewley SJ, Nelson-Piercy C. Primary antiphospholipid syndrome in pregnancy: an analysis of outcome in a cohort of 33 women treated with a rigorous protocol. J Thromb Haemost. 2005;3(2):243–5.

89. Verstraete M. Pharmacotherapeutic aspects of unfractionated and low molecular weight heparins. Drugs. 1990;40(4):498–530.

90. Vossen CY, Conard J, Fontcuberta J, Makris M, van der Meer FJM, Pabinger I, Palareti G, Preston FE, Scharrer I, Souto JC, Svensson P, Walker ID, Rosendaal FR. Risk of a first venous thrombotic event in carriers of a familial thrombophilic defect. The European Prospective Cohort on Thrombophilia (EPCOT). J Thromb Haemost. 2005;3:459–64.

91. Walker ID, Greaves M, Preston FE. British Society for Haematology Guideline. Investigation and management of heritable thrombophilia. Br J Haematol. 2001;114:512–28.

92. White RH, Chan WS, Zhou H, Ginsberg JS. Recurrent venous thromboembolism after pregnancy-associated versus unprovoked thromboembolism. Thromb Haemost. 2008;100(2):246–52.

93. Bates SM, Greer IA, Middeldorp S, Veenstra DL, Prabulos A-M, Vandvik PO. VTE, Thrombophilia, Antithrombotic Therapy, and Pregnancy. Antithrombotic Therapy and prevention of Thrombosis, 9th ed: American College of Chest Physicians Evidence-Based Clinical Practice Guidelines. Chest 2012;141(2)(Suppl):e691S–e736S.

Systemic Thromboembolism in Pregnancy: Venous Thromboembolism

4

Asma Khalil, Louise Bowles, and Pat O'Brien

Abstract

Pregnancy is a prothrombotic state, associated with a 5- to 10-fold increased risk of venous thromboembolism (VTE) compared with the non-pregnant state. VTE (which includes deep vein thrombosis, pulmonary embolus and cerebral vein thrombosis) remains a leading cause of maternal morbidity and mortality, despite improvements in prevention in recent years. Clinical diagnosis of VTE in pregnancy is difficult, and clinicians should have a low threshold for investigating women with suspected VTE in pregnancy. Low molecular weight heparin (LMWH) is the mainstay in the treatment of VTE. The primary aim in peripartum management is to balance the risk of major postpartum hemorrhage in a woman who is fully anticoagulated with the risk of extension or recurrence of VTE when anticoagulation is interrupted.

In general, being on treatment doses of anticoagulation is often an indication for timing delivery, but would not be an indication for elective Caesarean section; induction of labour is usually preferable. Once the immediate peripartum period has been negotiated, consideration is given to the duration of further therapeutic anticoagulation. Therapeutic anticoagulation should be continued for the duration of the pregnancy, and for at least 6 weeks postnatally and until at least 3 months of treatment has been given in total.

A. Khalil, MD, MRCOG, MSc. (✉)
St Georges Healthcare NHS Trust,
SW17 0QT, London, UK
e-mail: asmakhalil79@googlemail.com

L. Bowles, MRCP, FRCPath
Department of Hematology, Barts Health NHS Trust,
4th floor, Pathology and Pharmacy,
Building, 80 Newark Street,
Whitechapel E1 2ES, London, UK
e-mail: louise.bowles@bartshealth.nhs.uk

P. O'Brien, FRCOG, FFSRH, FICOG
Department of Obstetrics and Gynaecology,
University College London Hospitals, UK
e-mail: patrick.obrien@uclh.nhs.uk

4.1 Introduction

Venous thromboembolism (VTE) remains a leading cause of maternal mortality and morbidity worldwide, although the United Kingdom Centre for Maternal and Child Enquiries (CMACE) reported a significant fall in maternal death due to VTE [19, 43]. Physiological changes during pregnancy alter the balance in the hemostatic system in favor of thrombosis. The increased risk of VTE begins in early pregnancy and lasts throughout the puerperium. Pregnancy increases

H. Cohen, P. O'Brien (eds.), *Disorders of Thrombosis and Hemostasis in Pregnancy*,
DOI 10.1007/978-1-4471-4411-3_4, © Springer-Verlag London 2012

the risk of VTE 5- to 10-fold compared with the non-pregnant state, with VTE occurring in around 1 per 1,000 deliveries [3, 28, 44, 45, 48, 59]. While available data suggest that Caesarean section is associated with an increased risk of fatal and nonfatal VTE, in the four triennia between 1997–2008, half of all deaths followed vaginal delivery [19].

4.2 Epidemiology

The incidence of VTE in non-pregnant women of childbearing age is around 1 in 10,000 [4, 37, 52, 57, 70] compared with an incidence in pregnancy between 0.6 and 1.3 episodes per 1,000 births [3, 28, 44, 45, 48, 59]. The hypercoagulability of pregnancy confers benefit on the pregnant woman in that it helps to reduce the risk of death from hemorrhage after delivery of the baby and placenta. However, the price paid is an increased risk of thromboembolism throughout pregnancy and the puerperium (the 6 weeks after the birth). VTE can occur in any of the three trimesters, but the puerperium is the time of greatest risk [35]. This is consistent with the hypercoagulability providing the greatest protection against the risk of hemorrhage around the time of birth and immediately afterwards.

In the UK, CMACE reported that there were 18 deaths due to VTE in the triennium 2006–2008 [19]. This was notably fewer than the 41 deaths in the 2003–2005 report and by far the lowest since the UK-wide enquiry began in 1985. The fall in deaths from pulmonary embolism (PE), from 33 to 16, was mainly the result of a reduction in antenatal deaths and deaths following vaginal delivery, though deaths following Caesarean section also fell slightly. The CMACE report notes that "this is the first full triennium following publication of the 2004 RCOG guideline *Thromboprophylaxis during pregnancy, labour and after normal vaginal delivery* and it seems likely that the unprecedented fall in deaths is the result of better recognition of at-risk women and more widespread thromboprophylaxis."

In that CMACE report, 16 of the 18 deaths were due to PE; the remaining 2 were as a result of cerebral vein thrombosis (CVT). The United Kingdom Obstetric Surveillance System (UKOSS) reported that the incidence of antenatal PE in the UK was 13.1 per 100,000 maternities (95 % confidence intervals 10.6, 16) [39, 40], with a case fatality rate of 3.5 %. In the previous two Confidential Enquires into Maternal Deaths reports (2000–2002 and 2003–2005) [42, 43], there were 25 and 33 deaths, respectively, caused by PE, representing mortality rates of 1.56 and 1.2 per 100,000, respectively. These rates are similar to those published for the United States by the Centers for Disease Control and Prevention which monitors pregnancy mortality via the Pregnancy Mortality Surveillance System. They reported rates of deaths due to PE in pregnancy of 1.8 and 2.3 per 100,000 live births for the periods 1987–1990 and 1991–1999, respectively [13, 21]. Table 4.1 shows the numbers of direct deaths from VTE and rates per 100,000 maternities in the United Kingdom in the period 1985–2008.

The incidence of deep vein thrombosis (DVT) in pregnancy is 0.13–0.61 per 1,000 pregnancies [38]. In pregnancy, DVT occurs more commonly in the left leg (up to 90 %) in contrast to 55 % in the non-pregnant state [56]. This observation may be explained by compression of the left common iliac vein which is crossed by the right common iliac artery. The commonest sites for DVT in pregnancy are the iliac and femoral veins.

Compared with venous thromboembolism, arterial thrombosis is far less common in pregnancy, possibly reflecting the lower incidence of artherosclerotic plaques in women of this age. The incidence of stroke in pregnancy is reported as 0.18 per 1,000 births and myocardial infarction 0.1 per 1,000 births [67]. However, a proportion of stroke will be hemorrhagic, and myocardial infarction may be due to coronary artery dissection (the risk of which is increased in pregnancy). Some of the risk factors for VTE (see Table 3.1) also increase the risk of arterial thrombosis; these include older age, obesity and smoking. The risk of arterial thrombosis is also increased in

Table 4.1 Direct deaths from thrombosis and thromboembolism and rates per 100,000 maternities (United Kingdom, 1985–2008)

	Pulmonary embolism				Cerebral vein thrombosis				Thrombosis and thromboembolism			
	Number	Rate	95 % CI		Number	Rate	95 % CI		Number	Rate	95% CI	
1985–1987	30	1.32	0.83	1.89	2	0.09	0.02	0.32	32	1.41	1.00	1.99
1988–1990	24	1.02	0.68	1.51	9	0.38	0.20	0.72	33	1.40	1.00	1.96
1991–1993	30	1.30	0.91	1.85	5	0.22	0.09	0.51	35	1.51	1.09	2.10
1994–1996	46	2.09	1.57	2.79	2	0.09	0.02	0.33	48	2.18	1.65	2.90
1997–1999	31	1.46	1.03	2.07	4	0.19	0.07	0.48	35	1.65	1.19	2.29
2000–2002	25	1.25	0.85	1.85	5	0.25	0.11	0.59	30	1.50	1.05	2.14
2003–2005	33	1.56	1.11	2.19	8	0.38	0.19	0.75	41	1.94	1.43	2.63
2006–2008	16	0.70	0.43	1.14	2	0.09	0.02	0.35	18	0.79	0.49	1.25

Confidential Enquiry into Maternal and Child Health [24]

association with the antiphospholipid syndrome and with drugs which can cause arterial spasm such as ergometrine, cocaine, and marijuana.

The risk factors for VTE in pregnancy are shown in Table 3.1. The prevalence of many of these risk factors is increasing. For example, levels of obesity in the general and pregnant populations are rising in the UK and elsewhere. The average age of pregnancy is rising constantly, and, as a result, there are more pregnant women with coexisting medical morbidities such as heart, lung, or bowel disease. Because of the increasing availability of assisted reproduction technologies, multiple pregnancy is also on the rise. It is to be hoped that more widespread recognition and assessment of these risk factors will lead to more consistent use of thromboprophylactic measures (see Chap. 3).

Most women who die from PE will have identifiable risk factors. In the CMACE report of 2006–2008 [19], 16 of the 18 women who died from PE in the UK had recognized risk factors; in the UKOSS report of 143 fatal and nonfatal antenatal PE, 70 % had identifiable risk factors [40].

4.3 Pathophysiology of Venous Thromboembolism

The pathophysiology of VTE has classically been described in terms of Virchow's triad of venous stasis, hypercoagulability, and vascular damage. All three of these components are affected during pregnancy. Because of the vaso-

dilator effect of progesterone, relaxin, and other pregnancy-related hormones and because of the physical obstruction of the gravid uterus, there is increased venous stasis in the pelvic and lower limb veins. Doppler studies of venous blood flow in the lower limbs in pregnancy show that venous flow velocity is reduced by 50 % by the end of the second trimester and reaches a nadir at 36 weeks' gestation [46]. After delivery, flow velocity takes 6 weeks to return to normal. Pregnancy is a hypercoagulable state (as detailed in Chap. 1); hemostatic changes in coagulation factors, the fibrinolytic system, and natural anticoagulants prepare the body for the challenges of implantation, placentation, and delivery. A number of coagulation factor levels increase, including fibrinogen and factor VIII as well as von Willebrand factor, whilst other coagulation factor levels remain unchanged or decrease. The rise in factor VIII leads to a shortened activated partial thromboplastin time (APTT) in late pregnancy. These changes are not balanced by changes in the naturally occurring anticoagulants, with decreased free and total protein S. Although protein C levels remain normal or show a slight increase, there is an increase in activated protein C resistance (APCR), largely due to the increase in factor VIII and decrease in protein S levels. Antithrombin generally remains unchanged. Thrombin generation increases during pregnancy and, although global fibrinolytic activity is reduced, plasma D-dimer (a marker of activation of fibrinolysis) increases. Finally, delivery, whether vaginal (normal or instrumental) or abdominal (Caesarean section), inevitably causes a degree of injury to pelvic vessels.

4.4 Diagnosis of Venous Thromboembolism

The clinical diagnosis of acute VTE is often difficult, particularly in pregnancy when edema of the lower limbs is common, as is dyspnea (which occurs in up to 70 % of all pregnant women). The accuracy of clinical diagnosis of VTE is very low (approximately 8 % for DVT and 5 % for PE) [16, 56, 58]. It is important, therefore, to maintain a high index of suspicion in women presenting with some or all of the typical symptoms or signs of DVT (leg pain and swelling, usually unilateral lower abdominal pain) or PE (dyspnea, chest pain, hemoptysis, low grade pyrexia, collapse) or CVT (headache, clouding of consciousness or confusion, or other neurological symptoms). Any woman with suggestive symptoms and signs should undergo objective testing to confirm or rule out the diagnosis. Until the diagnosis is excluded, the woman should be started on a treatment dose of low-molecular-weight heparin (LMWH), unless there is a strong contraindication to anticoagulation. The symptoms, signs, and differential diagnoses of VTE are summarized in Tables 4.2 and 4.3, respectively.

4.4.1 Diagnosis of Deep Vein Thrombosis

When there is a clinical suspicion of DVT, the woman should undergo a venous duplex or compression ultrasound scan of the leg as soon as possible. If the scan confirms the presence of a DVT, anticoagulation therapy should be continued. If the scan is negative and clinical suspicion is low, anticoagulation should be stopped. However, if the scan is negative but the clinical suspicion remains high, anticoagulation should be continued and the duplex scan (or another

Table 4.2 Symptoms and signs of venous thromboembolism in pregnancy

Deep vein thrombosis
Painful warm leg
Swelling
Erythema
Tenderness
Lower abdominal pain

Pulmonary thromboembolism
Pleuritic chest pain
Dyspnea
Tachypnea
Cough
Hemoptysis
Tachycardia
Raised jugular venous pressure
Focal chest signs
Collapse
Shock

Cerebral vein thrombosis
Headache
Vomiting
Photophobia
Seizures
Impaired consciousness
Focal neurological signs

Table 4.3 Differential diagnosis of venous thromboembolism in pregnancy

Deep venous thrombosis
Muscle strain
Trauma
Cellulitis
Superficial thrombophlebitis
Ruptured Baker's cyst

Pulmonary thromboembolism
Myocardial infarction
Heart failure
Pericarditis
Dissecting aneurysm
Pneumothorax
Pneumonia
Lobar collapse

Cerebral vein thrombosis
Eclampsia
Subarachnoid hemorrhage
Encephalitis

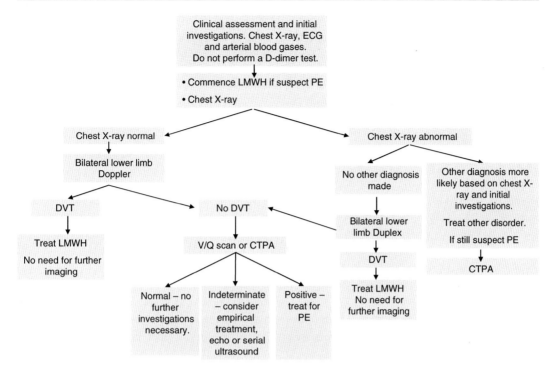

Fig. 4.1 Diagnostic algorithm for suspected non-high-risk pulmonary embolus in pregnant patients (i.e. without shock, hypotension, signs of pulmonary hypertension)

diagnostic test such as a venogram) repeated a week later. Persistently high clinical suspicion with negative duplex scans can be followed by either prophylactic or therapeutic dose LMWH for the remainder of the pregnancy, depending on the level of clinical suspicion. Diagnosis of iliac vein thrombosis may be more problematic, particularly in later pregnancy when the gravid uterus fills the pelvis. The diagnosis may be suggested by back pain and swelling of an entire lower limb; if duplex ultrasound cannot make the diagnosis, magnetic resonance venography or contrast venography may be used.

4.4.2   Diagnosis of Pulmonary Embolus

Oxygen saturation measured with a pulse oximeter may show resting hypoxia. Arterial blood gases (ABG) usually show a reduced PaO_2 and normal or low $PaCO_2$. Electrocardiogram (ECG) may be normal except for a sinus tachycardia. Large emboli may show features of acute right heart strain (right axis deviation, right bundle branch block, peaked P waves in lead II); the classical S1, Q3, T3 pattern is rare. ECG is also useful in excluding other diagnoses such as acute myocardial infarction and pericardial diseases.

In our practice, a woman in whom PE is suspected will have a definitive diagnostic investigation for example, ventilation perfusion (V/Q) scan or perfusion scan alone in the first instance. An alternative approach is to first have a chest X-ray and compression duplex Doppler scan of the legs (Fig. 4.1). Although chest X-ray may be normal in half of the pregnant women in whom PE is subsequently diagnosed, the X-ray may have features which suggest an alternative diagnosis, for example, pleural effusion, atelectasis, focal opacities, regional oligemia, or pulmonary edema. Therefore, a normal chest X-ray in a breathless hypoxic patient is highly suggestive of a diagnosis of PE. Furthermore, the dose of radiation received by the fetus from a plain chest X-ray is negligible (0.2 mRad while the maximum recommended radiation exposure in pregnancy is 5 Rad), particularly if lead screening of the abdomen is used. If the chest X-ray is abnormal, computed tomography pulmonary angiogram (CTPA) should be performed to establish the diagnosis. In some centers, if the chest X-ray is normal, bilateral duplex scans of the legs are performed. If this confirms a DVT, further imaging of the chest and therefore the extra radiation to mother and fetus may be avoided; the rationale is that the treatment of DVT and PE would be the same so diagnosing or excluding PE is unnecessary. If the chest X-ray is normal and the Doppler scan negative but the clinical suspicion remains high, a V/Q lung scan or CTPA should be performed. If the V/Q scan or CTPA is also normal but the clinical suspicion of PE remains, either prophylactic or therapeutic dose LMWH should be given for the remainder of the pregnancy, depending on the level of clinical suspicion.

The choice between V/Q scan and CTPA for the diagnosis of PE in pregnancy is controversial; each test has its advantages and disadvantages [56]. CTPA may have a lower diagnostic yield in pregnant women due to the hyperdynamic circulation. The advantage of CTPA is that the dose of radiation to the fetus is less than 10 % of that associated with a V/Q scan. As a result, there is a slightly lower risk of childhood cancer (up to the age of 15 years) associated with CTPA compared with a V/Q scan (1 in 280,000 vs. 1 in 1,000,000). On the other hand, CTPA delivers a higher dose of radiation to the maternal chest, and in particular to the maternal breast, compared with V/Q scan (20 mGy with CTPA). This increases the woman's lifetime risk of developing breast cancer; a frequently quoted estimate is that this risk is increased by 13.6 % against a background risk

of 1 in 200 [55]. Other studies [2] suggest that the risk is lower. Pregnant breast tissue is particularly sensitive to radiation, and every effort should be made to minimize radiation exposure during pregnancy.

In the UK, some authors recommend V/Q scan as the first-line investigation in pregnancy, as it has a high negative predictive value, lower radiation dose to the pregnant breast, and because most pregnant women in the UK will not have comorbid pulmonary pathology [25]. If the initial chest X-ray is normal, the ventilation portion of the V/Q scan may be omitted; the perfusion scan alone will often be enough to confirm or exclude PE.

Clearly, the choice of optimal test remains hotly debated and will be decided to some extent by local availability. The Royal College of Obstetricians and Gynaecologists recommends that "where feasible, women should be involved in the decision to undergo CTPA or V/Q scanning. Ideally, informed consent should be obtained before these tests are undertaken" [56]. It is essential, therefore, that these risk estimates are presented in a clear and balanced way. For example, rather than stating that V/Q scan increases the risk of childhood cancer by a factor of four compared with CTPA, the figures of 1 in 280,000 vs 1 in 1,000,000 should be presented. Similarly, with regard to the increased risk of breast cancer associated with a CTPA in pregnancy, the figure of a 13.6 % increased risk has been widely quoted. However, this represents an increase in the lifetime risk of breast cancer from a background risk of 1 in 200 to 1.1 in 200.

Pulmonary angiography exposes both mother and fetus to the highest level of radiation (5–30 mSv and 0.5 mSv, respectively). Iodinated contrast medium used with CTPA has the potential to affect fetal and neonatal thyroid function; when used, thyroid function should be checked in the neonate. Technetium-99, which is used for perfusion scans, is excreted in the urine and secreted into breast milk. A pregnant woman who has had a V/Q scan should be encouraged to drink plenty of fluids and empty her bladder frequently to reduce the small risk of continuing fetal exposure. Similarly, a lactating mother should be advised to avoid breast-feeding (i.e. express and discard her breast milk) for some time after a V/Q scan.

4.4.3   Diagnosis of Cerebral Vein Thrombosis

CT or MRI brain is diagnostic of CVT. All cases of suspected or confirmed CVT should be discussed with a neurologist.

4.4.4   D-dimer

Measurement of D-dimer is currently not recommended in the investigation of suspected acute VTE in pregnancy. This is because D-dimer levels may be raised in normal pregnancy, particularly in the third trimester and in the puerperium. They are also increased in other pregnancy-related pathologies such as preeclampsia [56]. However, a recent study reports that by using higher cut-off points than those used in non-pregnant patients, the specificity of D-dimer assays for the diagnosis of DVT in pregnancy can be improved without compromising sensitivity, and recommends that validation in prospective management studies is needed [20].

4.5   Management of Acute Venous Thromboembolism

As soon as the possibility of acute VTE is suspected, treatment dose LMWH should be started and appropriate investigations arranged. When the diagnosis is confirmed, the aim of anticoagulation therapy is to prevent extension and reduce the risk of recurrence in patients with established DVT and limit extension and prevent death in patients with established PE [9]. It is important to realize that, while there is good

(level 1) evidence guiding the treatment of acute VTE in non-pregnant patients, there is by comparison remarkably little good quality evidence in pregnancy. As a result, many of the guidelines relating to pregnant women are extrapolated from the non-pregnant population [22, 36, 51, 60].

The management of acute VTE will be primarily medical, that is, the use of anticoagulants, but nonmedical therapies must not be forgotten. Reversible risk factors for VTE, for example hyperemesis, wherever possible should be corrected, to enable optimal management.

4.5.1   Pharmacological Therapies: The Options in Patients with Acute Venous Thromboembolism

In non-pregnant patients, therapeutic options for VTE include unfractionated heparin (UFH), low-molecular-weight heparin (LMWH), and coumarins.

Coumarin derivatives such as warfarin cross the placenta; if taken in early pregnancy (6–12 weeks of gestation), they can cause a typical embryopathy, and later in pregnancy may cause microcephaly, probably secondary to small cerebral hemorrhages. There is also a risk of major fetal/neonatal intracerebral hemorrhage if the woman (and therefore the fetus) is anticoagulated around the time of delivery. Consequently, coumarins are avoided in pregnancy although they are an option in the highest-risk women, principally those with metallic heart valves.

Newer oral anticoagulants, such as dabigatran and rivaroxaban, are contraindicated in pregnancy. Fondaparinux and hirudin have not yet had their safety adequately established in pregnancy; hirudin is known to cross the placenta and may be teratogenic, and it is possible that fondaparinux may do the same. Although aspirin is safe in pregnancy it is not recommended as treatment for VTE [23]. Low-molecular-weight heparins are now the drugs of choice; in the UK and Ireland, over 95 % of centers use LMWH to treat acute VTE in pregnancy [66]. The only exception is massive pulmonary embolism with cardiovascular compromise, when thrombolysis should be considered. Selected patients, such as those with antiphospholipid syndrome, will be prescribed aspirin in addition to LMWH.

4.5.1.1 Unfractionated Heparin

Heparin is a natural product obtained from bovine or porcine mucosa; it cannot be manufactured in vitro. Naturally occurring heparin is comprised of a mix of molecules with differing molecular weights (range 5,000–35,000 Da). Only a third of these molecules contain the high-affinity pentasaccharide which mediates the primary anticoagulant effect of heparin. This accelerates the antithrombin inhibition of thrombin (factor IIa) and factors Xa. Because of its large molecular weight, high degree of ionization, and poor lipid solubility, heparin does not cross the placenta and is therefore safe to use in pregnancy [29, 32]. Neither is it secreted into breast milk, so it is safe to use in breast-feeding women. Heparin is cleared firstly by depolymerization after binding to macrophage receptors; this phase is rapid and can quickly become saturated. Heparin is then cleared by a much slower renal mechanism. When using concentrations of UFH in the therapeutic range, most is cleared by the rapid saturable mechanism; as a result, further rises in dosage can have a nonlinear effect on anticoagulant effect. In general, therapeutic doses of UFH have a half-life of less than 60 min [61].

The effect of UFH is generally monitored using the APTT, with a target range for the APTT ratio of 1.5–2.5 (although each laboratory should derive its own APTT ratio based on anti-Xa levels). In pregnancy, there is increased binding of UFH to plasma proteins and increased concentrations of factor VIII and fibrinogen; as a result, pregnant women require higher doses of UFH to achieve the same prolongation of APTT. As a result of the heterogeneous mix of molecules in

heparin, the clearance mechanisms discussed above, and the variable binding of heparin to plasma proteins, adjusting the dose of UFH in order to keep the APTT ratio in the therapeutic range can be problematic. Specific nomograms should be used and, if necessary, anti-factor-Xa assays (with a target anti-Xa range of 0.35–0.70 units/mL).

If prolonged UFH is used, platelet counts should be monitored from days 4–14. Heparin induced thrombocytopenia (HIT) should be suspected if the platelet count falls by 50 % or more and/or the patient develops new thrombosis or skin allergy between days 4 and 14 of heparin administration; in this situation, urgent hematological advice is needed [69].

Protamine sulfate rapidly reverses the anticoagulant effect of UFH. The dose of protamine is determined by the heparin exposure: 1 mg of protamine neutralises 80–100 U of UFH when administered within 15 min of the heparin dose. Less is required if protamine is given after a longer period because of the short half-life of intravenous UFH. Caution should be observed with higher doses because of a paradoxical risk of bleeding.

4.5.1.2 Low-Molecular-Weight Heparin

Low-molecular-weight heparins are produced synthetically by cleaving UFH either enzymatically (e.g. tinzaparin) or chemically (e.g. dalteparin, enoxaparin). This process yields low-molecular-weight heparins which have a molecular weight around 4,300–5,000 Da, around a third the molecular weight of UFH. Both LMWH and UFH bind to antithrombin, facilitating its anticoagulant effect. However, in all LMWHs the anti-Xa activity exceeds the anti-IIa activity.

Because LMWH has far less interaction with acute-phase proteins in the blood and because its clearance is primarily by the renal route, its pharmacokinetic characteristics are quite different to those of UFH and its anticoagulant activity much more predictable. This means that, particularly in non-pregnant patients, fixed weight-adjusted dosages can be used without the need for laboratory monitoring. However, in pregnancy, weight changes with gestation, the volume of distribution of the drug increases significantly, and there is a rise in renal clearance.

Glomerular filtration rate increases significantly in pregnancy, resulting in more rapid renal clearance of LMWH, that is, decreasing its half-life. Consequently, some centers prefer twice-daily therapeutic dosage regimens in pregnancy, in contrast to the once-daily regimens used in non-pregnant patients [5, 14, 18]. In non-pregnant subjects, LMWH has been shown to be at least as effective as UFH [30, 64]; and in one meta-analysis, more effective, when compared to UFH in the initial management of VTE [65]. In addition, LMWH and UFH use compare favorably to oral anticoagulation with warfarin [33, 54, 64]. Systematic reviews have shown that LMWH is safe in pregnancy and that it does not cross the placenta [27, 32]. LMWHs are also much less likely than UFH to cause HIT [68], and osteoporosis [8, 17, 26, 32, 49, 50, 53]. In a systematic review of the management of 2,777 pregnancies treated for acute VTE, the use of LMWH was safe and effective, associated with a recurrence rate of VTE of just 1.15 %. Similar studies in non-pregnant women using either LMWH or UFH followed by coumarins reported a VTE recurrence rate of between 5 % and 8 % up to 6 months after the initial event. Interestingly, in the 2,777 pregnancies treated with LMWH, not a single case of HIT was reported. The risk of heparin-induced osteoporosis also appears to be significantly lower with LMWH compared with UFH [17, 32, 49, 50, 53, 58]. Four cases of osteoporotic fractures in pregnant women using LMWH have been reported from one UK center, although each of these women had other significant risk factors for osteoporosis [55]. Although clearly more data are needed, the risk of this complication appears very low, in the order of 0.04 %. In spite of this apparently low incidence, it seems reasonable to encourage these women to take calcium supplements, plus vitamin D if the vitamin D level is suboptimal.

Although rare, skin reactions to LMWH are well recognized [7, 32]. These may be due to type 1 immediate hypersensitivity reaction or type 4 delayed hypersensitivity reaction. When they occur, treatment with the LMWH preparation being used should be discontinued, and an alternative LMWH preparation substituted. If a skin reaction occurs, HIT should be considered. If LMWH is not tolerated, options include vitamin K antagonists, UFH, or fondaparinux (although experience in pregnancy with fondaparinux is limited). Protamine sulfate incompletely reverses the effect of LMWH, although there is anecdotal evidence of clinical benefit.

4.5.2 Baseline Blood Investigations Prior to Initiating Anticoagulant Therapy

Before starting anticoagulant therapy, a full blood count, liver function tests, urea and electrolytes, and coagulation screen (APTT and prothrombin time) should be performed.

It is controversial whether thrombophilia screening should be performed at baseline or subsequently in a pregnant woman diagnosed with acute VTE and is not routinely recommended [6, 56]. Against testing is the fact that the results of thrombophilia testing are unlikely to influence management. Moreover, interpretation of the results can be misleading during pregnancy; for example, protein S levels are reduced in normal pregnancy, activated protein C resistance is found in up to 40 % of women in normal pregnancy and results of tests for antiphospholipid antibodies may not be representative. Antithrombin levels are reduced in conditions such as preeclampsia and nephrotic syndrome. Protein S and protein C are reduced in liver disease and vitamin K deficiency. For these reasons, careful consideration should be given to whether to perform thrombophilia testing and the results of thrombophilia screening tests in pregnancy should be interpreted by an experienced hematologist. The presence of a severe thrombophilia such as antithrombin deficiency may influence the management of anticoagulation during pregnancy.

4.5.3 Management During Pregnancy

Once VTE has been confirmed (either DVT or PE), anticoagulation should be continued. Low-molecular-weight heparin can be used in pregnancy for both initial and maintenance therapy.

As mentioned above, treatment with LMWH in non-pregnant patients is usually given once daily; however, a twice-daily regimen is recommended in pregnancy (Royal College of Obstetricians and Gynaecologists [56]) [14, 18]. In pregnancy, utilizing a twice-daily dosage regimen, the following doses are used: enoxaparin 1 mg/kg twice daily and dalteparin 100 units/kg twice daily. Although some early evidence suggests that once-daily administration of tinzaparin (175 units/kg) may be adequate in pregnancy, twice-daily dosing may be preferable until this regimen has been substantiated. Calculation of the initial dose is detailed in Table 4.4 by early pregnancy weight [56], although the dose may also be calculated according to current weight.

In pregnant, women on a treatment dose of LMWH for VTE, monitoring of anti-Xa activity is controversial and guidance is not evidence-based [31]. The Royal College of Obstetricians and Gynaecologists [56] recommends that periodic anti-Xa levels are indicated in women at extremes of weight (i.e. <50 kg or ≥90 kg), women who are bleeding (or are at increased risk of bleeding), who have recurrent VTE despite treatment with normal doses of LMWH, or who have renal disease. In such women, the target range for anti-Xa levels, measured 3–5 h after injection, depending on the type of LMWH is 0.5–1.0 units/mL.

In some studies of non-pregnant patients with acute VTE, the dose of LMWH has been reduced after an initial few weeks of therapeutic anticoagulation [41]. Currently, it is uncertain whether this would be adequate in pregnant women (bearing in mind that the prothrombotic state continues) and whether a reduction of dose would increase the risk of recurrence/propagation of the thrombosis. For the moment, therefore, until the safety of a reduced dose regimen

Table 4.4 Calculation of initial doses of drugs by early pregnancy weight

Initial dose	Early pregnancy weight (kg)			
	<50	50–69	70–89	>90
Enoxaparin (mg bd)	40	60	80	100
Dalteparin (iu bd)	5,000	6,000	8,000	10,000
Tinzaparin	175 units/kg once daily (all weights)			

Royal College of Obstetricians and Gynaecologists [57]
bd twice daily

in pregnancy is proved, it seems safer to continue the full therapeutic dose for at least six weeks after delivery.

Monitoring of the platelet count is not required when using treatment doses of LMWH during pregnancy, as LMWH is far less likely to cause HIT [32] when compared with UFH. Even in women who develop HIT when treated with LMWH, it is invariably the prior use of UFH which has sensitized them to heparin, even though the HIT does not develop until subsequent LMWH exposure. Consequently, if a woman is being treated with UFH or if she has had UFH treatment prior to treatment with LMWH, the platelet count should be checked every 3 days from day 4 to day 14, assuming heparin treatment is continued during that time.

When acute VTE is diagnosed in pregnancy, it is recommended that a treatment dose of LMWH should be continued throughout the pregnancy and for at least 6 weeks postpartum and until at least 3 months of treatment has been given in total [11, 12, 56]. These women can invariably be managed as outpatients; the patient or her partner can almost always be taught how to administer LMWH injections safely at home.

The initial management of lower limb DVT involves elevation of the leg and wearing graduated elastic compression stocking (GCS) on the affected leg (there is no need to wear a stocking on the unaffected leg). However, studies in the non-pregnant population have shown that once the patient is stable and anticoagulated, early mobilization is not associated with an increased risk of PE; it appears likely that the same applies in pregnancy. When used for thromboprophylaxis, antiembolism stockings have a pressure at the ankle of less than 20 mmHg; in contrast, GCS used in women with confirmed DVT have an ankle pressure of 30–40 mmHg. Accurate fitting is important and, as pregnancy progresses, repeat fittings with larger sizes may be necessary. If worn daily for 2 years following the initial DVT, the risk of post-thrombotic syndrome is reduced in non-pregnant patients (see below).

The use of a retrievable inferior vena cava (IVC) filter should be considered in a woman in whom anticoagulation is contraindicated or who has extensive DVT close to the time (within 2 weeks) of delivery, as full anticoagulation peripartum significantly increases the risk of hemorrhage, and the thrombotic risk is high. An IVC filter could also be considered in a woman with a DVT who has recurrent PE despite apparently adequate anticoagulation. However, it is preferable when possible to delay delivery and institute full anticoagulation rather than using an IVC filter; anticoagulation will then need to be managed around the time of delivery (see below). The use of an IVC filter is not without risk [6]. The IVC can be perforated during insertion. If inserted close to the time of delivery, there is a risk of filter migration due to the change in IVC pressure following delivery. On occasion, the filter may be difficult or impossible to retrieve, making long-term anticoagulation necessary.

Very rarely, DVT can lead to venous gangrene. Management in the non-pregnant patient includes elevation of the leg, anticoagulation, and possible surgical embolectomy or thrombolytic therapy. Thrombolytic therapy may increase the risk of placental abruption and, if used immediately postpartum, may increase the risk of postpartum hemorrhage. In pregnancy and peripartum, therefore, it is reserved for women with life-threatening PE.

Patients with CVT must have input from a neurologist. Principles of treatment are hydration, anticonvulsant therapy, and anticoagulation.

4.6   Acute Massive PE in Pregnancy

The differential diagnosis of acute maternal collapse in pregnancy includes PE, amniotic fluid embolus, myocardial infarct, and hemorrhage (concealed or revealed), among others. The immediate management is supportive, usually by a multidisciplinary team including an anesthetist, obstetrician, hematologist, nurses, and midwives. When PE is a possibility, an echocardiogram (bedside, if moving the patient is unfeasible) or CTPA should be arranged as a matter of urgency. Women with massive PE associated with hemodynamic compromise (low BP, tachycardia) should be managed on ITU and considered for thrombolysis, which can be lifesaving both during pregnancy and postpartum. The decision for thrombolysis should be made in conjunction with the multidisciplinary team. A suggested algorithm for management of women with clinically suspected massive PE is illustrated in Fig. 4.2. When the diagnosis of massive acute PE is established, intravenous UFH is generally preferred because of its rapid onset of action. Efficacy of the UFH is monitored by the APTT ratio, aiming for a range of 1.5–2.5 times the average laboratory control value, although each laboratory should define its own therapeutic range. APTT should be measured 4–6 h after the initial loading dose and 6 h after any change in dose. Once the APTT ratio is in the target range (usually 1.5–2.5), it should be rechecked at least every 24 h (more frequently if there are any issues with bleeding). A suggested algorithm for managing the infusion rate of UFH is shown in Table 4.5.

While adjustment of infusion rates of UFH on the basis of repeated APTT ratio measurements seems reasonable in theory, in practice it is problematic. This is partly because increased factor VIII levels in late pregnancy lead to apparent heparin resistance. This can lead to higher doses of UFH than necessary being used, which

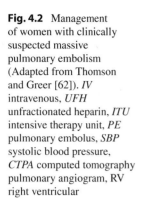

Fig. 4.2 Management of women with clinically suspected massive pulmonary embolism (Adapted from Thomson and Greer [62]). *IV* intravenous, *UFH* unfractionated heparin, *ITU* intensive therapy unit, *PE* pulmonary embolus, *SBP* systolic blood pressure, *CTPA* computed tomography pulmonary angiogram, *RV* right ventricular

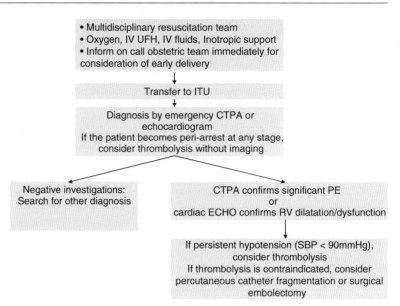

can cause bleeding problems. This increased risk of bleeding is particularly important soon after delivery, when the possibility of postpartum hemorrhage is a concern. In practice, in many maternity units, by the time a blood sample is taken, dispatched to the laboratory, analyzed, and the result received, several hours have usually passed. As a result, dose adjustments are delayed, and the risk (of either hemorrhage or thrombosis) has persisted during that time. An alternative approach is to measure anti-Xa activity; when UFH has been used, a lower level of anti-Xa is the aim (0.35–0.70 units/mL in a woman with PE which is not life-threatening; in a woman with life-threatening PE, the target is 0.5–1.0 units/mL). However, the laboratory turnaround time to measure anti-Xa activity is usually much longer than for APTT ratio measurement, making it less useful in clinical management.

There has always been a concern about the risk of using thrombolytic agents for the management of PE in pregnancy. The concern was that it might harm the fetus or increase the risk of placental abruption. In non-pregnant patients, several randomized controlled trials have shown that, while thrombolytic therapy is better than

Table 4.5 Infusion rates of unfractionated heparin (UFH) according to activated partial thromboplastin time (APTT)

APTT ratio	Dose change (units/kg/h)	Additional action	Next APTT (h)
<1.2	4	Rebolus 80 units/kg	6
1.2–1.5	2	Rebolus 40 units/kg	6
1.5–2.5	No change		24
2.5–3.0	−2		6
>3.0	−3	Stop infusion for 1 h	6

Royal College of Obstetricians and Gynaecologists [57]

heparin in reducing clot burden and improving hemodynamic function, there is no improvement in long-term survival. Because of the theoretical risks of placental abruption and the failure to demonstrate improvement in long-term outcome, it seems sensible to avoid thrombolytic agents in pregnancy except in life-threatening situations. Ahearn et al. [1] reviewed the many case reports of the use of thrombolytic agents in pregnancy. They found that bleeding complications occurred in 1–6 % of women, similar to the frequency in non-pregnant women receiving thrombolytic therapy. Of 172 women treated with thrombolysis, 5 had nonfatal maternal bleeding complications (2.9 %) and 3 suffered a fetal death (1.7 %). There were no maternal deaths and no reports of intracranial bleeding. Most bleeding complications were focused around catheter and puncture sites. In women whose life is threatened by massive PE, but in whom thrombolytic therapy also seems too risky (e.g. a woman immediately after Caesarean section), consideration should be given to urgent thoracotomy by a cardiothoracic surgeon. Another option is catheter-directed thrombolysis.

Such complicated patients clearly need the input of a hematologist experienced in anticoagulation in pregnancy. Ideally, management should be by a multidisciplinary team all familiar with the management of anticoagulation in pregnancy.

4.7 Planning for Delivery

Delivery planning should ideally take place well in advance of the due date and involve detailed discussion between the woman and her multidisciplinary team. The primary aim in peripartum management is to balance the risk of major postpartum hemorrhage in a woman who is fully anticoagulated with the risk of progressive or recurrent VTE when anticoagulation is interrupted. In general, being on treatment doses of anticoagulation would not be an indication for elective Caesarean section. However, in certain circumstances, it may be desirable to plan the timing of delivery (by induction of labor) for logistical reasons. Examples include the need to ensure delivery in the managing hospital of a woman who lives a long distance away or a woman who is certain that she wants an epidural for pain relief in labor.

In all cases, the woman should be kept well hydrated, wear antiembolism stockings, and stay as mobile as possible peri-delivery. In addition to the management of anticoagulation described below, in patients with congenital antithrombin deficiency, the peri-delivery use of antithrombin concentrate, either plasma derived or recombinant, should be considered. The use of antithrom-

bin concentrate in this situation provides thromboprophylaxis and thus enables reduction or interruption of LMWH. This approach minimizes the risk of both bleeding and venous thromboembolism. Until recently, antithrombin was available only as a pooled plasma-derived product which, despite effective viral inactivation, still carries a potential risk of transfusion-transmitted infection. A recombinant form of human antithrombin (ATryn®) is now licensed (Pan-European and USA).

4.7.1 Spontaneous Labor

Even in fully anticoagulated women, it is reasonable to aim for spontaneous labor and normal vaginal birth. The woman should be advised that, once she thinks her labor is starting, she should discontinue LMWH injections. If it turns out to be a false alarm and the contractions stop, the LMWH can be restarted. When she is admitted in labor, a blood sample should be sent for a coagulation screen, full blood count, and blood group and save. Assuming that the woman has a vaginal delivery and no postpartum hemorrhage, a prophylactic dose of LMWH can be started within 6 h after delivery and the full therapeutic dose recommenced 12 h later. A post-delivery weight should be checked to guide LMWH dosing.

4.7.2 Elective Caesarean Section

If elective Caesarean section is indicated for obstetric reasons, the last dose of (therapeutic dose) LMWH should be given 24 h before the planned operation. In practice, this will usually be the morning of the day before the Caesarean section.

After delivery by Caesarean section, if there is no problem with controlling bleeding, the first *prophylactic* dose of LMWH can be given within 6 h after the procedure. However, LMWH should not be given for at least four hours after an epidural catheter has been removed. In many units, an epidural or a combined spinal epidural (CSE) is used for elective Caesarean sections, and the epidural catheter is removed immediately at the end of the operation; in this case, the first dose of LMWH will be given 6 h after the Caesarean section (which is also 6 h after removal of the epidural catheter). After the first dose, assuming there is no issue with bleeding, the first *treatment* dose of LMWH can be given 12 h later. The new treatment dose should be recalculated on the basis of the woman's postpartum weight.

Anticoagulated women who have a Caesarean section are at increased risk of wound hematoma (in the order of 2 %) whether they are managed with UFH or LMWH. Consequently, there should be a lower threshold for using wound drains (either pelvic or rectus sheath), and consideration should be given to using interrupted staples or sutures for closing the skin as this will allow easier drainage of any subcutaneous hematoma.

4.7.3 Induction of Labor

Labor may be induced for obstetric indications (e.g. postdates) or for logistical reasons, for example, if the woman lives distant from the hospital yet it is desirable that she delivers in the hospital because of her anticoagulation. When admitted to hospital, a blood sample should be taken for a coagulation screen, full blood count, and blood group and save. Regional anesthesia (epidural for labor or spinal anesthesia for Caesarean section) is not considered safe until 24 h after the last *treatment* dose of LMWH, with dosing on a 12-hourly basis, (in comparison to 12 h after the last *prophylactic* dose). In practice, women taking therapeutic dose LMWH who go into spontaneous labor are unlikely to have the option of regional anesthesia for labor or Caesarean section.

When induction of labor is planned, a judgment needs to be made by an experienced obstetrician as to how long it is likely to take from the commencement of the induction process until labor is established. For example, in a primi-

gravid woman at 38 weeks' gestation, this could easily take up to 24 h. On the other hand, in a woman who has had two previous vaginal births and is now at 40 weeks' gestation, labor is likely to start within 6–8 h after the first dose of prostaglandin induction agent. This estimate will help to decide when the last treatment dose of LMWH should be given. The other factor influencing this decision is whether the woman wishes to have an epidural for pain relief in labor or not. If she does, it should be borne in mind that epidural anesthesia is not considered safe until 24 h after her last treatment dose of LMWH.

In practice, this means that when inducing labor in an unfavorable primigravid woman, the last dose of treatment LMWH could be given 12 h before the first dose of prostaglandin-inducing agent. For example, she could have her final dose of LMWH at the usual time the night before induction. The following morning, induction of labor is commenced. Consideration should be given to using misoprostol rather than the usual dinoprostone in these women. Misoprostol is a stronger prostaglandin which speeds up the induction process although carries a small increased risk of hyperstimulation.

In a multiparous woman with a favorable cervix, the last dose of treatment LMWH should be given 24 h prior to commencement of the induction process, in the expectation that labor will establish quickly once induction is commenced. In practice, this would normally mean that the woman injects her last dose of LMWH on the morning of the day prior to induction. Induction commences the following morning.

Six hours after vaginal delivery, assuming there is no issue with bleeding, a *prophylactic* dose of LMWH can be given and, 12 h later, the first *therapeutic* dose restarted.

4.7.4 Regional Anesthesia and Heparin

Regional anesthesia (epidural or spinal) is not considered safe until at least 24 h after the last therapeutic dose of LMWH (administered on a 12-hourly basis) or 12 h after the last prophylactic dose of LMWH. This is because of the risk of spinal hematoma, a potentially serious complication. The patient may have an epidural/spinal 24 h following a therapeutic dose of LMWH (administered 12 hourly) provided that the coagulation screen is normal and the platelet count >80 × 10^9/L. After the birth, in general the woman should be given her first dose of LMWH within 6 h after the delivery and at least 4 h after the epidural catheter has been removed. Epidural catheters are often removed soon after vaginal delivery or at the end of a Caesarean section, as the woman is being moved from the operating table; in this case, the next dose of LMWH should not be given until at least four hours later. If the epidural catheter is retained after delivery (it may, for example, be retained for further analgesia for 24 h after Caesarean section, by which time injections of LMWH have resumed), the epidural catheter should not be removed until 12 h have passed since the last injection of LMWH. In practice, this means that once the epidural catheter is removed (12 h after the previous dose of LMWH), the next dose of LMWH (which would have been due around the same time) will need to be delayed for a further 4 h.

Subcutaneous intermittent injections of UFH (which is uncommon in current management strategies for VTE in pregnancy) should be stopped 12 h before regional anesthesia can be given; a treatment dose intravenous infusion of UFH should be stopped 6 h before regional anesthesia.

4.8 Management After Delivery

If there is a problem with continued postpartum bleeding or the woman remains at high risk of bleeding, it is better to delay resumption of LMWH. If there is active bleeding, all anticoagulation should be stopped. If the risk of bleeding remains high but there is currently no active bleeding, it may be safer to continue an IV infusion of UFH. This is because UFH has a shorter half-life than LMWH and because this activity can be more completely reversed with protamine sulfate. If the woman is actively bleeding, all heparin should be stopped and expert hematological advice sought; other methods of stopping the bleeding, for example, surgical, should be pursued.

Once the immediate peripartum period has been negotiated, consideration is given to the duration of further therapeutic anticoagulation. Therapeutic anticoagulation should be continued for at least six weeks postnatally and for a total of at least three months' anticoagulation [10, 12, 34, 56, 63].

There are two common options for this postpartum anticoagulation, namely, LMWH or warfarin. The treatment regimen of LMWH that was used antenatally may be continued, but the dose recalculated on the basis of the woman's postpartum weight. Consideration could be given to changing to once-daily injections, similar to the regimen used in non-pregnant patients. The second option is to change to warfarin anticoagulation. The choice will depend on the woman's preference and the proposed duration of further anticoagulation. When this is just a further 6 weeks, a woman who is already used to administering LMWH may prefer to continue with this regimen rather than the regular testing and hospital visits that are often necessary when warfarin is initiated.

Warfarin should not be commenced until at least three days after the birth because there may be an increased risk of postpartum hemorrhage if started early [56]. Warfarin should be interrupted in the event of postpartum hemorrhage and should not be restarted until the bleeding has abated. In women who suffer a postpartum hemorrhage while on warfarin, consideration should be given to reversing the effect of warfarin with prothrombin complex concentrate plus intravenous vitamin K in consultation with a hematologist.

The woman should be made aware that changing to warfarin will require frequent testing of the international normalized ratio (INR), initially daily, over the first few weeks until a stable INR (target 2.5, range 2–3) is achieved. When long-term anticoagulation is proposed, this effort is worth it; when anticoagulation is planned for only a further 6 weeks, the inconvenience generally outweighs the benefits. In practice, the process of starting warfarin is often undertaken after discharge from hospital, usually in an outpatient anticoagulation clinic. LMWH is continued until an INR of 2 or more is achieved on two successive days.

Women should be advised that heparin and warfarin are safe during breast-feeding. Few data are available on whether LMWH crosses into breast milk. However, absorption of heparins from the gastrointestinal tract is minimal, so, even if some is ingested by the baby in breast milk, systemic absorption is likely to be negligible.

When it is time for anticoagulation to be stopped (often 6 weeks postnatally, assuming that the woman has had at least three months of anticoagulation), any continuing risk of thrombosis should be assessed. This should include a review of personal and family history of VTE. The results of any thrombophilia screen should be reviewed, on or off anticoagulation, and repeated if necessary. Where a significant thrombotic risk persists, anticoagulation may need to be continued for a further three months or longer.

Thromboprophylaxis in any future pregnancy and at other times of increased risk, for example, long-haul flights, should be discussed. The safety or otherwise of hormonal contraception should also be addressed.

4.9 Post-thrombotic Syndrome

Post-thrombotic syndrome (PTS) is relatively common following DVT, occurring in over 60 % of cases [47]. Symptoms and signs include persistent leg swelling and pain, chronic pigmentation, eczema and telangiectasis, persistent varicose veins, and sometimes chronic ulceration and dependant cyanosis. The risk of PTS can be halved by wearing class II graduated elastic compression stockings on the affected limb for a period of 2 years [15, 56].

Learning Points
- VTE is the leading direct cause of maternal mortality in many developed countries, including the UK.
- Pregnancy is a prothrombotic state, associated with a 5- to 10-fold increased risk of VTE compared with the non-pregnant state.
- Clinicians should have a low threshold for investigating women with suspected VTE in pregnancy.
- Healthcare professionals should be aware of the risk factors for venous and arterial thromboembolism.
- LMWH is the mainstay in the treatment of VTE in pregnancy.

References

1. Ahearn GS, Hadjiliadis MD, Govert JA, Tapson VF. Massive pulmonary embolism during pregnancy successfully treated with recombinant tissue plasminogen activator. Arch Intern Med. 2002;162:1221–7.
2. Allen C, Demetriades T. Radiation risk overestimated. Radiology. 2006;240:613–4.
3. Andersen BS, Steffensen FH, Sorensen HT, Nielsen GL, Olsen J. The cumulative incidence of venous thromboembolism during pregnancy and puerperium – an 11 year Danish population-based study of 63,300 pregnancies. Acta Obstet Gynecol Scand. 1998;77(2):170–3.
4. Anderson F, Wheeler H, Goldberg R, et al. A population-based perspective of the hospital incidence and case-fatality rates of deep vein thrombosis and pulmonary embolism. The Worcester DVT study. Arch Intern Med. 1991;151(5):933–8.
5. Baglin T, British Committee for Standard in Haematology (BCSH), et al. Guidelines on the use and monitoring of heparin. Br J Haematol. 2006;133:19–34.
6. Baglin T, Gray E, Greaves M, et al. Clinical guidelines for testing for heritable thrombophilia. Br J Haematol. 2010;149:209–20.
7. Bank I, Libourel EJ, Middeldorp S, Van Der Meer J, Buller HR. High rate of skin complications due to low-molecular-weight heparins in pregnant women. J Thromb Haemost. 2003;1:859–61.
8. Barbour LA, Kick SD, Steiner JF, et al. A prospective study of heparin-induced osteoporosis in pregnancy using bone densitometry. Am J Obstet Gynecol. 1994; 170:862–9.

9. Bates SM, Ginsberg JS. How we manage venous thromboembolism in pregnancy. Blood. 2002;100:3470–8.

10. Bates SM, Greer IA, Hirsh J, Ginsberg JS. Use of antithrombotic agents during pregnancy: the seventh ACCP conference on antithrombotic and thrombolytic therapy. Chest. 2004;163:627S–44.

11. Bates SM, Greer IA, Pabinger I, Sofaer S, Hirsh J. Venous thromboembolism, thrombophilia, antithrombotic therapy, and pregnancy: American College of Chest Physicians (ACCP) guidelines (8th edition). Chest. 2008;133:844–86.

12. Bates SM, Greer IA, Middeldorp S, Veenstra DL, Prabulos A-M, Vandvik PO. VTE, thrombophilia, antithrombotic therapy, and pregnancy. Antithrombotic Therapy and prevention of Thrombosis, 9th ed: American College of Chest Physicians Evidence-Based Clinical Practice Guidelines. Chest. 2012; 141(2)(Suppl):e691S–e736S.

13. Berg CJ, Atrash HK, Koonin LM, Tucker M. Pregnancy-related mortality in the United States, 1987–1990. Obstet Gynecol. 1996;88:161–7.

14. Blomback M, Bremme K, Hellgren M, Lindberg H. A pharmacokinetic study of dalteparin (Fragmin) during late pregnancy. Blood Coagul Fibrinolysis. 1998;9:343–50.

15. Brandjes DP, Buller HR, Heijboer H, Huisman MV, de Rijk M, Jagt H, et al. Randomised trial of effect of compression stockings in patients with symptomatic proximal–vein thrombosis. Lancet. 1997;349: 759–62.

16. British Thoracic Society Standards of Care Committee Pulmonary Embolism Guideline Development Group. British Thoracic Society guidelines for the management of suspected acute pulmonary embolism. Thorax. 2003;58:470–84.

17. Carlin AJ, Farquharson RG, Quenby SM, Topping J, Fraser WD. Prospective observational study of bone mineral density during pregnancy: low molecular weight heparin versus control. Hum Reprod. 2004;19:1211–4.

18. Casele HL, Laifer SA, Woelkers DA, Venkataramanan R. Changes in the pharmacokinetics of the low molecular weight heparin enoxaparin sodium during pregnancy. Am J Obstet Gynecol. 1999;181:1113–7.

19. Centre for Maternal and Child Enquiries (CMACE). Saving mothers' lives: reviewing maternal deaths to make motherhood safer: 2006–08. The eighth report on confidential enquiries into maternal deaths in the United Kingdom. BJOG. 2011;118 Suppl 1:57–65. 71–76.

20. Chan WS, Lee A, Spencer FA, Chunilal S, Crowther M, Wu W, Johnston M, Rodger M, Ginsberg JS. D-dimer testing in pregnant patients: towards determining the next 'level' in the diagnosis of deep vein thrombosis. J Thromb Haemost. 2010;8(5):1004–11.

21. Chang J, Elam-Evans LD, Berg CJ, et al. Pregnancy-related mortality surveillance – United States, 1991–1999. MMWR Surveill Summ. 2003;52:1–8.

22. Che Yaakob CA, Dzarr AA, Ismail AA, Zuky Nik Lah NA, Ho JJ. Anticoagulant therapy for deep vein thrombosis (DVT) in pregnancy. Cochrane Database Syst Rev. 2010;(6):CD007801.

23. CLASP Collaborative Group. CLASP: a randomised trial of low-dose aspirin for the prevention and treatment of pre-eclampsia among 9364 pregnant women. Lancet. 1994;343:619–29.

24. Confidential Enquiry into Maternal and Child Health. Saving mothers' lives: reviewing maternal deaths to make motherhood safer, 2006–2008. The eighth report of the confidential enquiries into maternal deaths in the United Kingdom. London: CEMACH; 2011. www.cmace.org.uk/Publications/CEMACHPublications/Maternal-and-Perinatal-Health.aspx.

25. Cook JV, Kyriou J. Radiation from CT and perfusion scanning in pregnancy. Br Med J. 2005;221:350.

26. Douketis JD, Ginsberg JS, Burrows RF, et al. The effects of long-term heparin therapy during pregnancy on bone density. A prospective matched cohort study. Thromb Haemost. 1996;75:254–7.

27. Forestier F, Daffos F, Capella-Pavlovsky M. Low molecular weight heparin (PK 10169) does not cross the placenta during the second trimester of pregnancy: study by direct fetal blood sampling under ultrasound. Thromb Res. 1984;34:557–60.

28. Gherman RB, Goodwin TM, Leung B, et al. Incidence, clinical characteristics, and timing of objectively diagnosed venous thromboembolism during pregnancy. Obstet Gynecol. 1999;94(5 Part 1):730–4.

29. Ginsberg JS, Kowalchuk G, Hirsh J, Brill-Edwards P, Burrows R. Heparin therapy during pregnancy. Risks to the fetus and mother. Arch Intern Med. 1989;149: 2233–6.

30. Gould MK, Dembitzer AD, Doyle RL, Hastie TJ, Garber AM. Low-molecular-weight heparins compared with unfractionated heparin for treatment of acute deep venous thrombosis: a meta-analysis of randomized, controlled trials. Ann Intern Med. 1999;130:800–9.

31. Greer I, Hunt BJ. Low molecular weight heparin in pregnancy: current issues. Br J Haematol. 2005;128: 593–601.

32. Greer IA, Nelson-Piercy C. Low-molecular-weight heparins for thromboprophylaxis and treatment of venous thrombo-embolism in pregnancy: a systematic review of safety and efficacy. Blood. 2005;106:401–7.

33. Hull R, Delmore T, Carter C, et al. Adjusted subcutaneous heparin versus warfarin sodium in the long-term treatment of venous thrombosis. N Engl J Med. 1982;306:189–94.

34. Hyers TM, Hull RD, Weg JG. Antithrombotic therapy for venous thromboembolic disease. Chest. 1995;108: 335s–51.

35. Jacobsen AF, Skjeldestad FE, Sandet PM. Incidence and risk patterns of venous thromboembolism in pregnancy and puerperium – a register-based case–control study. Am J Obstet Gynecol. 2008;198:223–34.

36. James AH. Prevention and management of venous thromboembolism in pregnancy. Am J Med. 2007;120(10 Suppl 2):S26–34.

37. James AH, Jamison MG, Brancazio LR, Myers ER. Venous thromboembolism during pregnancy and the postpartum period: incidence, risk factors, and the mortality. Am J Obstet Gynecol. 2006;194:1311–5.
38. Kieregaard A. Incidence and diagnosis of deep vein thrombosis associated with pregnancy. Acta Obstet Gynecol Scand. 1983;62(3):239–43.
39. Knight M, Kurinczuk JJ, Spark P, Brocklehurst P. United Kingdom Obstetric Surveillance System (UKOSS) annual report. 2007. National Perinatal Epidemiology Unit, Oxford.
40. Knight M, on behalf of UKOSS. Antenatal pulmonary embolism: risk factors, management and outcomes. BJOG. 2008;115:453–61.
41. Lee AY, Levine MN, Baker RI, Bowden C, Kakkar AK, Prins M, Randomized Comparison of Low-Molecular-Weight Heparin versus Oral Anticoagulant Therapy for the Prevention of Recurrent Venous Thromboembolism in Patients with Cancer (CLOT) Investigators, et al. Low-molecular-weight heparin versus a coumarin for the prevention of recurrent venous thromboembolism in patients with cancer. N Engl J Med. 2003;349:146–53.
42. Lewis G, editor. Why mothers die 2000–2002. Sixth report of the confidential enquiries into maternal death. London: Royal College of Obstetricians and Gynaecologists Press; 2004.
43. Lewis G, editor. Mothers' lives 2003–2005. Seventh report of the confidential enquiries into maternal death. London: Royal College of Obstetricians and Gynaecologists Press; 2007.
44. Lindqvist P, Dahlback B, Marsal K. Thrombotic risk during pregnancy: a population study. Obstet Gynecol. 1999;94(4):595–9.
45. Macklon NS, Greer IA. Venous thromboembolic disease in obstetrics and gynaecology: the Scottish experience. Scott Med J. 1996;41(3):83–6.
46. Macklon NS, Greer IA, Bowman AW. An ultrasound study of gestational and postural changes in the deep venous system of the leg in pregnancy. BJOG. 1997;104:191–7.
47. McColl MD, Ellison J, Greer IA, Tait RC, Walker ID. Prevalence of the post thrombotic syndrome in young women with previous venous thromboembolism. Br J Haematol. 2000;108:272–4.
48. Mcoll MD, Ramsay JE, Tait RC, et al. Risk factors for pregnancy associated venous thromboembolism. Thromb Haemost. 1997;78(4):1183–8.
49. Melissari E, Parker CJ, Wilson NV, Monte G, Kanthou C, Pemberton KD, et al. Use of low molecular weight heparin in pregnancy. Thromb Haemost. 1992;68:652–6.
50. Monreal M. Long-term treatment of venous thromboembolism: the place of low molecular weight heparin. Vessels. 1997;3:18–21.
51. Nelson S, Greer I. Thromboembolic events in pregnancy: pharmacological prophylaxis and treatment. Expert Opin Pharmacother. 2007;8(17):2917–31.
52. Nordstrom M, Lindblad B, Bergqvist D, Kjellstrom T. A prospective study of the incidence of deep-vein thrombosis within a defined urban population. J Intern Med. 1992;232(2):155–60.
53. Pettila V, Leinonen P, Markkola A, Hiilesmaa V, Kaaja R. Postpartum bone mineral density in women treated for thromboprophylaxis with unfractionated heparin or LMW heparin. Thromb Haemost. 2002;87:182–6.
54. Pini M, Aiello S, Manotti C, et al. Low molecular weight heparin versus warfarin in the prevention of recurrences after deep vein thrombosis. Thromb Haemost. 1994;72:191–7.
55. Remy-Jardin M, Remy J. Spiral CT angiography of the pulmonary circulation. Radiology. 1999;212:615–36.
56. Royal College of Obstetricians and Gynaecologists. Thromboembolic disease in pregnancy and the puerperium: acute management. Green-top guideline no. 37b. London: RCOG; 2007. www.rcog.org.uk/womens-health/clinicalguidance/thromboembolic-disease-pregnancy-andpuerperium-acute-management-gre.
57. Samuelsson E, Hagg S. Incidence of venous thromboembolism in young Swedish women and possibly preventable cases among combined oral contraceptive users. Acta Obstet Gynecol Scand. 2004;83(7):674–81.
58. Scarsbrook AF, Evans AL, Owen AR, Gleeson FV. Diagnosis of suspected venous thromboembolic disease in pregnancy. Clin Radiol. 2006;61(1):1–12.
69. Simpson EL, Lawrenson RA, Nightingale AL, Farmer RD. Venous thromboembolism in pregnancy and the puerperium: incidence and additional risk factors from a London perinatal database. BJOG. 2001;108(1):56–60.
60. The Task Force for the Diagnosis and Management of Acute Pulmonary Embolism of the European Society of Cardiology. Guidelines on the diagnosis and management of acute pulmonary embolism. Eur Heart J. 2008;29:2276–315.
61. Thomson AJ, Greer IA. Advances in low molecular weight heparin use in pregnancy. In: Garg HG, Linhardt RJ, Hales CA, editors. Chemistry and biology of heparin and heparan sulfate. Elsevier: Amsterdam; 2005. p. 745–68.
62. Thomson AJ, Greer IA. Acute management of suspected thromboembolic disease in pregnancy. In: Sue Pavord S, Hunt B, editors. The obstetric hematology manual. Cambridge: Cambridge University Press; 2010.
63. Toglia MR, Weg JG. Venous thromboembolism during pregnancy. N Engl J Med. 1996;335:108–14.
64. Van Der Heijden JF, Hutten BA, Buller HR, Prins MH. Vitamin K antagonists or low-molecular-weight heparin for the long-term treatment of symptomatic venous thromboembolism. Cochrane Database Syst Rev. 2002;(1):CD002001.
65. Van Dongen CJ, Van Den Belt AG, Prins MH, Lensing AW. Fixed dose subcutaneous low molecular weight heparins versus adjusted dose unfractionated heparin for venous thromboembolism. Cochrane Database Syst Rev. 2004;(4):CD001100.

66. Voke KM, Keidan J, Parvod S, Spencer NH, Hunt BJ. The management of antenatal venous thromboembolism in the UK and Ireland: a prospective multi-centre survey. Br J Haematol. 2007;139: 545–58.
67. Walker ID. Venous and arterial thrombosis during pregnancy: epidemiology. Semin Vasc Med. 2003;3:25–32.
68. Warkentin TE, Levine MN, Hirsh J, et al. Heparin-induced thrombocytopenia in patients treated with low-molecular-weight heparin or unfractionated heparin. N Engl J Med. 1995;332:1330–5.
69. Warkentin TE, Greinacher A, Koster A, Lincoff AM. Treatment and prevention of heparin-induced thrombocytopenia. American College of Chest Physicians (ACCP) guidelines (8th edition). Chest. 2008;133: 340–80.
70. White R. The epidemiology of venous thromboembolism. Circulation. 2003;107:I-4–8.

Pregnancy Morbidity Associated with Hereditary and Acquired Thrombophilias: Recurrent Miscarriage

5

Raj Rai and Lesley Regan

Abstract

Components of the haemostatic pathways play a key role in the establishment and maintenance of pregnancy. Pregnancy itself is a hypercoaguable state. An exaggerated haemostatic response is associated with an increased risk nor only for recurrent miscarriage but for adverse pregnancy outcome at all gestational stages. Antiphospholipid antibodies (aPL) are the most important treatable cause for recurrent miscarriage. Recent advances have allowed us to escape from the restrictive concept of pregnancy loss being purely related to thrombosis to now emphasising the role of these antibodies in decidualisation of the endometrium and in trophoblast biology. Concurrently emphasis is now placed on the non-anticoagulant effects of heparin on improving pregnancy in those with a thrombophilic defect.

5.1 Background

Miscarriage, the loss of a pregnancy before viability, is the commonest complication of pregnancy. The term therefore includes all pregnancy losses from the time of conception, which is shortly after ovulation, until 24 weeks of gestation [39].

R. Rai, MD, MRCOG (✉)
Department of Surgery & Cancer, Imperial College Hospitals NHS Trust, St Mary's Hospital, Mint Wing, South Wharf Road, London W2 1PL, UK
e-mail: r.rai@imperial.ac.uk

L. Regan, MD, FRCOG
Department of Surgery & Cancer, St Mary's Hospital, Mint Wing, South Wharf Road, London W2 1PL, UK
e-mail: l.regan@imperial.ac.uk

Although 15 % of clinically recognized pregnancies miscarry, total reproductive losses are closer to 50 %. The vast majority of miscarriages occur early in pregnancy, before 10 weeks gestation. The incidence of late- or second-trimester pregnancy loss, between 10 and 24 weeks of gestation, is no more than 2 % [15].

Miscarriage may be divided into two types – sporadic and recurrent. Approximately 25 % of all couples will experience a single sporadic miscarriage. The most common cause of such miscarriages is a random fetal chromosome abnormality, the incidence of which increases with advancing maternal age. In contrast, only 1–2 % of couples will be diagnosed with recurrent miscarriages, the accepted definition of which is the loss of three or more consecutive pregnancies. Three strands of evidence suggest that recurrent miscarriage is a distinct clinical problem rather than one which occurs by chance alone: (a) the observed incidence is significantly higher than that expected by chance alone (0.3 %), (b) a woman's risk of miscarriage is directly related to the outcome of her previous pregnancies – the risk of miscarriage increasing with the number of previous miscarriages she has experienced, and (c) women with recurrent miscarriage tend to lose chromosomally normal rather than abnormal pregnancies [39].

Recurrent miscarriage is associated with significant psychological sequelae for both women and their partners and considerable economic cost for the state. Among the 6,000 new couples/year diagnosed with recurrent miscarriage in the UK, pronounced emotional responses, such as anxiety, depression, denial, anger, marital disruption, and a sense of loss and inadequacy, are common [10]. While the financial burden to the UK health service is in the region of £30 million/year, this does not include the much larger cost of treatment of depressive illness and of lost productivity.

5.1.1 Recurrent Miscarriage: A Defect in the Hemostatic Response?

In preparation for pregnancy, the uterine endometrium undergoes a process of "decidualization" in which the endometrium becomes receptive to implantation of an embryo. The processes of implantation of the embryo into the uterine decidua and subsequent formation of the placenta are key events in pregnancy. Defects in this process underlie adverse pregnancy outcome at all gestational ages. Implantation of the embryo can be divided into three stages – apposition of the embryo with the uterine decidua, adhesion of the embryo to the decidua, and finally invasion of primitive placental cells (trophoblast) through the decidua into the maternal uterine spiral arteries which lie within the myometrium (Fig. 5.1). Subsequent formation of the placenta in humans is termed "hemochorial placentation," as the placenta is in contact with the maternal blood supply. Components of both the coagulation and the fibrinolytic pathways are intimately involved in these processes.

Pregnancy itself is a prothrombotic state – characterized by an increase in the levels of procoagulant factors, a simultaneous decrease in the levels of anticoagulant proteins, and activation of fibrinolysis [8, 32, 49]. The evolutionary advantage of this is thought to counteract the inherent instability of hemochorial placentation. Over the last 20 years, the hypothesis has been developed that many cases of recurrent miscarriage are due to an abnormal or exaggerated hemostatic response in pregnancy [36]. This hypothesis is supported by data reporting increased markers of thrombin generation among women with recurrent miscarriage outside of pregnancy [36, 53], an increased prevalence of coagulation defects among women with recurrent miscarriage [40, 44, 55], and histological evidence of placental

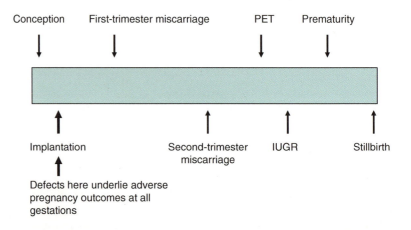

Fig. 5.1 Implantation spectrum

thrombosis in some cases of recurrent miscarriage [20, 43].

Remarkably few studies have reported the placental histological findings among the pregnancies of women with recurrent miscarriage. Nayar and Lage [29] were the first to reported massive infarction in the first-trimester placenta from a pregnancy of a woman with antiphospholipid antibodies (aPL) and recurrent miscarriage. Our own unit reported a significantly increased prevalence of placental infarction among the pregnancies of women with recurrent miscarriage (10 %), irrespective of the presence of aPL, versus 1 % using the same criteria to assess infarction, among those with a previously uncomplicated reproductive history [20].

This chapter examines the role of thrombophilic defects – both heritable and acquired – in the pathogenesis of recurrent miscarriage.

5.2 Antiphospholipid Syndrome

5.2.1 Introduction

Antiphospholipid syndrome (APS) is the most important treatable cause of recurrent miscarriage. Antiphospholipid antibodies are also associated with adverse pregnancy outcome at later gestational ages including preeclampsia and preterm delivery (Table 5.1). In relation to adverse pregnancy outcome, lupus anticoagulant and anticardiolipin antibodies (both IgG and IgM) together with anti-β2GPI appear to be the most important members of the family of antiphospholipid anti-

Table 5.1 Pregnancy morbidity associated with antiphospholipid syndrome

One or more unexplained deaths of a morphologically healthy fetus at or beyond the 10th week of gestation, with healthy fetal morphology documented by ultrasound or by direct examination of the fetus

One or more premature births of a morphologically healthy newborn baby before the 34th week of gestation because of eclampsia or severe preeclampsia defined according to standard definitions or recognized features of placental failure

Three or more unexplained consecutive spontaneous abortions before the 10th week of gestation, with maternal anatomical or hormonal abnormalities and paternal and maternal chromosomal causes excluded

bodies. In accordance with the revised Sapporo (Sydney) International consensus criteria [27], a diagnosis of obstetric antiphospholipid syndrome demands the presence of one of the defining criteria listed in Table 5.1 together with persistently positive tests for one or more of lupus anticoagulant, anticardiolipin antibodies and anti-β2GPI.

5.2.2 Prevalence

Approximately 15 % of women with recurrent miscarriage have APS [42, 44]. In contrast, the prevalence of aPL in women with a "low-risk" obstetric history is less than 2 % [25, 34]. The largest prevalence study (500 consecutive women with recurrent miscarriage attending a specialist recurrent miscarriage clinic) reported the prevalence of persistently positive tests for lupus anticoagulant to be 9.6 %, IgG anticardiolipin 3.3 %, and IgM anticardiolipin 2.2 %. Importantly, among the miscarriage population there appears to be little crossover between lupus anticoagulant and anticardiolipin positivity and a large number of women have only transiently positive tests (66 % lupus anticoagulant and 37 % for either IgG or IgM anticardiolipin).

5.2.3 Outcome of Untreated Pregnancies

The outcome of pregnancy in untreated women with aPL and a history of recurrent miscarriage is poor. The earliest studies reported that the fetal loss rate in women with APS was in the range of 50–70 % [25, 35]. It was subsequently realized that these figures underestimated the scale of the problem because recruitment only took place after these women had presented for antenatal care (at approximately 12 weeks) by which time the majority of miscarriages have already occurred. A prospective observational study in which women with APS were identified prior to pregnancy and followed from the time of a positive pregnancy test reported the miscarriage rate to be 90 % with no pharmacological treatment [42, 44]. In contrast, the miscarriage rate among a control group of aPL-negative women with recurrent miscarriage was significantly lower – in the region of 40 %. In untreated pregnancies, women with APS are also at significant increased risk for later pregnancy complications. In a population-based analysis of 141,286 deliveries in Florida, USA, positivity for aPL increased the risk for both preeclampsia and placental insufficiency (adjusted odds ratio 2.93 [95 % CI 1.51–5.61] and 4.58 [2.0–10.5]), respectively [31].

5.2.4 Mechanisms of aPL Pregnancy Loss

Pregnancy loss associated with aPL has tradition-ally been attributed to thrombosis of the placental vasculature [11, 18, 33]. However, thrombosis is neither a universal nor a specific feature in antiphos-pholipid-associated miscarriages [33]. Advances in our understanding of early pregnancy development and phospholipid biology have highlighted alterna-tive mechanisms of action of these antibodies in the pathogenesis of pregnancy loss.

In vitro studies demonstrate that antiphospho-lipid antibodies have a direct deleterious effect on implantation by affecting both the function of the uterine decidua and of the trophoblast. Antiphospholipid antibodies (a) impair signal transduction mechanisms controlling endometrial cell decidualization and impair endometrial angio-genesis [13, 26], (b) increase trophoblast apopto-sis [5], and (c) decrease trophoblast fusion and impair trophoblast invasion [4, 5]. Interestingly, the effects of aPL on trophoblast function are reversed, at least in vitro, by low-molecular-weight heparin (LMWH) [4, 5, 12].

More recently, attention has focused on the role of complement activation in aPL related pregnancy loss. Injection of aPL into pregnant mice results in antibody and C3 deposition in the decidua, along with focal necrosis and apop-tosis and neutrophil infiltration [19]. These effects are accompanied by a fourfold increase in the frequency of fetal resorption; fetal loss can be reversed by simultaneous treatment with soluble recombinant complement receptor 1-related gene/protein y (Crry), which also pre-vents C3 deposition and neutrophil infiltration. Finally, a causative role for complement activa-tion was shown conclusively by injecting aPL

antibodies into C3-deficient mice, which became resistant to aPL antibody-mediated fetal loss. To reevaluate the link between aPL and thrombo-sis, the authors showed that aPL induce throm-bus formation following local vascular injury and that soluble Crry significantly decreases the size of the thrombi. Thus, complement activa-tion is likely to be an important upstream medi-ator in both aPL IgG-induced vascular thrombosis and fetal loss.

5.2.5 Management of Recurrent Miscarriage Associated with aPL

The management of women with APS depends on comprehensive investigation prior to preg-nancy, definition of the management plan and counseling regarding (a) the live birth rate with treatment; (b) treatment not preventing the loss of a genetically abnormal pregnancy; (c) the increased risk of later pregnancy complications such as preeclampsia and placental insufficiency necessitating preterm delivery; (d) risks of an APS-related complication in the neonate; and (e) increased risk to the mother herself dur-ing pregnancy and postpartum and the need for thromboprophylaxis.

5.2.5.1 Treatment of Obstetric Antiphospholipid Syndrome
Over the last 25 years, a variety of pharmaceuti-cal agents have been used, either individually or in combination, in attempts to improve the preg-nancy outcome of women with antiphospholipid syndrome. Low-dose aspirin (LDA) in combina-tion with heparin remains the mainstay of treat-ment, as confirmed in two meta-analyses [16, 26]. This treatment combination leads to a 70 % live birth rate [23, 38].

Two randomized trials [23, 38] have reported that LDA and unfractionated heparin (UFH) improve the live birth rate in women with APS when compared to aspirin alone. In the trial reported by Rai et al [38], 90 women were ran-domized at the time of a positive urinary pregnancy test to receive either LDA or LDA and heparin daily until the time of miscarriage or 34 weeks gestation. The live birth rate with LDA and heparin was 71 % compared to 42 % with LDA alone (OR 3.37, 95 % CI 1.40–8.10). Importantly, there was no difference in live birth rates between the two treatment groups in those pregnancies which advanced beyond 13 weeks. This implies that the beneficial effect of adjuvant heparin therapy is conferred in the first trimester of pregnancy, at a time when the intervillous circulation has not been fully established and hence cannot be due to the anticoagulant actions of heparin. It appears that the combination of LDA and heparin promotes successful embryonic implantation in the early stages of pregnancy by protecting the trophoblast from attack by aPL. Later in pregnancy, the combination therapy helps protect against subsequent thrombosis of the uteroplacental vasculature.

Treatment with LDA and heparin significantly reduces the severity of the defective endovascular trophoblastic invasion in women with APS, allowing them to achieve a live birth. However, it is important to remember that a proportion of pregnant women with aPL will remain at risk for late pregnancy complications due to the underlying uteroplacental vasculopathy. In a prospective series of 150 treated women with APS, a high risk for preterm delivery, placental abruption, fetal growth restriction, and the development of pregnancy-induced hypertension was found [2]. Once the pregnancy advances beyond the first trimester, specialist antenatal surveillance is required. Uterine artery Doppler ultrasonography at 22–24 weeks, followed by serial fetal growth and Doppler scans during the third trimester are useful tools with which to predict preeclampsia and intrauterine growth restriction in APS pregnancies [52]. Women with a circulating lupus anticoagulant or high titers of IgG anticardiolipin antibodies are at particularly high risk of these complications.

Two studies have challenged the view that LDA and heparin is the treatment of choice for pregnant women with APS. Farquhaon et al. [17] reported that LDA alone is as effective as LMWH, but they included women with low positive titers for anticardiolipin antibodies, who were randomly assigned to treatment at a late stage in the first trimester, when pregnancy outcome was more likely to be successful. In addition, nearly 25 % of the study participants switched treatment groups. The more recent study by Laskin et al. [24] aimed to investigate whether treatment with LMWH plus LDA results in an increased rate of live births compared to treatment with LDA alone, but the study group was highly heterogeneous. The authors included women with two or more unexplained pregnancy losses prior to 32 weeks of gestation, accompanied by one or more of the following: positive aPL, positive antinuclear antibodies (ANA), or an inherited thrombophilic defect. A total of 88 women were recruited to the study over a 4-year period, but the RCT was then stopped prematurely when an interim analysis showed no difference in live birth rates in the two groups and a lower rate of pregnancy loss in the aspirin group than expected.

The relative effectiveness of UFH versus LMWH as regards the prevention of recurrent pregnancy loss in women with APS is not established. The results of two recent pilot studies suggest that the combination of LMWH and LDA might be equivalent to UFH and LDA in preventing recurrent pregnancy loss [30, 48]. The American College of Chest Physicians (ACCP) recommends prophylactic or intermediate dose UFH or prophylactic dose LMWH in combination with LDA for the treatment of obstetric APS associated with a history of recurrent miscarriages [1].

While treatment with LDA and heparin leads to a high live birth rate, some women do experience further miscarriages despite treatment. The single most important investigation to perform if a women miscarries while taking treatment is to obtain fetal tissue for karyotype analysis. If the fetal karyotype is abnormal, pregnancy loss was not a failure of treatment and the woman can be offered treatment with LDA and heparin again in a future pregnancy. However, if the fetal karyotype was normal, one has to assume that pregnancy loss was a failure of treatment. This situation, although uncommon, has led to the use of other adjuvant therapies including intravenous immunoglobulin (IVIg). There is however considerable evidence that IVIg is of no benefit in the treatment of obstetric APS and its use is not to be recommended [7, 51]. Potential novel therapeutic agents that may be of benefit include complement inhibitors and hydroxychloroquine. With respect to the latter, it has recently been reported that hydroxychloroquine protects the anticoagulant annexin A5 shield which surrounds the trophoblast from damage induced by antiphospholipid antibodies [45]. Bramham et al. suggest that the addition of first trimester low-dose prednisolone to conventional treatment may be useful in the management of refractory aPL-related loss(es), although complications remain increased [6].

5.2.5.2 Neonatal Complications

Babies born to mothers with antiphospholipid syndrome are at risk of the consequences of preterm delivery. A Pan-European study reported that among 138 pregnancies, 16.3 % of babies were delivered at less than 37 weeks of gestation, 17 % were low birth weight, and, in addition, 11.3 % of neonates were small for gestational age. During the follow-up period of 6 years, 5 of the 141 babies exhibited behavioral abnormalities [3]. Almost 30 % of babies will passively acquire aPL [50]. There have been individual case reports of neonatal stroke – both hemorrhagic secondary to thrombocytopenia and thrombotic – as well as thrombosis of the renal and axillary veins.

5.2.6   Heritable Thrombophilias

The relationship between heritable thrombophilias and recurrent first-trimester miscarriage is controversial. Indeed, many studies have been of a small size, prone to stratification and admixture bias, in which there has been poor matching of cases and controls as a result of racial heterogeneity. In addition, publication bias is evident, as judged by the discrepancy between the number of published abstracts reporting a lack of association between congenital thrombophilia and the number of peer-reviewed papers reporting an association.

A meta-analysis of pooled data from 31 retrospective studies suggested that the magnitude of the association between inherited thrombophilias and fetal loss varies according to type of fetal loss and type of thrombophilia [46]. The association between thrombophilia and late pregnancy loss has been consistently stronger than for early pregnancy loss. In this meta-analysis, factor V Leiden was associated with recur-

rent first-trimester fetal loss (OR 2.01, 95 % CI 1.13–3.58), recurrent fetal loss after 22 weeks (OR 7.83, 95 % CI 2.83–21.67), and nonrecurrent fetal loss after 19 weeks (OR 3.26, 95 % CI 1.82–5.83). Activated protein C resistance was associated with recurrent first-trimester fetal loss (OR 3.48, 95 % CI 1.58–7.69). The G202310A the G20210A prothrombin gene mutation was associated with recurrent first-trimester fetal loss (OR 2.32, 95 % CI 1.12–4.79), recurrent fetal loss before 25 weeks (OR 2.56, 95 % CI 1.04–6.29), and late nonrecurrent fetal loss (OR 2.3, 95 % CI 1.09–4.87).

Similarly, another meta-analysis of 16 case–control studies reported that carriers of factor V Leiden or the G20210A prothrombin gene mutation have doubled the risk of experiencing recurrent miscarriage compared to women without these thrombophilic mutations [22].

Prospective data on the outcome of untreated pregnancies in women with such thrombophilias are scarce. One small study of six hereditary thrombophilias reported no adverse effects on the live birth rate of women with recurrent miscarriage [9]. In contrast, two small prospective studies reported an increased risk of miscarriage in untreated pregnancies for women with recurrent miscarriage who carry the factor V Leiden mutation compared to those with a normal factor V genotype [21, 37].

The importance of the fetal genetic thrombophilia status in governing pregnancy outcome has not been explored in large studies. Dizon-Townson et al. reported that fetal carriage of the factor V Leiden mutation is associated with a significantly increased risk of miscarriage. This area of research demands further attention [14].

While some centers advocate the use of thromboprophylactic therapy – typically LDA in combination with heparin – for those with recurrent miscarriage and hereditary thrombophilias, there is little evidence base for this. Indeed the Habenox study, a multicenter randomized study, reported no difference in live birth rates among those with an inherited thrombophilia who were treated with heparin, heparin and LDA, or LDA alone [54]. The results of this study however have to be treated with some caution as the sample population was small (26 women with thrombophilia, including 17 women with factor V Leiden and 5 with prothrombin G20210A) and the study was stopped prematurely due to slow recruitment.

5.3 Tests of Global Haemostasis and Coagulation Activation

Conventional hemostasis tests are expensive, time-consuming, and take no account of the fact that hemostasis in vivo is a dynamic process which involves the interaction of coagulation and fibrinolytic pathways together with cellular elements such as endothelial cell surfaces. Hence, the measurement of individual coagulation factors is of limited use in establishing an individual's thrombotic risk, particularly during pregnancy. These limitations have prompted us to investigate the value of global tests of hemostasis in the investigation and treatment of women with recurrent miscarriage.

5.3.1 Thrombin-Antithrombin Levels

We studied levels of thrombin-antithrombin (TAT) complexes, a marker of thrombin generation, in nonpregnant women with recurrent miscarriage, with and without aPL [53]. TAT concentrations were significantly raised in both aPL-positive and aPL-negative women with a history of recurrent miscarriage compared with normal controls. There was no significant difference in TAT values between aPL-positive and aPL-negative women or between women with early or late miscarriage. This study of 130 women demonstrated that even outside of pregnancy there is a cohort of women with recurrent miscarriage who are in an identifiable prothrombotic state [53].

5.3.2 Activated Protein C Resistance

Activated protein C resistance (APCR) testing examines the protein C/S anticoagulant pathway together with the level of coagulation factor VIII. Resistance to activated protein C may be either genetic (usually due to factor V Leiden) or acquired.

Individuals with an impaired response to activated protein C are at increased risk of thrombosis.

A large observational study including more than 1,000 consecutive nonpregnant women attending a specialist recurrent miscarriage clinic reported that acquired APC resistance is significantly more common among women with recurrent early miscarriage (80/904, 8.8 %: $p = 0.02$) and those with a previous late miscarriage (18/207, 8.7 %: $p = 0.04$) compared to parous controls (17/150, 3.3 %) [40]. Furthermore, those women with acquired APC resistance were significantly less likely to have had a previous live birth ($p < 0.01$) compared to those with a normal APC ratio. These data suggest that acquired APC resistance contributes to the burden of recurrent pregnancy loss, the mechanism of which is likely to be thrombosis of the placental vasculature. Since a degree of APC resistance develops during normal pregnancy, it is possible that among women who are APC resistant prior to pregnancy, this effect is amplified when they become pregnant. This theory has prompted the use of thromboprophylactic treatment regimens for women with recurrent miscarriage and APC resistance (both the inherited and acquired forms) during the next pregnancy in order to improve the live birth rate and protect the mother from the risk of venous thrombosis during the pregnancy and puerperium. Although it has not been possible to conduct a randomized controlled therapeutic trial to assess the potential benefits of low-dose heparin therapy during pregnancy in these women, current clinical practice favors the use of thromboprophylaxis from early in the first trimester until 6–12 weeks postpartum.

5.4 Thromboelastography

Thromboelastography (TEG) is a reproducible near-patient test of global haemostasis which measures the rate of formation of a blood clot, its maximum strength, and fibrinolysis [28]. An important advantage of thromboelastography over conventional hemostasis testing is that it is a dynamic test, which yields information relating to the cumulative effect of the many components of coagulation including platelet function.

Our studies have shown that TEG is a useful tool with which to identify a prothrombotic state in women with a history of previously unexplained recurrent miscarriage [36]. The maximum clot amplitude (MA) was significantly greater among recurrent miscarriage women compared with normal parous controls. Furthermore, increases in the MA were more marked in women with a history of late miscarriage compared with women with a history of only early pregnancy losses. None of the women in these studies smoked, was taking the oral contraceptive pill or had a history of thromboembolic disease.

The MA is a reflection of the absolute strength of the fibrin clot formed and hence is a dynamic test of fibrin and platelet function. Some 30 % of nonpregnant recurrent miscarriage women have an MA that is more than two standard deviations above the mean of a control parous population, adding further weight to the hypothesis that a significant proportion of RM women are in a prothrombotic state outside of pregnancy. Furthermore, the prepregnancy MA was predictive of future pregnancy outcome, being significantly higher among those RM women whose next pregnancy ended in a further miscarriage as opposed to a live birth. Once pregnancy is confirmed, serial TEG testing during the first trimester can identify increases in the MA that precede the clinical evidence of impending miscarriage by several weeks. Our initial studies suggest that variable doses of aspirin can normalize the raised MA levels in early pregnancy and improve the live birth rate.

Conclusions

There is a substantial body of evidence that thrombophilic disorders are associated with adverse pregnancy outcome at all gestational ages. Antiphospholipid syndrome remains the most important treatable cause of recurrent miscarriage. Low dose aspirin together with heparin (LMWH being the most widely used) is the first-line treatment for this condition. The relationship between heritable thrombophilias and early pregnancy loss remains controversial. Large well-designed prospective studies are needed in order to clarify the relationship or lack of relationship between these defects and pregnancy outcome and the efficacy of treatment. The ongoing TIPPS (Thrombophilia in Pregnancy Prophylaxis Study; ClinicalTrials.gov identifier: NCT00967382) seeks to determine the safety and effectiveness of LMWH in preventing placenta-mediated pregnancy complications and venous thromboembolism in women with thrombophilia, and includes women with recurrent miscarriages.

Tests of global of hemostasis identify a subgroup of women with recurrent miscarriage who are in a prothrombotic state prior to pregnancy. Prospective data suggest that such women are at increased risk of further miscarriages in untreated pregnancies. The long-term health consequences of this hypercoagulability are increasingly recognized. A retrospective study of 130,000 women reported that a history of first-trimester spontaneous miscarriage is associated with a significant increased risk of maternal ischemic heart disease (IHD). This risk increased with the number of miscarriages such that among those with three or more miscarriages, the risk of death or hospital admission for IHD was 2.3 times greater than that among those with no previous history of miscarriage. In contrast, there was no association between therapeutic abortion and the subsequent risk of IHD [47]. Clearly, if these retrospective data are confirmed in a large prospective study, pregnancy history will become an important criterion in the risk assessment of IHD.

Learning Points

- Antiphospholipid syndrome is the most important treatable cause for recurrent miscarriage. Low dose aspirin in combination with heparin leads to a significant increase in the live birth rate.
- Both in vitro and in vivo data demonstrate that the major mechanisms by which antiphospholipid antibodies cause pregnancy loss are via excessive complement-mediated inflammatory damage; an increased rate of trophoblast apoptosis; decreased trophoblast fusion, and a direct deleterious effect on endometrial receptivity. These effects are decreased by subanticoagulant doses of heparin.

- Tests of global haemostasis suggest that women with recurrent miscarriage are in a prothrombotic state outside of pregnancy. This may have implications for their health beyond their reproductive years.
- Apart from antiphospholipid antibodies, the relationship between individual thrombophilic defects and recurrent miscarriage is controversial.
- The use of aspirin and or aspirin together with heparin in the treatment of women with recurrent miscarriage who have no demonstrable thrombophilia remains unknown.

Pregnancy 5:
Miscarriage at 7 weeks gestation
Fetal karyotype Trisomy 13, i.e., not a failure of treatment
Pregnancy 6:
Treatment with aspirin (75 mg/day)+ low-molecular-weight heparin (enoxaparin 20 mg daily)
Outcome:
Spontaneous vaginal delivery at 39 weeks gestation
Pregnancy course uncomplicated

Case Study

Patient details:
  Mrs AF
  Age 34
  Parity 0+4
  Miscarriage history:

Pregnancy 1	Miscarriage at 10 weeks gestation
Pregnancy 2	Miscarriage at 8 weeks gestation
Pregnancy 3	Miscarriage at 6 weeks gestation
Pregnancy 4	Miscarriage at 10 weeks gestation. Fetal karyotype 46 XY

Medical history:
Unremarkable. No personal or family history of thrombosis
Investigations:
Lupus anticoagulant +ve on two consecutive occasions 8 weeks apart
IgG and IgM anticardiolipin antibodies and anti-beta2GPI−ve
Factor V Leiden and prothrombin G20210A negative
Parental karyotypes normal – 46 XX and 46 XY
Normal uterine anatomy
Plan of management:
Aspirin (75 mg/day) and low-molecular-weight heparin (enoxaparin 20 mg daily) to commence from time of positive pregnancy test

References

1. Bates SM, Greer IA, Middeldorp S, Veenstra DL, Prabulos A-M, Vandvik PO. VTE, thrombophilia, antithrombotic therapy, and pregnancy: antithrombotic therapy and prevention of thrombosis, 9th ed: American College of Chest Physicians Evidence-Based Clinical Practice Guidelines. Chest. 2012;141 (2 Suppl):e691S–736S.
2. Backos M, Rai R, Baxter N, Chilcott IT, Cohen H, Regan L. Pregnancy complications in women with recurrent miscarriage associated with antiphospholipid antibodies treated with low dose aspirin and heparin. Br J Obstet Gynaecol. 1999;106:102–7.
3. Boffa MC, Lachassinne E, Boinot C, De CS, Rovere-Querini P, Avcin T, Biasini-Rebaioli C, Le TP, Aurousseau MH, Tincani A. European registry of babies born to mothers with antiphospholipid syndrome: a result update. Lupus. 2009;18:900–4.
4. Bose P, Black S, Kadyrov M, Bartz C, Shlebak A, Regan L, Huppertz B. Adverse effects of lupus anticoagulant positive blood sera on placental viability can be prevented by heparin in vitro. Am J Obstet Gynecol. 2004;191:2125–31.
5. Bose P, Black S, Kadyrov M, Weissenborn U, Neulen J, Regan L, Huppertz B. Heparin and aspirin attenuate placental apoptosis in vitro: implications for early pregnancy failure. Am J Obstet Gynecol. 2005;192:23–30.
6. Bramham K, Thomas M, Nelson-Piercy C, Khamashta M, Hunt BJ. First-trimester low-dose prednisolone in refractory antiphospholipid antibody–related pregnancy loss. Blood. 2011;117:6948–51.
7. Branch DW, Peaceman AM, Druzin M, Silver RK, El-Sayed Y, Silver RM, Esplin MS, Spinnato J, Harger J. A multicenter, placebo-controlled pilot study of intravenous immune globulin treatment of antiphospholipid syndrome during pregnancy. The Pregnancy Loss Study Group. Am J Obstet Gynecol. 2000; 182:122–7.

8. Bremme KA. Haemostatic changes in pregnancy. Best Pract Res Clin Haematol. 2003;16:153–68.

9. Carp H, Dolitzky M, Tur-Kaspa I, Inbal A. Hereditary thrombophilias are not associated with a decreased live birth rate in women with recurrent miscarriage. Fertil Steril. 2002;78:58–62.

10. Craig M, Tata P, Regan L. Psychiatric morbidity among patients with recurrent miscarriage. J Psychosom Obstet Gynaecol. 2002;23:157–64.

11. De WF, Carreras LO, Moerman P, Vermylen J, Van AA, Renaer M. Decidual vasculopathy and extensive placental infarction in a patient with repeated thromboembolic accidents, recurrent fetal loss, and a lupus anticoagulant. Am J Obstet Gynecol. 1982;142:829–34.

12. Di SN, Caliandro D, Castellani R, Ferrazzani S, De CS, Caruso A. Low-molecular weight heparin restores in-vitro trophoblast invasiveness and differentiation in presence of immunoglobulin G fractions obtained from patients with antiphospholipid syndrome. Hum Reprod. 1999;14:489–95.

13. Di SN, Di NF, D'Ippolito S, Castellani R, Tersigni C, Caruso A, Meroni P, Marana R. Antiphospholipid antibodies affect human endometrial angiogenesis. Biol Reprod. 2010;83:212–9.

14. Dizon-Townson DS, Meline L, Nelson LM, Varner M, Ward K. Fetal carriers of the factor V Leiden mutation are prone to miscarriage and placental infarction. Am J Obstet Gynecol. 1997;177:402–5.

15. Drakeley AJ, Quenby S, Farquharson RG. Midtrimester loss – appraisal of a screening protocol. Hum Reprod. 1998;13:1975–80.

16. Empson M, Lassere M, Craig J, et al. Prevention of recurrent miscarriage for women with antiphospholipid antibody or lupus anticoagulant. Cochrane Database Syst Rev 2005; Apr 18;(2):CD002859.

17. Farquharson RG, Quenby S, Greaves M. Antiphospholipid syndrome in pregnancy: a randomized, controlled trial of treatment. Obstet Gynecol. 2002;100:408–13.

18. Hanly JG, Gladman DD, Rose TH, Laskin CA, Urowitz MB. Lupus pregnancy. A prospective study of placental changes. Arthritis Rheum. 1988;31:358–66.

19. Holers VM, Girardi G, Mo L, Guthridge JM, Molina H, Pierangeli SS, Espinola R, Xiaowei LE, Mao D, Vialpando CG, et al. Complement C3 activation is required for antiphospholipid antibody-induced fetal loss. J Exp Med. 2002;195:211–20.

20. Jindal P, Regan L, Fourkala EO, Rai R, Moore G, Goldin RD, Sebire NJ. Placental pathology of recurrent spontaneous abortion: the role of histopathological examination of products of conception in routine clinical practice: a mini review. Hum Reprod. 2007;22:313–6.

21. Jivraj S, Makris M, Saravelos S, Li TC. Pregnancy outcome in women with factor V Leiden and recurrent miscarriage. BJOG. 2009;116:995–8.

22. Kovalevsky G, Gracia CR, Berlin JA, Sammel MD, Barnhart KT. Evaluation of the association between hereditary thrombophilias and recurrent pregnancy loss: a meta-analysis. Arch Intern Med. 2004;164:558–63.

23. Kutteh WH. Antiphospholipid antibody-associated recurrent pregnancy loss: treatment with heparin and low-dose aspirin is superior to low-dose aspirin alone. Am J Obstet Gynecol. 1996;174:1584–9.

24. Laskin CA, Spitzer KA, Clark CA, Crowther MR, Ginsberg JS, Hawker GA, Kingdom JC, Barrett J, Gent M. Low molecular weight heparin and aspirin for recurrent pregnancy loss: results from the randomized, controlled HepASA Trial. J Rheumatol. 2009;36:279–87.

25. Lockwood CJ, Romero R, Feinberg RF, Clyne LP, Coster B, Hobbins JC. The prevalence and biologic significance of lupus anticoagulant and anticardiolipin antibodies in a general obstetric population. Am J Obstet Gynecol. 1989;161:369–73.

26. Mak IY, Brosens JJ, Christian M, Hills FA, Chamley L, Regan L, White JO. Regulated expression of signal transducer and activator of transcription, Stat5, and its enhancement of PRL expression in human endometrial stromal cells in vitro. J Clin Endocrinol Metab. 2002;87:2581–8.

27. Miyakis S, Lockshin MD, Atsumi T, Branch DW, Brey RL, Cervera R, Derksen RH, De Groot PG, Koike T, Meroni PL, et al. International consensus statement on an update of the classification criteria for definite antiphospholipid syndrome (APS). J Thromb Haemost. 2006;4:295–306.

28. Nair SC, Dargaud Y, Chitlur M, Srivastava A. Tests of global haemostasis and their applications in bleeding disorders. Haemophilia. 2010;16 Suppl 5:85–92, 85–92.

29. Nayar R, Lage JM. Placental changes in a first trimester missed abortion in maternal systemic lupus erythematosus with antiphospholipid syndrome; a case report and review of the literature. Hum Pathol. 1996;27:201–6.

30. Noble LS, Kutteh WH, Lashey N, et al. Antiphospholipid antibodies associated with recurrent pregnancy loss: prospective, multicenter, controlled pilot study comparing treatment with low-molecular-weight heparin versus unfractionated heparin. Fertil Steril. 2005;83:684–90.

31. Nodler J, Moolamalla SR, Ledger EM, Nuwayhid BS, Mulla ZD. Elevated antiphospholipid antibody titers and adverse pregnancy outcomes: analysis of a population-based hospital dataset. BMC Pregnancy Childbirth. 2009;9(11):11.

32. O'Riordan MN, Higgins JR. Haemostasis in normal and abnormal pregnancy. Best Pract Res Clin Obstet Gynaecol. 2003;17:385–96.

33. Out HJ, Kooijman CD, Bruinse HW, Derksen RH. Histopathological findings in placentae from patients with intrauterine fetal death and anti-phospholipid antibodies. Eur J Obstet Gynecol Reprod Biol. 1991;41:179–86.

34. Pattison NS, Chamley LW, McKay EJ, Liggins GC, Butler WS. Antiphospholipid antibodies in pregnancy: prevalence and clinical associations. Br J Obstet Gynaecol. 1993;100:909–13.
35. Perez MC, Wilson WA, Brown HL, Scopelitis E. Anticardiolipin antibodies in unselected pregnant women. Relationship to fetal outcome. J Perinatol. 1991;11:33–6.
36. Rai R. Is miscarriage a coagulopathy? Curr Opin Obstet Gynecol. 2003;15:265–8.
37. Rai R, Backos M, Elgaddal S, Shlebak A, Regan L. Factor V Leiden and recurrent miscarriage-prospective outcome of untreated pregnancies. Hum Reprod. 2002;17:442–5.
38. Rai R, Cohen H, Dave M, Regan L. Randomised controlled trial of aspirin and aspirin plus heparin in pregnant women with recurrent miscarriage associated with phospholipid antibodies (or antiphospholipid antibodies). BMJ. 1997;314:253–7.
39. Rai R, Regan L. Recurrent miscarriage. Lancet. 2006;368:601–11.
40. Rai R, Shlebak A, Cohen H, Backos M, Holmes Z, Marriott K, Regan L. Factor V Leiden and acquired activated protein C resistance among 1000 women with recurrent miscarriage. Hum Reprod. 2001;16:961–5.
41. Rai R, Tuddenham E, Backos M, Jivraj S, El'Gaddal S, Choy S, Cork B, Regan L. Thromboelastography, whole-blood haemostasis and recurrent miscarriage. Hum Reprod. 2003;18:2540–3.
42. Rai RS, Clifford K, Cohen H, Regan L. High prospective fetal loss rate in untreated pregnancies of women with recurrent miscarriage and antiphospholipid antibodies. Hum Reprod. 1995;10:3301–4.
43. Rai RS, Regan L, Chitolie A, Donald JG, Cohen H. Placental thrombosis and second trimester miscarriage in association with activated protein C resistance. Br J Obstet Gynaecol. 1996;103:842–4.
44. Rai RS, Regan L, Clifford K, Pickering W, Dave M, Mackie I, McNally T, Cohen H. Antiphospholipid antibodies and beta 2-glycoprotein-I in 500 women with recurrent miscarriage: results of a comprehensive screening approach. Hum Reprod. 1995;10:2001–5.
45. Rand JH, Wu XX, Quinn AS, Taatjes DJ. The annexin A5-mediated pathogenic mechanism in the antiphospholipid syndrome: role in pregnancy losses and thrombosis. Lupus. 2010;19:460–9.
46. Rey E, Kahn SR, David M, Shrier I. Thrombophilic disorders and fetal loss: a meta-analysis. Lancet. 2003;361:901–8.
47. Smith GC, Pell JP, Walsh D. Spontaneous loss of early pregnancy and risk of ischaemic heart disease in later life: retrospective cohort study. BMJ. 2003;326(423–424326): 423–4.
48. Stephenson MD, Ballem PJ, Tsang P, et al. Treatment of antiphospholipid antibody syndrome (APS) in pregnancy: a randomized pilot trial comparing low molecular weight heparin to unfractionated heparin. J Obstet Gynaecol Can. 2004;26:729–34.
49. Stirling Y, Woolf L, North WR, Seghatchian MJ, Meade TW. Haemostasis in normal pregnancy. Thromb Haemost. 1984;52:176–82.
50. Tincani A, Rebaioli CB, Andreoli L, Lojacono A, Motta M. Neonatal effects of maternal antiphospholipid syndrome. Curr Rheumatol Rep. 2009;11:70–6.
51. Triolo G, Ferrante A, Ciccia F, Accardo-Palumbo A, Perino A, Castelli A, Giarratano A, Licata G. Randomized study of subcutaneous low molecular weight heparin plus aspirin versus intravenous immunoglobulin in the treatment of recurrent fetal loss associated with antiphospholipid antibodies. Arthritis Rheum. 2003;48:728–31.
52. Venkat-Raman N, Backos M, Teoh TG, Lo WT, Regan L. Uterine artery Doppler in predicting pregnancy outcome in women with antiphospholipid syndrome. Obstet Gynecol. 2001;98:235–42.
53. Vincent T, Rai R, Regan L, Cohen H. Increased thrombin generation in women with recurrent miscarriage. Lancet. 1998;352:116.
54. Visser J, Ulander VM, Helmerhorst FM, Lampinen K, Morin-Papunen L, Bloemenkamp KW, Kaaja RJ. Thromboprophylaxis for recurrent miscarriage in women with or without thrombophilia. HABENOX: a randomised multicentre trial. Thromb Haemost. 2011;105:295–301.
55. Yenicesu GI, Cetin M, Ozdemir O, Cetin A, Ozen F, Yenicesu C, Yildiz C, Kocak N. A prospective case-control study analyzes 12 thrombophilic gene mutations in Turkish couples with recurrent pregnancy loss. Am J Reprod Immunol. 2010;63:126–36.

Pregnancy Morbidity Associated with Hereditary and Acquired Thrombophilias: Late Obstetric Complications

6

Sukrutha Veerareddy and Donald Peebles

Abstract

As well as being associated with recurrent miscarriage (RM), antiphospholipid antibodies (aPL) are associated with late placental vascular-mediated pregnancy complications such as severe pre-eclampsia, intrauterine growth restriction (IUGR), abruptio placentae, late fetal loss, and stillbirth. There are also associations between heritable thrombophilias and these late pregnancy complications. Finally, venous thromboembolism (VTE) in pregnancy, as in the non-pregnant state, is linked to thrombophilia. In this review, potential adverse effects of thrombophilia in late pregnancy are discussed. Preliminary data suggest that maternal antithrombotic prophylaxis may result in improved pregnancy outcome in selected cases. Randomized trials are needed to evaluate treatment strategies.

6.1 Introduction

Thrombophilic risk factors are common and can be found in approximately 20 % of Caucasian populations. Since pregnancy is an acquired hypercoagulable state, women harboring thrombophilia may present with clinical symptoms of vascular complications for the first time during gestation or the postpartum period. This chapter will focus on different types of thrombophilia and their association with placental vascular complications including preeclampsia, IUGR, placental abruption, and late fetal loss (fetal loss above 24 weeks' gestation is defined as stillbirth and fetal loss between 20 and 24 weeks is generally described as late fetal loss). The reader should also refer to Chap. 2. on heritable and acquired thrombophilias.

6.2 Hemostatic Changes in Normal Pregnancy

For a detailed description, the reader should refer to Chap. 1. There is a marked increase in blood pro coagulant activity, characterized by an elevation of factors VII, X, VIII; fibrinogen; and von Willebrand factor [14], especially at

S. Veerareddy, MRCOG
Consultant in Obstetrics and Gynaecology
Queen Elizabeth Hospital,
South London Healthcare Trust,
Stadium Road, Woolwich, London SE18 4QH, UK
e-mail: sukrutha.veerareddy@nhs.net

D. Peebles, MD, FRCOG (✉)
Consultant in Fetal Medicine,
University College London Hospitals,
250 Euston Road, London, NW1 2PG, UK
e-mail: d.peebles@ucl.ac.uk

Table 6.1 Classification and prevalence of thrombophilia

	Thrombophilia	% of general population
Inherited	Antithrombin deficiency	0.07
	Protein C deficiency	0.3
	Protein S deficiency	0.2
	Factor V Leiden (heterozygous)	4
	Factor V Leiden (homozygous)	0.06
	Prothrombin gene mutation	2
Acquired	Antiphospholipid antibodies (Lupus anticoagulant Anticardiolipin antibodies)	2
	Acquired APC resistance without factor V Leiden	3.3

term in normal pregnancy. This is associated with an increase in prothrombin fragment F1.2 and thrombin-antithrombin complexes [15, 87]. There is a decrease in physiologic anticoagulants manifested by a significant reduction in protein S activity and [21] by acquired activated protein C resistance (APCR) [23]. The overall fibrinolytic activity is impaired during pregnancy but rapidly returns to normal following delivery [110]. This is largely due to placenta-derived plasminogen activator inhibitor type 2 (PAI-2), which is present in substantial quantities during pregnancy [55]. D-dimer, a specific marker of fibrinolysis resulting from breakdown of cross-linked fibrin polymer by plasmin, increases as pregnancy progresses [35]. Overall, there is a five- to ten-fold increased risk of VTE throughout gestation and the postpartum period.

Thrombophilias can be either inherited or acquired. The prevalence of these thrombophilias in the general population is depicted in Table 6.1.

6.3 Heritable Thrombophilia

Table 6.1 lists the congenital thrombophilic factors most frequently associated with obstetric complications. For details on heritable thrombophilias, the reader should refer to Chap. 2. The prevalence of the factor V Leiden (FVL) mutation is very low in Asian and African populations, and around 4% higher in Caucasians. However,

APCR may be present in pregnancy without FVL; the reported prevalence ranges from 50 % [107] to 95 % [8]. The frequency of the prothrombin gene mutation increases geographically from Northern to Southern Europe [119]. The prevalence of heterozygosity for the G20210A prothrombin gene mutation is 2 % [117]. Protein S and protein C deficiencies are quite rare, and carriers have a significantly increased risk of thrombosis when the inhibitory effect on coagulation is lost [22, 67]. Antithrombin (AT) deficiency may be the result of many different mutations and has a prevalence of 0.07 %. It is the most thrombogenic of the inherited thrombophilias, with a reported 70–90 % lifetime risk of thromboembolism in individuals with type 1 AT deficiency [22, 67]. Homozygosity for the C677T methylenetetrahydrofolate reductase (MTHFR) polymorphism has an observed prevalence varying from 15.2 % in Hispanic populations to 10.2 % in Caucasians, 8.8 % in Asians, and 2.4 % in African Americans [117]. Several alleles (C and T) have been described. Homozygosity for the T variant results in elevated homocysteine levels, which can cause vascular injury [117]. The plasminogen activator inhibitor (PAI) 4G/4G polymorphism has a reported prevalence of around 25 % [35]. PAI 4G/4G inhibits the activation of plasminogen to the fibrinolytic enzyme plasmin. The resulting decreased fibrinolytic activity would potentially increase the risk of thrombosis [35], but the clinical significance of this polymorphism remains uncertain.

6.4 Acquired Thrombophilia

6.4.1 The Antiphospholipid Syndrome and Late Pregnancy Complications

The international consensus statement on revised criteria (Sapporo) for the diagnosis of obstetric antiphospholipid syndrome (APS) is based on clinical criteria for the diagnosis of APS with laboratory findings of persistent medium- or high-titer antiphospholipid antibodies (aPL) that are present on two or more occasions at least 12 weeks apart [75]. Women with aPL may present with

Table 6.2 Revised Sapporo criteria (international consensus statement) for the diagnosis of antiphospholipid syndrome [75]

Clinical criteria (one or more)

1. *Vascular thrombosis*: One or more objectively confirmed episodes of arterial, venous or small vessel thrombosis occurring in any tissue or organ

2. *Pregnancy morbidity*:

   (a) One or more unexplained deaths of a morphologically normal fetus ≥10th week of gestation; or

   (b) One or more premature births of a morphologically normal neonate <34th week of gestation because of eclampsia, pre-eclampsia or placental insufficiency; or

   (c) Three or more unexplained consecutive miscarriages <10th week of gestation

Laboratory criteria (one or more, present on two or more occasions at least 12 weeks apart using recommended procedures)

1. Lupus anticoagulant (LA), detected according to the guidelines of the International Society on Thrombosis and Haemostasis

2. Anticardiolipin antibody (aCL) of IgG and/or IgM isotype, present in medium or high titre (>40 GPL or MPL, or >99th percentile), measured by a standardized ELISA

3. Anti-β2-glycoprotein-1 antibody (anti-β2-GP1) of IgG and/or IgM isotype, present in titre >99th percentile, measured by a standardized ELISA

either recurrent miscarriage (RM) [86, 95] (in up to 20 %) [11, 86, 96] or fetal demise beyond 10 weeks of gestation [84], and aPL are also associated with one or more of the following: eclampsia, pre-eclampsia or IUGR, with the criteria for late obstetric morbidity in APS in Table 6.2. In a study of 60 pregnancies in women with APS, the most specific clinical features were reported to be thrombosis (both venous and arterial), RM, fetal loss in the second and third trimesters, and autoimmune thrombocytopenia [64].

Pregnancy morbidity in the form of fetal loss or premature birth is a relatively common finding in women with APS [85]. The mechanism of fetal loss is believed to be due to binding of antiphospholipid antibodies to trophoblast cells, resulting in defective placentation [27]. Thrombotic complications within the uteroplacental circulation have also been proposed as a contributing mechanism [42, 96]. APS is associated with placental vascular thrombosis, decidual vasculopathy, intervillous fibrin deposition, and placental infarction [49, 96]. These pathological changes

in the placenta may result in RM, early severe pre-eclampsia, IUGR, or stillbirth. A positive test result for anticardiolipin antibodies (aCL) or presence of lupus anticoagulant (LA) may be found in 10–15 % of women with fetal death beyond 20 weeks of gestation [9, 13, 84].

The relation between APS and pre-eclampsia has been shown in several studies [13, 26, 108]. aCL were detected in 21 % of more than 300 patients with severe pre-eclampsia [112], with a 27.4 % incidence in the group who delivered before 28 weeks' gestation and a 19.3 % incidence in the group who delivered after 28 weeks. As low positive IgG and/or IgM titers were noted in 20 % of controls, the authors concluded that 16 % is a realistic estimate of the incidence of aCL-positivity in patients with a history of severe pre-eclampsia, which is concordant with the findings of other studies [10, 56, 89]. Most studies found an association with positive tests for aCL and early-onset severe pre-eclampsia, and testing in these patients may have therapeutic implications for future pregnancies. Conversely, other investigators did not find a correlation between APS and pre-eclampsia [68, 85]. Women with APS are also at substantial risk (increased by approximately 30 %) of IUGR [10, 90]. In one study, 24 % of mothers who delivered an IUGR infant had medium or high positive test results for aCL [90].

6.5   Placental Findings Associated with Thrombophilias and Pregnancy Complications

A research group from Tel Aviv [70] described placental findings in women who had severe complications during pregnancy and were carriers of thrombophilias, and compared them to women with severe complications during pregnancy without thrombophilia. The study population consisted of 68 women with singleton pregnancies who had severe pre-eclampsia, IUGR, abruptio placentae, or stillbirth. They were evaluated after delivery for the presence of mutations of FVL, C677T MTHFR, prothrombin G20210A, and deficiencies of protein S, protein C, and AT. All were negative for aPL. Thirty-two women carried a thrombophilia and 36 women did not. All placentas were evaluated by a single pathologist who was blinded to the results of the thrombophilia assessment. There was no difference in the maternal age, parity, type of pregnancy complication, and fetoplacental weight ratio between the groups. The proportion of women with villous infarcts was significantly higher in women with thrombophilias (72 % vs. 39 %, $p<0.01$), as was the proportion of women with multiple infarcts or fibrinoid necrosis of decidual vessels. Conversely, in a recent study with a very similar design which also examined the relationship between placental histology and thrombophilia in women with severe complications, no specific histological pattern could be identified when thrombophilia-positive and thrombophilia-negative groups were compared [77]. Nevertheless, a high rate of placental infarcts (50 %) and thrombosis was confirmed in women both with and without thrombophilias. Likewise, placental pathology in early-onset pre-eclampsia and IUGR was similar in women with and without thrombophilia although a high rate of placental abnormalities was found [109, 118]. Arias et al. (1999) evaluated 13 women with thrombotic lesions of the placenta [4]. All women had obstetric complications such as pre-eclampsia, preterm labor, IUGR, or stillbirth. In 10 of the 13 (77 %), an inherited thrombophilia was found; 7 were heterozygous for the FV Leiden mutation and 3 had protein S deficiency. The most promi-

nent placental lesions were fetal stem vessel thrombosis, infarcts, hypoplasia, spiral artery thrombosis, and perivillous fibrin deposition [4].

6.6 Thrombophilia and IUGR

IUGR is an important cause of perinatal morbidity and mortality. Growth-restricted infants are at increased risk of developing neuropsychological defects and suffering educational disadvantages later in childhood [46, 98]. Moreover, there is epidemiological evidence that children whose intrauterine growth was restricted have a higher risk of cardiovascular and endocrine diseases in adulthood [5]. An association between obstetric complications and heritable causes of thrombophilia has been reported [40, 114] (Table 6.3). Kupferminc et al. (1999) reported an association between inherited thrombophilia (FVL, prothrombin G20210A, MTHFR) and IUGR (defined as a birth weight below the 5th percentile for gestational age) [56]; an association was demonstrated in women with severe IUGR but not in milder cases. Martinelli et al. (2001) compared 63 women with a history of IUGR, defined as birth weight below the 10th percentile, and 93 parous women with uneventful pregnancies. Among women with IUGR, 13 % had FVL compared with 2.2 % of controls (OR, 6.9; 95 % CI 1.4–33.5), and 12 % had the

Table 6.3 Association of thrombophilia with placental vascular complications

	IUFD	Severe IUGR	Severe pre-eclampsia	Abruption
Antithrombin deficiency	I+ (98, 105)	II+	II+	III+
Protein C deficiency	II+ (98, 106)	ND	ND	II+ 4
Protein S deficiency	I+ (98, 105, 106)	II+ (28)	II+ (28)	III+ (25)
APC resistance	I+ (116)	II+	II+	II+ (116)
Factor V Leiden	I+ (107, 116)	II+ (40, 114)	I+ (28, 30, 54, 65, 78)	II (53, 116)
MTHFR 677TT	I– (28)	II– (28, 113)	II– (27, 28, 41, 82, 113)	II–
Hyperhomocysteinemia	I+ (28, 113)	II+ (28, 113)	II+	II+ (25, 113)
Factor II 20210G_A	I+ (77, 107)	II+ (43, 54, 59)	II+ (47, 76)	II+ (59, 99)
Antiphospholipid antibodies	I+ (45)	II+ (58)	II+ (9, 27, 58)	II+ (58)
Combined defects	I+ (47, 69, 98)	II+ (58)	II+ (58)	II+ (58)

Reference numbers are listed in parentheses

Level I (*I*) indicates that the recommendation is based on one or more well-designed prospective studies or two or more well-designed retrospective studies; level II (*II*), the recommendation is based on retrospective studies that reach consensus; level III (*III*), the recommendation is based on isolated anecdotal studies and/or the consensus of expert practitioners

+ association present, – association not present, *ND* no data, *MTHFR* methylenetetrahydrofolate reductase

G20210A prothrombin mutation compared with 2.2 % of controls (OR, 5.9; 95 % CI 1.2–29.4). In a regression-analysis model, these thrombophilias were independently associated with IUGR [72]. A later report from the same group [40] tested for these mutations in neonates weighing less than 2.5 kg. Neonates delivered by mothers with FVL or prothrombin mutations accounted for 30 % of newborns weighing less than 1 kg, 18.7 % of those ranging from 1.001 to 2.499 kg, and only 9.5 % of those weighing 2.5 kg or more. Overall, 27.6 % of neonates of mothers with the mutations weighed less than 2.5 kg compared with 13.9 % of neonates of mothers without mutations (OR, 2.4; 95 % CI 1.5–3.7). However, other studies failed to confirm an association between IUGR and thrombophilic mutations [50]. In one such study [50], the prevalence of thrombophilia in mothers of 493 newborns with IUGR (<10th percentile) and 472 controls did not differ significantly. However, one third of the study population was not Caucasian and the degree of IUGR was mild, with mean birth weight of 2.393 ± 0.606 kg and 83 % of newborns delivered at 36–40 weeks' gestation. In contrast, in the study by Kupferminc et al. (1999), the mean birth weight was 1.387 ± 0.616 kg and mean gestational week at delivery was 33 ± 4.0 [56]. Similarly, Martinelli et al. (2001) reported a mean gestational week at delivery of 35 ± 3 and a mean birth weight of 1.584 ± 0.586 kg [72]. It is therefore suggested that these studies are dealing with noncomparable fetal and neonatal populations with different clinical relevance. Several meta-analyses suggest a strong association between thrombophilia and IUGR [1, 30, 48, 53, 102]. On the other hand, a large cohort study and prospective studies found no significant association [19, 29, 66, 73].

6.7 Thrombophilia and Pre-eclampsia

The association of pre-eclampsia with thrombophilia is similarly controversial; a number of case–control studies demonstrate an association, while others fail to do so. Women with FVL and severe pre-eclampsia may have a higher risk of serious maternal complications and adverse perinatal outcomes than those without thrombophilia [28, 32, 38, 74, 105] (Table 6.3). An association between the presence of FVL and a history of severe forms of pre-eclampsia has been reported [30]. One study demonstrated an increased prevalence of thrombophilia (65 %) in women with severe pre-eclampsia compared with controls (18 %) [56]. There was a higher prevalence of thrombophilic polymorphisms including FVL, prothrombin G20210A, and MTFHR in women presenting with pre-eclampsia [47, 52, 56]. The same study also highlighted that women with other obstetric complications had a significantly higher incidence of combined thrombophilias. In a sample of 140 Italian women with a history of gestational hypertension, with or without significant proteinuria, a significantly higher prevalence of thrombophilias was documented regardless of the presence of proteinuria [39]. Logistic regression showed that FVL and prothrombin G20210A mutations were independently associated with occurrence of gestational hypertension.

A recent meta-analysis has confirmed an association between FVL or prothrombin G20210A and severe early-onset pre-eclampsia [76]. Several studies have reported an association between HELLP syndrome and thrombophilia (and the FVL mutation in particular), with a frequency (compared with controls) of 7.9 % vs. 1.8 % [78], 7.2 % vs. 4.5 % [41], and 20 % vs. 6 % ($p = 0.003$) [7, 78, 83]. In larger meta-analyses, heterozygosity for the FVL mutation was associated with a twofold increased risk [30, 54, 65, 102]. However, these risk estimates were based on pooled data from contradictory studies. These conflicting results may be due at least in part to differences in the severity of pre-eclampsia [74, 76]. A more recent meta-analysis of six cohort studies found a modest but statistically significant increase in the risk of pre-eclampsia in women with a FVL mutation (OR = 1.49) [29]. Many studies suggest that FVL has a stronger association with severe and early-onset pre-eclampsia than with milder forms of the disease [50, 72, 78]. Furthermore, a recent prospective cohort study suggests that FVL was associated with a six- to seven-fold increased risk of recurrent severe pre-eclampsia, which occurred in 59 % of heterozygous women [32].

In contrast, several studies found no association between FVL and pre-eclampsia [2, 76]. FVL did not increase the risk of pre-eclampsia in six prospective studies of unselected women screened during pregnancy [19, 29, 52, 66, 79]. Histopathologic features of placental insufficiency were found in 63 % of women with pre-eclampsia but were not associated with the FVL mutation [52].

The G20210A prothrombin gene mutation has been variously reported in 11.4 % of women with pre-eclampsia vs. 4.1 % of controls (OR = 2.96) [51], 10 % vs. 3 % ($p = 0.03$) [7], and 13 % vs. 3.2 % ($p = 0.001$) [59]. This mutation was more prevalent in women with IUGR ($p = 0.0009$), placental abruption ($p = 0.01$), and second-trimester loss ($p = 0.001$), but not in women with severe pre-eclampsia, third-trimester loss, and recurrent early fetal loss [59].

Women with FVL appear to be at a small absolute increased risk of late pregnancy loss. Women with FVL and PGM appear not to be at increased risk of pre-eclampsia or birth of a small for gestational age (SGA) infant [103].

Homozygosity for the MTHFR polymorphism was found in 22 % of cases of pre-eclampsia compared with 8 % of controls ($p = 0.005$) [7]. The frequency of any inherited thrombophilia in pre-eclamptic women has been estimated to be as high as 56 % [59] and 52 % [7] vs. 19 % in controls, and as high as 69 % in women with severe IUGR in the second trimester vs. 4 % in controls ($p = 0.001$) [58]. Other studies failed to find an association between a common genetic risk factor for thrombosis and the occurrence of pre-eclampsia [24]. However, these studies seem to differ in selection of controls and in ethnic backgrounds. The size of these studies of pre-eclampsia is generally small, especially if the aim was to detect any possible association between the less frequent thrombophilias, such as protein S, protein C, and AT deficiencies, and obstetric complications. Those studies reporting a significant association are generally smaller (31–140 study subjects) than those reporting a lack of association (15–707 subjects). In many of the studies, groups of different thrombophilias or complications are pooled together, which sometimes results in significant associations that do not remain significant when the relevant subgroups are analyzed separately. The pooling of study subjects can lead to inaccuracy in determining the exact impact of a specific mutation on each of the complications.

Nonetheless, overall these data suggest that, while prothrombotic genotypes might not be causative factors for pre-eclampsia, they could be linked to the severity of disease expression once the condition arises.

6.8 Thrombophilia and Placental Abruption

Van der Molen et al. (2000) investigated coagulation inhibitors and abnormalities of homocysteine metabolism as risk factors for placental vasculopathy [111]. They compared non-pregnant women with a history of placental vasculopathy with non-pregnant controls. Protein C activity was noted to be significantly lower in women that had adverse pregnancy outcome. Homozygotes for the MTHFR polymorphism and carriers of the FVL mutation were significantly more common in the study group. The median levels of homocysteine, APCR ratio, protein S, and AT were not different between the groups. However, homocysteine levels above 14.4 μmol/L (the 80th percentile of control values) were associated with a significant increase in OR. Also, combination of risk factors such as homocysteine levels above 14.4 μmol and protein S deficiency resulted in a significantly increased OR for placental vasculopathy. The risk factors for placental vasculopathy which emerge in this study are APCR and decreased levels of protein C, elevated homocysteine, and the C677T MTHFR polymorphism, or a combination of these.

Wiener-Megnagi et al. (1998) studied 27 women who had placental abruption and 29 controls and found that 63 % of cases had an APCR ratio ≤ 2.5 compared with 17 % of controls (OR 8.16, $p = 0.001$) [116]. Eight of 15 patients

(53 %) tested were found to have the FVL mutation (5 heterozygous and 3 homozygous) compared with 1 heterozygote among the control subjects (3.4 %). Similarly, Kupferminc et al. (1999) found a 70 % incidence of thrombophilias in women with placental abruption [56], of which 60 % had thrombophilic mutations and 10 % had AT deficiency or APS. Of the 20 women who had an abruption, 3 also had mild pre-eclampsia, 7 had antepartum or postpartum hypertension, and 11 of the neonates were below the 10th percentile for gestational age. In this study, which was the first to examine the G20210A prothrombin gene mutation in women with pregnancy complications, the OR for abruption with this mutation was 8.9 (95 % CI 1.8–43.6), whereas the ORs for the FVL mutation and MTHFR polymorphism were 4.9 (95 % CI 1.0–17.4) and 2 (95 % CI 0.5–8.1), respectively. In another study, the incidence of the prothrombin gene mutation in 27 women with placental abruption was 18.5 % compared to 3.2 % of controls (OR, 5.8; 95 % CI 1.8–18.6, $p = 0.01$) [59]. In the study by de Vries et al. (1997), 26 % of women with placental abruption had hyperhomocysteinemia and 29 % protein S deficiency [25, 36, 113].

Prochazka et al. (2003) reported that FVL carrier status was not significantly different in women with placental abruption but was associated with a positive family history of venous thrombosis [92]. However, the same group reported that 20 of 142 (14.1 %) women with placental abruption were heterozygous for FVL, compared to 10 of 196 (5.1 %) of controls (OR 3.0, 95 % CI 1.4–6.7) [93]. Association with FVL may be stronger for placental abruption that occurs at earlier gestations [53]. In a meta-analysis, heterozygosity for FVL was associated with a nearly fivefold increased risk of placental abruption [33, 102]. Several other studies found no significant association [3, 66, 81].

Analysis of The New Jersey-Placental Abruption Study (2002–2007) suggests that women with lower protein C levels (<5th centile) had an increased risk of abruption, with an OR of 3.2 (95 % CI 1.2–9.9) [4]. Reduction in both protein S and APCR ratio was not associated with abruption (Table 6.3).

6.9 Thrombophilia and Late Fetal Loss

Preston et al. (1996) reported increased fetal loss in women with heritable thrombophilic defects [88, 91, 100] (Table 6.3). The authors studied 1,384 women enrolled in the European Prospective Cohort on Thrombophilia (EPCOT). Of 843 women with thrombophilia, 571 had 1,524 pregnancies; of 541 control women, 395 had 1,019 pregnancies. The authors analyzed the frequency of fetal loss (<28 weeks of gestation) and stillbirth (>28 weeks of gestation) jointly and separately. The risk of fetal loss was increased in women with thrombophilia (OR, 1.35, 95 % CI 1.01–1.82). The OR was higher for stillbirth than for miscarriage (3.6; 95 % CI 1.4–9.4 vs. 1.27; 95 % CI 0.94–1.71). The highest OR for stillbirth was in women with combined defects (OR, 14.3; 95 % CI 2.4–86.0) compared with 5.2 (1.5–18.1) in AT deficiency, 2.3 (0.6–8.3) in protein C deficiency, 3.3 (1.0–11.3) in protein S deficiency, and 2.0 (0.5–7.7) with FVL. The authors concluded that women with familial thrombophilia, especially those with combined defects or AT deficiency, have an increased risk of fetal loss, particularly stillbirth.

Gris et al. (1999) performed a case–control study in 232 women with a history of one or more second- or third-trimester losses and no history of thrombosis who were matched with 464 controls and tested for thrombophilias and APS [45]. They found at least one thrombophilia in 21.1 % of the patients and in 3.9 % of the controls ($p < 0.0001$), with an OR of 5.5 (95 % CI 3.4–9.0) for stillbirth in women positive for any thrombophilia. After logistic regression analysis, four adjusted risk factors for stillbirth remained: protein S deficiency, anti-beta2 glycoprotein IgG antibodies, aCL IgG antibodies, and the FVL mutation.

Multiple other studies and four meta-analyses suggest that FVL heterozygotes have a higher relative risk of late pregnancy loss than early first-trimester loss [30, 53, 99, 103, 107]. A meta-analysis found that heterozygosity for FVL is associated with a twofold increased risk of late unexplained fetal loss and a fourfold higher risk of loss in the second trimester compared to the first trimester [102]. One possible explanation is that late pregnancy losses reflect thrombosis of the placental vessels, in contrast to first-trimester losses, which are more commonly attributable to other causes, in particular fetal chromosome abnormality. In several studies, the majority of placentas from women heterozygous for FVL and with a late fetal loss had evidence of thrombotic vasculopathy or infarction, supporting this hypothesis [45, 71].

In a study of 18 pregnancies with AT deficiency [105, 106], 10 suffered an adverse outcome (55.6 %), including stillbirth (11.1 %), IUGR (33.3 %), abruption (6.7 %), and pre-eclampsia (6.7 %). A lower incidence of pregnancy complications was observed among women with anti-thrombotic treatment [105].

Kupferminc et al. (1999) found a 50 % prevalence of thrombophilias in women with intrauterine fetal death (IUFD) occurring after 23 weeks' gestation [56]. A recent study tested 67 women with fetal loss after 20 weeks of pregnancy and 232 controls, for FVL, prothrombin gene mutation, and MTHFR mutation. Sixteen percent of the 67 women with fetal loss and 6 % of the controls had either the FVL or the prothrombin gene mutation. The relative risks of late fetal loss in carriers of the FVL and prothrombin gene mutations were 3.2 (95 % CI 1.0–10.9) and 3.3 (95 % CI 1.1–10.3), respectively. Placental

investigation showed histological evidence of thrombosis in 76 % of placentas examined [71]. A study that investigated women with IUFD at 27 weeks' gestation or more found that, in 40 women with unexplained IUFD, the prevalence of inherited thrombophilias was 42.5 % compared with 15 % in controls (OR, 2.8; 95 % CI 1.5–5.3, $p = 0.001$) [69].

6.10 Management of Adverse Pregnancy Outcome Associated with Thrombophilia

The management of the obstetric patient with thrombophilia is complex [20, 104, 115] (Table 6.4). Many women with an underlying thrombophilia are healthy, while many others without any known thrombophilia experience medical and obstetric complications. The risk of thromboembolism and adverse pregnancy outcomes seems to arise from an interplay of medical, obstetric, and family history, along with genetic and environmental factors. Futhermore, current treatment with low molecular weight heparin (LMWH) when used as prophylactic or therapeutic anticoagulation , is not without risks such as the potential for bleeding and allergies, and is inconvenient.

Table 6.4 Observational studies on prevention of poor gestational outcome in carriers of thrombophilia

Patients, n	Thrombophilia	Obstetric history	Treatment	Live birth with normal outcome	Reference no.
60	APS	RFL	LMWH LDA	70 %	Lima et al. [64]
50	Inherited and acquired	RFL	Enoxaparin (LDA for APS)	46/61 (75 %)	Brenner et al. [17]
25	Factor V Leiden or factor II 20210GA	RFL pre-eclampsia IUGR	UFH or LMWH or LDA	29/31 (93 %)	Grandone et al. [37]
33	Not specified	Pregnancy complications	40 mg enoxaparin LDA	30/33 (91 %)	Kupferminc et al. [57]
26 Patients vs. birth weight	Inherited and acquired	Pregnancy complications	40 mg enoxaparin LDA	Higher birthweight with LMWH	Riyazi et al. [101]
160	Inherited and acquired	Pregnancy complications	40 mg enoxaparin LDA	Higher birth weight with LMWH	Gris et al. [44]
160	Inherited	Abruption	40 mg enoxaparin	Lower incidence of pregnancy complications	Gris et al. [43]

APS antiphospholipid syndrome, *LDA* low-dose aspirin, *RFL* recurrent fetal loss, *IUGR* intrauterine growth restriction

Screening for acquired thrombophilia (APS) is recommended in women who suffer recurrent first-trimester miscarriage or who have had late fetal losses, particularly if associated with features of placental thrombosis or infarction, and those who suffer one or more premature births of a morphologically normal neonate <34th week of gestation because of eclampsia, pre-eclampsia, or IUGR [75]. This is because evidence is accumulating for a beneficial effect of aspirin and heparin to prevent RM [60, 94] and fetal loss [13, 61, 64] in APS. Prospective studies of women with previous poor pregnancy outcome, including late fetal death and neonatal death, demonstrate that the use of aspirin and/or heparin combined with judicious monitoring and timely intervention results in an improved live birth rate from 12 to 69 % [13] and from 19 to 70 % [64].

A Cochrane review [51] revealed a paucity of studies on the efficacy and safety of aspirin and heparin in women with a history of RM without apparent causes other than inherited thrombophilia. Therefore, the use of anticoagulants in unexplained RM is not recommended. Conversely, in heritable thrombophilia, our knowledge of the optimal treatment (except for the role of low-dose aspirin: see below) during pregnancy is limited. The data suggest that certain risk groups should be screened for thrombophilia, as the evidence suggests that there is a high recurrence rate of complications in future pregnancies in women who previously experienced adverse pregnancy outcome and carry a thrombophilia [37]. These at-risk groups include women with a personal or family history of thromboembolism, recurrent first- and second-trimester loss, severe pre-eclampsia, IUGR, stillbirth, or abruptio placentae. Ideally, testing should take place between pregnancies since protein S levels fall and APCR increases during normal pregnancy [18].

The Cochrane Collaboration (2001) demonstrated that the use of low-dose aspirin is associated with a 17 % reduction in the risk of pre-eclampsia (32 trials with 29,331 women, relative risk [RR] 0.85; 95 % CI 0.78–0.92) and a 14 % reduction in the risk of fetal or neonatal death (30 trials with 30,093 women, RR, 0.86; 95 % CI 0.75–0.99). This reduction in fetal and neonatal death was greatest among high-risk women (4,134 women, RR, 0.73; 95 % CI 0.56–0.96) [31]. However, the combined role of low-dose aspirin and heparin treatment in inherited thrombophilia, particularly in later pregnancy, has not been evaluated in randomized controlled trials. Many studies suggest that they may have a complementary role.

In a large retrospective cohort study performed by North et al. (1995), women with renal disease in pregnancy were allocated to a "no-treatment" control group, a low-dose aspirin group, or a group that received prophylactic heparin combined with aspirin and/or dipyridamole [82]. Pre-eclampsia was less common in the heparin group compared with the no-treatment group and the aspirin group.

Another study by Kupferminc et al. (2001) included women with known thrombophilia and a history of severe pre-eclampsia, abruption, IUGR, or stillbirth [57]. Women were treated with enoxaparin 40 mg/day and aspirin 100 mg/day from 8 to 12 weeks' gestation onward. The mean gestational age at delivery in the untreated women was 32.1 ± 5.0 weeks as compared to 37.6 ± 2.3 weeks in women treated with enoxaparin ($p < 0.001$). The mean birth weight of the infants from the control group was 1.175 ± 0.59 kg compared to 2.719 ± 0.526 kg in the treated women ($p < 0.001$). Pregnancy complications occurred in only 9 % of women, and neither severe pre-eclampsia nor perinatal deaths occurred in the treated women [57].

Similarly, favorable effects were suggested in a small study that evaluated treatment with LMWH combined with aspirin in pregnant women with thrombophilia and a history of early-onset pre-eclampsia and/or IUGR [101]. Pregnant women with thrombophilia were randomized to low-dose aspirin and LMWH ($n = 26$) or aspirin alone ($n = 19$). There was no difference in the overall birth weight between the groups. However, when considering the 18 patients with a single thrombophilia (i.e. excluding 8 patients with multiple thrombophilias), birth weights were significantly higher ($p = 0.019$) compared to the 19 with no coagulation abnormality. In addition, two perinatal deaths occurred in the aspirin group vs. no perinatal death in the aspirin plus LMWH group. These preliminary studies suggest that LMWH may have an additional beneficial effect on the pregnancy outcome of women with a history of severe pre-eclampsia and/or IUGR and documented thrombophilia.

In the Live-Enox study, the incidence of pre-eclampsia, placental abruption, and IUGR was substantially lower with LMWH prophylaxis than in prior untreated pregnancies [16, 17]. A favorable effect on birth weight was noted in women with thrombophilia and prior fetal loss that were treated with LMWH and aspirin [44]. A randomized trial studied the effect of LMWH prophylaxis in women with thrombophilia and previous adverse pregnancy outcome. LMWH significantly reduced the incidence of the severe pre-eclampsia, IUGR, abruption, and IUFD after 20 weeks [99].

A pilot study investigated the effectiveness of enoxaparin in women with a previous placental abruption and inherited thrombophilia. Women were randomized to either a prophylactic daily dose of enoxaparin starting from the time of a positive pregnancy test ($n=80$) or no enoxaparin ($n=80$). Enoxaparin was safe, with no obvious side-effects such as thrombocytopenia or major bleeding events. Furthermore, enoxaparin reduced the occurrence of placental vascular complications [43].

Leeda et al. (1998) studied the effects of folic acid and vitamin B6 supplementation in women with hyperhomocysteinemia and a history of pre-eclampsia or IUGR [63]. A total of 207 consecutive patients with a history of pre-eclampsia or IUGR were tested for hyperhomocysteinemia. Thirty-seven were found to have raised levels and were treated with folic acid and vitamin B6, and 27 had a second methionine-loading test after vitamin supplementation. This showed that 14 patients became pregnant while receiving vitamin B6, folic acid, and aspirin; 7 of these 14 were complicated by pre-eclampsia. Birth weights were 2.867 ± 0.648 kg compared with 1.088 ± 0.57 kg in the previous pregnancies ($p < 0.001$). Therefore, in women with hyperhomocysteinemia and a history of pre-eclampsia or IUGR, vitamin B6 and folic acid can correct the methionine-loading test and appear to have a favorable effect on birth weight, but not pre-eclampsia.

Presence of moderate quality evidence, the American College of Chest Physicians (ACCP) guidelines recommend low-dose aspirin throughout pregnancy for women at risk of pre-eclampsia. Unfractionated or LMWH are not recommended for thrombophilic women with a history of pre-eclampsia or other adverse pregnancy outcomes [6].

The findings of the FRUIT trial, (FRactionated heparin in pregnant women with a history of Utero-placental Insufficiency and Thrombophilia), a randomized controlled trial, have been published. This study found that adding LMWH to aspirin before 12 weeks of gestation reduces the risk of recurrence of pre-eclampsia with onset before 34 weeks' gestation in women with inheritable thrombophilia and prior delivery for pre-eclampsia/IUGR before 34 weeks [26].

In summary, although combined treatment with aspirin and LMWH appears to have improved perinatal outcome in some women with a poor obstetric history and inherited thrombophilias, there is a lack of clear evidence from large trials. Large adequately powered randomized controlled trials are needed before definitive recommendations can be made about the treatment of thrombophilias in pregnancy. The Thrombophilia in Pregnancy Prophylaxis Study (TIPPS) is underway (ClinicalTrials.gov identifier: NCT00967382). This trial seeks to determine the safety and effectiveness of LMWH in preventing placenta-mediated pregnancy complications and venous thromboembolism in women with thrombophilia. Until the uncertainties surrounding the management of thrombophilias are resolved, decisions about anti-thrombotic therapy in women with thrombophilia and pregnancy complications should be based on an individual risk/benefit assessment. Assessment of the maternal thrombotic risk during pregnancy should also be incorporated into the decision-making process regarding prophylaxis.

6.11 Unresolved Issues

6.11.1 Fetal Genotype

While there have been some reports that fetal thrombophilia status is important for the outcome of pregnancy [28], there are a several reasons to suggest that this may not be the case. First, most thrombophilic polymorphisms are mild risk factors for gestational vascular complications and gestational thromboembolism. Second, thrombotic changes are noted mainly on the maternal side of the uteroplacental unit. Third, LMWH that does not cross the placenta is beneficial. Thus, unless there is a severe thrombophilic defect (i.e. homozygous protein C deficiency), fetal thrombophilic state is probably not a major contributor to gestational vascular complications or thromboembolism. However, further data from studies addressing the triad of mother, father and fetus are needed to clarify this issue.

6.11.2 Women with Unexplained Pregnancy Loss

When evaluation for the current known thrombophilias is negative, it is theoretically possible that an as yet undiscovered thrombophilia may be implicated in placental thrombotic changes found in women with gestational vascular complications. Following preliminary experience with antithrombotic therapy in these women [99], prospective randomized multicenter trials are currently underway.

6.12 Future Perspectives

A number of issues in this field need to be addressed. First, 30–50 % of vascular gestational pathologies cannot be accounted for by the currently available tests for thrombophilia. Whether other genetic or acquired thrombophilias will be found to play a role remains to be determined. Polymorphisms at the thrombomodulin and endothelial protein C receptor genes [34, 80] may be associated with recurrent fetal loss. It has also been suggested that circulating microparticles may play a role in unexplained fetal loss [62]. While the mechanism(s) involved in the development of vascular gestational pathologies has(ve) not been established, it is intriguing to speculate whether antithrombotic strategies will be of value in this setting [41].

Management of the obstetric patient with thrombophilia, or an obstetric history that could be associated with thrombophilia, is controversial due to the fact that there are no evidence-based guidelines directing all aspects of management. Finally, the role of antithrombotic treatment should continue to be explored in prospective clinical trials, in the hope of improving gestational outcomes in this large population of women.

References

1. Agorastos T, Karavida A, Lambropoulos A, Constantinidis T, Tzitzimikas S, Chrisafi S, et al. Factor V Leiden and prothrombin G20210A mutations in pregnancies with adverse outcome. J Matern Fetal Neonatal Med. 2002;12(4):267–73.
2. Alfirevic Z, Mousa HA, Martlew V, Briscoe L, Perez-Casal M, Toh CH. Postnatal screening for thrombophilia in women with severe pregnancy complications. Obstet Gynecol. 2001;97(5 Pt 1):753–9.
3. Alfirevic Z, Roberts D, Martlew V. How strong is the association between maternal thrombophilia and adverse pregnancy outcome? A systematic review. Eur J Obstet Gynecol Reprod Biol. 2002;101(1):6–14.
4. Arias F, Romero R, Joist H, Kraus FT. Thrombophilia: a mechanism of disease in women with adverse pregnancy outcome and thrombotic lesions in the placenta. J Matern Fetal Med. 1998;7(6):277–86.
5. Barker DJ. The fetal and infant origins of adult disease. BMJ. 1990;301(6761):1111.
6. Bates SM, Greer IA, Middeldorp S, Veenstra DL, Prabulos A-M, Vandvik PO. VTE, thrombophilia, antithrombotic therapy, and pregnancy: antithrombotic therapy and prevention of thrombosis, 9th ed: American College of Chest Physicians Evidence-Based Clinical Practice Guidelines. Chest. 2012;141 (2 Suppl):e691S–736S.
7. Benedetto C, Marozio L, Salton L, Maula V, Chieppa G, Massobrio M. Factor V Leiden and factor II G20210A in preeclampsia and HELLP syndrome. Acta Obstet Gynecol Scand. 2002;81(12):1095–100.
8. Bloomenthal D, von Dadelszen P, Liston R, Magee L, Tsang P. The effect of factor V Leiden carriage on maternal and fetal health. CMAJ. 2002;167(1):48–54.
9. Bocciolone L, Meroni P, Parazzini F, Tincani A, Radici E, Tarantini M, et al. Antiphospholipid antibodies and risk of intrauterine late fetal death. Acta Obstet Gynecol Scand. 1994;73(5):389–92.
10. Branch DW, Andres R, Digre KB, Rote NS, Scott JR. The association of antiphospholipid antibodies with severe preeclampsia. Obstet Gynecol. 1989;73(4): 541–5.
11. Branch DW, Scott JR, Kochenour NK, Hershgold E. Obstetric complications associated with the lupus anticoagulant. N Engl J Med. 1985;313(21):1322–6.

12. Branch DW, Silver R, Pierangeli S, van Leeuwen I, Harris EN. Antiphospholipid antibodies other than lupus anticoagulant and anticardiolipin antibodies in women with recurrent pregnancy loss, fertile controls, and antiphospholipid syndrome. Obstet Gynecol. 1997;89(4):549–55.

13. Branch DW, Silver RM, Blackwell JL, Reading JC, Scott JR. Outcome of treated pregnancies in women with antiphospholipid syndrome: an update of the Utah experience. Obstet Gynecol. 1992;80(4):614–20.

14. Bremme K, Ostlund E, Almqvist I, Heinonen K, Blomback M. Enhanced thrombin generation and fibrinolytic activity in normal pregnancy and the puerperium. Obstet Gynecol. 1992;80(1):132–7.

15. Bremme KA. Haemostatic changes in pregnancy. Best Pract Res Clin Haematol. 2003;16(2):153–68.

16. Brenner B, Hoffman R, Blumenfeld Z, Weiner Z, Younis JS. Gestational outcome in thrombophilic women with recurrent pregnancy loss treated by enoxaparin. Thromb Haemost. 2000;83(5):693–7.

17. Brenner B, Hoffman R, Carp H, Dulitsky M, Younis J. Efficacy and safety of two doses of enoxaparin in women with thrombophilia and recurrent pregnancy loss: the LIVE-ENOX study. J Thromb Haemost. 2005;3(2):227–9.

18. Clark P, Brennand J, Conkie JA, McCall F, Greer IA, Walker ID. Activated protein C sensitivity, protein C, protein S and coagulation in normal pregnancy. Thromb Haemost. 1998;79(6):1166–70.

19. Clark P, Walker ID, Govan L, Wu O, Greer IA. The GOAL study: a prospective examination of the impact of factor V Leiden and ABO(H) blood groups on haemorrhagic and thrombotic pregnancy outcomes. Br J Haematol. 2008;140(2):236–40.

20. Cleary-Goldman J, Bettes B, Robinson JN, Norwitz E, Schulkin J. Thrombophilia and the obstetric patient. Obstet Gynecol. 2007;110(3):669–74.

21. Comp PC, Thurnau GR, Welsh J, Esmon CT. Functional and immunologic protein S levels are decreased during pregnancy. Blood. 1986;68(4):881–5.

22. Conard J, Horellou MH, Van DP, Lecompte T, Samama M. Thrombosis and pregnancy in congenital deficiencies in AT III, protein C or protein S: study of 78 women. Thromb Haemost. 1990;63(2):319–20.

23. Cumming AM, Tait RC, Fildes S, Yoong A, Keeney S, Hay CR. Development of resistance to activated protein C during pregnancy. Br J Haematol. 1995;90(3): 725–7.

24. De Groot CJ, Bloemenkamp KW, Duvekot EJ, Helmerhorst FM, Bertina RM, Van Der Meer F, et al. Preeclampsia and genetic risk factors for thrombosis: a case–control study. Am J Obstet Gynecol. 1999; 181(4):975–80.

25. de Vries JI, Dekker GA, Huijgens PC, Jakobs C, Blomberg BM, van Geijn HP. Hyperhomocysteinaemia and protein S deficiency in complicated pregnancies. Br J Obstet Gynaecol. 1997;104(11):1248–54.

26. de Vries JIP, Van Pampus MG, Hague WM, Bezemer PD, Joosten JH, On Behalf of Fruit Investigators. Low-molecular-weight heparin added to aspirin in the pre-vention of recurrent early-onset pre-eclampsia in women with inheritable thrombophilia: the FRUIT-RCT. J Thromb Haemost. 2012;10:64–72.

27. Di SN, Luigi MP, Marco D, Fiorella DN, Silvia D, Clara DM, et al. Pregnancies complicated with antiphospholipid syndrome: the pathogenic mechanism of antiphospholipid antibodies: a review of the literature. Ann N Y Acad Sci. 2007;1108:505–14.

28. Dizon-Townson DS, Meline L, Nelson LM, Varner M, Ward K. Fetal carriers of the factor V Leiden mutation are prone to miscarriage and placental infarction. Am J Obstet Gynecol. 1997;177(2):402–5.

29. Dudding T, Heron J, Thakkinstian A, Nurk E, Golding J, Pembrey M, et al. Factor V Leiden is associated with pre-eclampsia but not with fetal growth restriction: a genetic association study and meta-analysis. J Thromb Haemost. 2008;6(11):1869–75.

30. Dudding TE, Attia J. The association between adverse pregnancy outcomes and maternal factor V Leiden genotype: a meta-analysis. Thromb Haemost. 2004;91(4):700–11.

31. Duley L, Henderson-Smart D, Knight M, King J. Antiplatelet drugs for prevention of pre-eclampsia and its consequences: systematic review. BMJ. 2001;322(7282):329–33.

32. Facchinetti F, Marozio L, Frusca T, Grandone E, Venturini P, Tiscia GL, et al. Maternal thrombophilia and the risk of recurrence of preeclampsia. Am J Obstet Gynecol. 2009;200(1):46–5.

33. Facco F, You W, Grobman W. Genetic thrombophilias and intrauterine growth restriction: a meta-analysis. Obstet Gynecol. 2009;113(6):1206–16.

34. Franchi F, Biguzzi E, Cetin I, Facchetti F, Radaelli T, Bozzo M, et al. Mutations in the thrombomodulin and endothelial protein C receptor genes in women with late fetal loss. Br J Haematol. 2001;114(3):641–6.

35. Giavarina D, Mezzena G, Dorizzi RM, Soffiati G. Reference interval of D-dimer in pregnant women. Clin Biochem. 2001;34(4):331–3.

36. Glueck CJ, Kupferminc MJ, Fontaine RN, Wang P, Weksler BB, Eldor A. Genetic hypofibrinolysis in complicated pregnancies. Obstet Gynecol. 2001;97(1):44–8.

37. Grandone E, Brancaccio V, Colaizzo D, Scianname N, Pavone G, Di MG, et al. Preventing adverse obstetric outcomes in women with genetic thrombophilia. Fertil Steril. 2002;78(2):371–5.

38. Grandone E, Margaglione M, Colaizzo D, Cappucci G, Paladini D, Martinelli P, et al. Factor V Leiden, C > T MTHFR polymorphism and genetic susceptibility to preeclampsia. Thromb Haemost. 1997;77(6):1052–4.

39. Grandone E, Margaglione M, Colaizzo D, Cappucci G, Scianname N, Montanaro S, et al. Prothrombotic genetic risk factors and the occurrence of gestational hypertension with or without proteinuria. Thromb Haemost. 1999;81(3):349–52.

40. Grandone E, Margaglione M, Colaizzo D, Pavone G, Paladini D, Martinelli P, et al. Lower birth-weight in neonates of mothers carrying factor V G1691A and factor II A(20210) mutations. Haematologica. 2002; 87(2):177–81.

41. Greer IA. Procoagulant microparticles: new insights and opportunities in pregnancy loss? Thromb Haemost. 2001;85(1):3–4.
42. Greer IA. Thrombophilia: implications for pregnancy outcome. Thromb Res. 2003;109(2–3):73–81.
43. Gris JC, Chauleur C, Faillie JL, Baer G, Mares P, Fabbro-Peray P, et al. Enoxaparin for the secondary prevention of placental vascular complications in women with abruptio placentae. The pilot randomised controlled NOH-AP trial. Thromb Haemost. 2010;104(4):771–9.
44. Gris JC, Mercier E, Quere I, Lavigne-Lissalde G, Cochery-Nouvellon E, Hoffet M, et al. Low-molecular-weight heparin versus low-dose aspirin in women with one fetal loss and a constitutional thrombophilic disorder. Blood. 2004;103(10):3695–9.
45. Gris JC, Quere I, Monpeyroux F, Mercier E, Ripart-Neveu S, Tailland ML, et al. Case–control study of the frequency of thrombophilic disorders in couples with late foetal loss and no thrombotic antecedent – the Nimes Obstetricians and Haematologists Study5 (NOHA5). Thromb Haemost. 1999;81(6):891–9.
46. Hack M, Flannery DJ, Schluchter M, Cartar L, Borawski E, Klein N. Outcomes in young adulthood for very-low-birth-weight infants. N Engl J Med. 2002;346(3):149–57.
47. Higgins JR, Kaiser T, Moses EK, North R, Brennecke SP. Prothrombin G20210A mutation: is it associated with pre-eclampsia? Gynecol Obstet Invest. 2000; 50(4):254–7.
48. Howley HE, Walker M, Rodger MA. A systematic review of the association between factor V Leiden or prothrombin gene variant and intrauterine growth restriction. Am J Obstet Gynecol. 2005;192(3):694–708.
49. Infante-Rivard C, David M, Gauthier R, Rivard GE. Lupus anticoagulants, anticardiolipin antibodies, and fetal loss. A case–control study. N Engl J Med. 1991; 325(15):1063–6.
50. Infante-Rivard C, Rivard GE, Yotov WV, Genin E, Guiguet M, Weinberg C, et al. Absence of association of thrombophilia polymorphisms with intrauterine growth restriction. N Engl J Med. 2002;347(1):19–25.
51. Kaandorp S, Di NM, Goddijn M, Middeldorp S. Aspirin or anticoagulants for treating recurrent miscarriage in women without antiphospholipid syndrome. Cochrane Database Syst Rev. 2009;(1): CD004734.
52. Kahn SR, Platt R, McNamara H, Rozen R, Chen MF, Genest Jr J, et al. Inherited thrombophilia and preeclampsia within a multicenter cohort: the Montreal Preeclampsia Study. Am J Obstet Gynecol. 2009; 200(2):151–9.
53. Kist WJ, Janssen NG, Kalk JJ, Hague WM, Dekker GA, de Vries JI. Thrombophilias and adverse pregnancy outcome – A confounded problem! Thromb Haemost. 2008;99(1):77–85.
54. Kosmas IP, Tatsioni A, Ioannidis JP. Association of Leiden mutation in factor V gene with hypertension in pregnancy and pre-eclampsia: a meta-analysis. J Hypertens. 2003;21(7):1221–8.
55. Kruithof EK, Tran-Thang C, Gudinchet A, Hauert J, Nicoloso G, Genton C, et al. Fibrinolysis in pregnancy: a study of plasminogen activator inhibitors. Blood. 1987;69(2):460–6.
56. Kupferminc MJ, Eldor A, Steinman N, Many A, Bar-Am A, Jaffa A, et al. Increased frequency of genetic thrombophilia in women with complications of pregnancy. N Engl J Med. 1999;340(1):9–13.
57. Kupferminc MJ, Fait G, Many A, Lessing JB, Yair D, Bar-Am A, et al. Low-molecular-weight heparin for the prevention of obstetric complications in women with thrombophilias. Hypertens Pregnancy. 2001; 20(1):35–44.
58. Kupferminc MJ, Many A, Bar-Am A, Lessing JB, Ascher-Landsberg J. Mid-trimester severe intrauterine growth restriction is associated with a highprevalence of thrombophilia. BJOG. 2002;109(12):1373–6.
59. Kupferminc MJ, Peri H, Zwang E, Yaron Y, Wolman I, Eldor A. High prevalence of the prothrombin gene mutation in women with intrauterine growth retardation, abruptio placentae and second trimester loss. Acta Obstet Gynecol Scand. 2000;79(11):963–7.
60. Kutteh WH. Antiphospholipid antibody-associated recurrent pregnancy loss: treatment with heparin and low-dose aspirin is superior to low-dose aspirin alone. Am J Obstet Gynecol. 1996;174(5):1584–9.
61. Laskin CA, Bombardier C, Hannah ME, Mandel FP, Ritchie JW, Farewell V, et al. Prednisone and aspirin in women with autoantibodies and unexplained recurrent fetal loss. N Engl J Med. 1997;337(3):148–53.
62. Laude I, Rongieres-Bertrand C, Boyer-Neumann C, Wolf M, Mairovitz V, Hugel B, et al. Circulating procoagulant microparticles in women with unexplained pregnancy loss: a new insight. Thromb Haemost. 2001;85(1):18–21.
63. Leeda M, Riyazi N, de Vries JI, Jakobs C, van Geijn HP, Dekker GA. Effects of folic acid and vitamin B6 supplementation on women with hyperhomocysteinemia and a history of preeclampsia or fetal growth restriction. Am J Obstet Gynecol. 1998;179(1):135–9.
64. Lima F, Khamashta MA, Buchanan NM, Kerslake S, Hunt BJ, Hughes GR. A study of sixty pregnancies in patients with the antiphospholipid syndrome. Clin Exp Rheumatol. 1996;14(2):131–6.
65. Lin J, August P. Genetic thrombophilias and preeclampsia: a meta-analysis. Obstet Gynecol. 2005; 105(1):182–92.
66. Lindqvist PG, Svensson PJ, Marsaal K, Grennert L, Luterkort M, Dahlback B. Activated protein C resistance (FV:Q506) and pregnancy. Thromb Haemost. 1999;81(4):532–7.
67. Lockwood CJ. Inherited thrombophilias in pregnant patients: detection and treatment paradigm. Obstet Gynecol. 2002;99(2):333–41.
68. Lynch A, Marlar R, Murphy J, Davila G, Santos M, Rutledge J, et al. Antiphospholipid antibodies in predicting adverse pregnancy outcome. A prospective study. Ann Intern Med. 1994;120(6):470–5.
69. Many A, Elad R, Yaron Y, Eldor A, Lessing JB, Kupferminc MJ. Third-trimester unexplained intra-

uterine fetal death is associated with inherited thrombophilia. Obstet Gynecol. 2002;99(5 Pt 1):684–7.

70. Many A, Schreiber L, Rosner S, Lessing JB, Eldor
A, Kupferminc MJ. Pathologic features of the placenta in women with severe pregnancy complications and thrombophilia. Obstet Gynecol. 2001;
98(6):1041–4.

71. Martinelli I, Taioli E, Cetin I, Marinoni A, Gerosa S,
Villa MV, et al. Mutations in coagulation factors in
women with unexplained late fetal loss. N Engl J
Med. 2000;343(14):1015–8.

72. Martinelli P, Grandone E, Colaizzo D, Paladini D,
Scianname N, Margaglione M, et al. Familial thrombophilia and the occurrence of fetal growth restriction. Haematologica. 2001;86(4):428–31.

73. McCowan LM, Craigie S, Taylor RS, Ward C,
McLintock C, North RA. Inherited thrombophilias
are not increased in "idiopathic" small-for-gestation-
al-age pregnancies. Am J Obstet Gynecol. 2003;
188(4):981–5.

74. Mello G, Parretti E, Marozio L, Pizzi C, Lojacono A,
Frusca T, et al. Thrombophilia is significantly associated with severe preeclampsia: results of a large-scale,
case-controlled study. Hypertension. 2005;46(6):
1270–4.

75. Miyakis S, Lockshin MD, Atsumi T, Branch DW,
Brey RL, Cervera R, Derksen RH, De Groot PG,
Koike T, Meroni PL, Reber G, Shoenfeld Y, Tincani
A, Vlachoyiannopoulos PG, Krilis SA. International
consensus statement on an update of the classification
criteria for definite antiphospholipid syndrome (APS).
J Thromb Haemost. 2006;4(2):295–306.

76. Morrison ER, Miedzybrodzka ZH, Campbell DM,
Haites NE, Wilson BJ, Watson MS, et al. Prothrombotic
genotypes are not associated with pre-eclampsia and
gestational hypertension: results from a large population-based study and systematic review. Thromb
Haemost. 2002;87(5):779–85.

77. Mousa HA, Alfirevic Z. Do placental lesions reflect
thrombophilia state in women with adverse pregnancy
outcome? Hum Reprod. 2000;15(8):1830–3.

78. Muetze S, Leeners B, Ortlepp JR, Kuse S, Tag CG,
Weiskirchen R, et al. Maternal factor V Leiden
mutation is associated with HELLP syndrome in
Caucasian women. Acta Obstet Gynecol Scand. 2008;
87(6):635–42.

79. Murphy RP, Donoghue C, Nallen RJ, D'Mello M,
Regan C, Whitehead AS, et al. Prospective evaluation
of the risk conferred by factor V Leiden and thermolabile methylenetetrahydrofolate reductase polymorphisms in pregnancy. Arterioscler Thromb Vasc Biol.
2000;20(1):266–70.

80. Nakabayashi M, Yamamoto S, Suzuki K. Analysis of
thrombomodulin gene polymorphism in women with
severe early-onset preeclampsia. Semin Thromb Hemost.
1999;25(5):473–9.

81. Nath CA, Ananth CV, DeMarco C, Vintzileos AM.
Low birthweight in relation to placental abruption and
maternal thrombophilia status. Am J Obstet Gynecol.
2008;198(3):293–5.

82. North RA, Ferrier C, Gamble G, Fairley KF,
Kincaid-Smith P. Prevention of preeclampsia with
heparin and antiplatelet drugs in women with renal
disease. Aust N Z J Obstet Gynaecol. 1995;35(4):
357–62.

83. Nurk E, Tell GS, Refsum H, Ueland PM, Vollset SE.
Factor V Leiden, pregnancy complications and
adverse outcomes: the Hordaland Homocysteine
Study. QJM. 2006;99(5):289–98.

84. Oshiro BT, Silver RM, Scott JR, Yu H, Branch DW.
Antiphospholipid antibodies and fetal death. Obstet
Gynecol. 1996;87(4):489–93.

85. Out HJ, Bruinse HW, Christiaens GC, van Vliet M,
De Groot PG, Nieuwenhuis HK, et al. A prospective,
controlled multicenter study on the obstetric risks of
pregnant women with antiphospholipid antibodies.
Am J Obstet Gynecol. 1992;167(1):26–32.

86. Out HJ, Bruinse HW, Christiaens GC, van Vliet M,
Meilof JF, De Groot PG, et al. Prevalence of antiphos-
pholipid antibodies in patients with fetal loss. Ann
Rheum Dis. 1991;50(8):553–7.

87. Pabinger I, Schneider B. Thrombotic risk in heredi-
tary antithrombin III, protein C, or protein S deficiency.
A cooperative, retrospective study. Gesellschaft fur
Thrombose- und Hamostaseforschung (GTH) Study
Group on Natural Inhibitors. Arterioscler Thromb
Vasc Biol. 1996;16(6):742–8.

88. Pasquier E, Bohec C, Mottier D, Jaffuel S, Mercier B,
Ferec C, et al. Inherited thrombophilias and unexplained pregnancy loss: an incident case–control
study. J Thromb Haemost. 2009;7(2):306–11.

89. Pattison NS, Chamley LW, McKay EJ, Liggins GC,
Butler WS. Antiphospholipid antibodies in pregnancy:
prevalence and clinical associations. Br J Obstet
Gynaecol. 1993;100(10):909–13.

90. Polzin WJ, Kopelman JN, Robinson RD, Read JA,
Brady K. The association of antiphospholipid antibodies with pregnancies complicated by fetal growth
restriction. Obstet Gynecol. 1991;78(6):1108–11.

91. Preston FE, Rosendaal FR, Walker ID, Briet E,
Berntorp E, Conard J, et al. Increased fetal loss in
women with heritable thrombophilia. Lancet. 1996;
348(9032):913–6.

92. Prochazka M, Happach C, Marsal K, Dahlback B,
Lindqvist PG. Factor V Leiden in pregnancies
complicated by placental abruption. BJOG. 2003;
110(5):462–6.

93. Prochazka M, Lubusky M, Slavik L, Hrachovec P,
Zielina P, Kudela M, et al. Frequency of selected
thrombophilias in women with placental abruption.
Aust N Z J Obstet Gynaecol. 2007;47(4):297–301.

94. Rai R, Cohen H, Dave M, Regan L. Randomised controlled trial of aspirin and aspirin plus heparin in pregnant women with recurrent miscarriage associated
with phospholipid antibodies (or antiphospholipid
antibodies). BMJ. 1997;314(7076):253–7.

95. Rai RS, Clifford K, Cohen H, Regan L. High prospective fetal loss rate in untreated pregnancies of women
with recurrent miscarriage and antiphospholipid antibodies. Hum Reprod. 1995;10(12):3301–4.

96. Rand JH, Wu XX, Andree HA, Lockwood CJ, Guller S, Scher J, et al. Pregnancy loss in the antiphospholipid-antibody syndrome – a possible thrombogenic mechanism. N Engl J Med. 1997;337(3):154–60.

97. Rees DC, Cox M, Clegg JB. World distribution of factor V Leiden. Lancet. 1995;346(8983):1133–4.

98. Resnik R. Intrauterine growth restriction. Obstet Gynecol. 2002;99(3):490–6.

99. Rey E, Garneau P, David M, Gauthier R, Leduc L, Michon N, et al. Dalteparin for the prevention of recurrence of placental-mediated complications of pregnancy in women without thrombophilia: a pilot randomized controlled trial. J Thromb Haemost. 2009;7(1):58–64.

100. Rey E, Kahn SR, David M, Shrier I. Thrombophilic disorders and fetal loss: a meta-analysis. Lancet. 2003;361(9361):901–8.

101. Riyazi N, Leeda M, de Vries JI, Huijgens PC, van Geijn HP, Dekker GA. Low-molecular-weight heparin combined with aspirin in pregnant women with thrombophilia and a history of preeclampsia or fetal growth restriction: a preliminary study. Eur J Obstet Gynecol Reprod Biol. 1998;80(1):49–54.

102. Robertson L, Wu O, Langhorne P, Twaddle S, Clark P, Lowe GD, et al. Thrombophilia in pregnancy: a systematic review. Br J Haematol. 2006;132(2):171–96.

103. Rodger MA, Betancourt MT, Clark P, Lindqvist PG, Dizon-Townson D, Said J, et al. The association of factor V Leiden and prothrombin gene mutation and placenta-mediated pregnancy complications: a systematic review and meta-analysis of prospective cohort studies. PLoS Med. 2010;7(6):e1000292.

104. Rodger MA, Carrier M, Keely E, Karovitch A, Nimrod C, Walker M, et al. The management of thrombophilia during pregnancy: a Canadian survey. J Obstet Gynaecol Can. 2002;24(12):946–52.

105. Sabadell J, Casellas M, Alijotas-Reig J, Arellano-Rodrigo E, Cabero L. Inherited antithrombin deficiency and pregnancy: maternal and fetal outcomes. Eur J Obstet Gynecol Reprod Biol. 2010; 149(1):47–51.

106. Sanson BJ, Friederich PW, Simioni P, Zanardi S, Hilsman MV, Girolami A, et al. The risk of abortion and stillbirth in antithrombin-, protein C-, and protein S-deficient women. Thromb Haemost. 1996; 75(3):387–8.

107. Sarig G, Younis JS, Hoffman R, Lanir N, Blumenfeld Z, Brenner B. Thrombophilia is common in women with idiopathic pregnancy loss and is associated with late pregnancy wastage. Fertil Steril. 2002;77(2):342–7.

108. Scott RA. Anti-cardiolipin antibodies and pre-eclampsia. Br J Obstet Gynaecol. 1987;94(6):604–5.

109. Sikkema JM, Franx A, Bruinse HW, van der Wijk NG, de Valk HW, Nikkels PG. Placental pathology in early onset pre-eclampsia and intra-uterine growth restriction in women with and without thrombophilia. Placenta. 2002;23(4):337–42.

110. Stirling Y, Woolf L, North WR, Seghatchian MJ, Meade TW. Haemostasis in normal pregnancy. Thromb Haemost. 1984;52(2):176–82.

111. van der Molen EF, Verbruggen B, Novakova I, Eskes TK, Monnens LA, Blom HJ. Hyperhomocysteinemia and other thrombotic risk factors in women with placental vasculopathy. BJOG. 2000;107(6):785–91.

112. van Pampus MG, Dekker GA, Wolf H, Huijgens PC, Koopman MM, von Blomberg BM, et al. High prevalence of hemostatic abnormalities in women with a history of severe preeclampsia. Am J Obstet Gynecol. 1999;180(5):1146–50.

113. Vollset SE, Refsum H, Irgens LM, Emblem BM, Tverdal A, Gjessing HK, et al. Plasma total homocysteine, pregnancy complications, and adverse pregnancy outcomes: the Hordaland Homocysteine study. Am J Clin Nutr. 2000; 71(4):962–8.

114. von Kries R, Junker R, Oberle D, Kosch A, Nowak-Gottl U. Foetal growth restriction in children with prothrombotic risk factors. Thromb Haemost. 2001;86(4):1012–6.

115. Walker ID, Kujovich JL, Greer IA, Rey E, David M, Salmon JE, et al. The use of LMWH in pregnancies at risk: new evidence or perception? J Thromb Haemost. 2005;3(4):778–93.

116. Wiener-Megnagi Z, Ben-Shlomo I, Goldberg Y, Shalev E. Resistance to activated protein C and the leiden mutation: high prevalence in patients with abruptio placentae. Am J Obstet Gynecol. 1998;179(6 Pt 1):1565–7.

117. Wilson ML, Goodwin TM, Pan VL, Ingles SA. Molecular epidemiology of preeclampsia. Obstet Gynecol Surv. 2003;58(1):39–66.

118. Younis JS, Samueloff A. Gestational vascular complications. Best Pract Res Clin Haematol. 2003;16(2):135–51.

119. Zoller B, de Garcia FP, Hillarp A, Dahlback B. Thrombophilia as a multigenic disease. Haematologica. 1999;84(1):59–70.

Antithrombotic Therapy for Cardiac Disorders in Pregnancy

7

Anna Herrey, Hannah Cohen, and Fiona Walker

Abstract

Pregnancy is a prothrombotic state and it is therefore essential that women with heart disease embarking on pregnancy have an assessment of cardiac risk as well as their risk of venous thromboembolism. Even in the non-pregnant state many women with heart disease require thromboprophylaxis with antiplatelet agents or oral vitamin K antagonists. In this chapter we discuss how these prior treated patients are managed during pregnancy, as well as highlighting other patient groups that should be considered for thromboprophylaxis only while pregnant.

7.1 Introduction

It is well recognized that pregnancy is a prothrombotic state (discussed in detail in Chap. 1) due to the many changes in the coagulation cascade (discussed in Chapter 1), which in the presence of lower limb venous stasis and hypertension create a favorable environment for thrombus formation.

A. Herrey, MD, PhD, MRCP
The Heart Hospital, 16-18 Westmoreland St,
University College London Hospitals NHS Trust,
London, UK
e-mail: anna.herrey@uclh.nhs.uk

H. Cohen, MD, FRCP, FRCPath
Department of Haematology,
University College London Hospitals NHS
Foundation Trust, London NW1 2PG, UK
e-mail: hannah.cohen@uclh.nhs.uk

F. Walker, BM(Hons), FRCP, FESC (✉)
The Heart Hospital, University College London Hospitals
NHS Foundation Trust, 16-18 Westmoreland Street,
London W1G 8PH, UK
e-mail: fiona.walker@uclh.nhs.uk

It is therefore essential that women with heart disease embarking on pregnancy have not only an assessment of cardiac risk but are also assessed for venous thromboembolic (VTE) risk (detailed in Chapter 3). This risk assessment must take account of not only the usual VTE risk factors (such as hyperemesis/dehydration, age >35 years, multiparity, pre-eclampsia, obesity, smoking, inherited or acquired thrombophilia) but also thromboembolic risks associated with the underlying cardiac malformation, for example, chamber dilatation, sluggish intracardiac blood flow, and arrhythmias.

Even in the nonpregnant state, many women with heart disease require thromboprophylaxis with antiplatelet agents or oral vitamin K antagonists. In this chapter, we will discuss how these prior treated patients are managed during pregnancy and will highlight other patient groups that should be considered for thromboprophylaxis only when pregnant. It is, however, important to note that it is only in recent years that there have been sizable numbers of women with such complex heart disease embarking

Table 7.1 Hierarchy of care for adults with Congenital Heart Disease (CHD)

Level I	*Highly complex lesions*
Exclusive care in a specialist unit	Repairs with conduits, Rastelli, Fontan, MFS, Ebstein's, pulmonary atresia, Eisenmenger syndrome, repaired TGA (arterial switch or atrial switch), CCTGA, PHT, cyanotic CHD
Level II	*Lesions of moderate complexity*
Shared care with regional adult cardiology unit	CoA (repaired/native), repaired AVSD, AS, PS/PR, TOF, VSD+AR, mechanical valves, HCM, DCM
Level III	*Simple lesions*
Care predominantly in general adult cardiology unit	Repaired PDA/VSD/TAPVD/ASD, mild PS/PR, small VSD

Adapted from Heart Disease and Pregnancy – study group statement (http://www.rcog.org.uk/womens-health/clinical-guidance/heart-disease-and-pregnancy-study-group-statement)
TGA complete transposition of great arteries, *CCTGA* congenitally corrected transposition of great arteries, *ASD* atrial septal defect, *AVSD* atrioventricular septal defect, *AS* aortic stenosis, *PS* pulmonary stenosis, *PR* pulmonary regurgitation, *TOF* tetralogy of Fallot, *VSD* ventricular septal defect, *AR* aorta regurgitation, *PDA* patent ductus arteriosus, *MFS* Marfan syndrome, *HCM* hypertrophic cardiomyopathy, *DCM* dilated cardiomyopathy, *CoA* coarctation of the aorta, *TAPVD* total anomalous pulmonary venous drainage

on pregnancy, so scientific data on this subject are sparse. This new and unique cohort of women will define their pregnancy outcome not only with regard to thromboembolic risk and its prevention but also as regards their underlying heart disease. This chapter is therefore based largely on our single-center experience, using scientific data if and when available.

7.2 Background

Cardiovascular disease complicates around 1–3 % of pregnancies in the developed world [1]. The improved survival of patients with complex congenital disease well into childbearing age has contributed a large number to the cohort of women with heart disease embarking on pregnancy. Another important but smaller group are women with acquired heart disease, including rheumatic heart disease (RHD) and ischemic heart disease (IHD). RHD nowadays is confined to immigrant populations, but the numbers of younger women with IHD have increased, due to advancing maternal age and an increase in risk factors for IHD (smoking, obesity, and diabetes) in this younger age group. Although accurate prevalence data for maternal heart disease in the UK are not available, heart disease is now the single leading cause of maternal death in the UK, with the majority of deaths in those with undiagnosed acquired heart disease [2].

In the largest prospective study of pregnancy outcome in women with heart disease (CARPREG study), the outcome of 562 pregnancies was reported. Around 75 % of women had congenital heart disease and 25 % acquired heart disease. There were three deaths and four pregnancies were complicated by embolic stroke [3]. Both this study and the UK Centre for Maternal and Child Enquiries (CMACE) highlight the fact that there are risks for women with heart disease during pregnancy. A pre-pregnancy risk assessment, which allows stratification of antenatal care to an appropriate level of surveillance and specialist input, should be undertaken where possible. [4, 5] (Table 7.1).

7.3 Thromboprophylactic Agents Commonly Used in Heart Disease

Aspirin is the most widely used antithrombotic agent in patients with cardiovascular disease. It is given to patients with coronary artery disease and those with low thromboembolic risk conditions. It crosses the placenta but at a thromboprophylactic dose (75–150 mg once daily) is considered safe during all trimesters of pregnancy. Higher anti-inflammatory and analgesic doses are not recommended.

Clopidogrel is mostly used at a dose of 75 mg od in combination with aspirin (75 mg od) as part of a dual antiplatelet regimen following coronary (or other vascular) interventions. For bare metal coronary stents, dual antiplatelet therapy is given for 1 month, with aspirin lifelong thereafter, and for drug-eluting coronary stents, dual therapy (doses as above) is recommended for a minimum of 12 months with aspirin lifelong (75 mg od). It crosses the placenta and, although there are no reliable safety data available for its use during pregnancy, case reports and anecdotal evidence suggest that it may be safe [6, 7].

Dipyridamole is an antiplatelet agent often used alone or in combination with aspirin for secondary thromboprophylaxis most commonly in patients with cerebrovascular disease. The usual dose is 200 mg twice daily. There are no safety data for its use during pregnancy, but it has been used in combination with aspirin or warfarin, during both pregnancy and breastfeeding [8].

Warfarin (or oral coumarol derivatives) is the most commonly used oral vitamin K antagonist. It is used in patients at high risk of thromboembolism, for example, patients with prosthetic valves, a previous history of thrombosis (pulmonary embolism or deep vein thrombosis), atrial fibrillation, or dilated cardiomyopathy with poor systolic function. The dose is adjusted to achieve a target international normalized ratio (INR), which is determined by the indication for treatment. Warfarin crosses the placental barrier and increases the risk of spontaneous miscarriage [9–11]. It also causes an embryopathy [12–14] and fetal coagulopathy, which may lead to spontaneous fetal intracerebral hemorrhage [15, 16]. The risk of warfarin embryopathy (WE) is particularly high between gestational weeks 6 and 12. It is characterized by nasal hypoplasia and epiphyseal changes, and some evidence of a lower intelligence in the long term [17, 18]. The reported incidence of WE is between 0 and 20 % [19] and appears to be greater if the warfarin dose is in excess of 5 mg per day [20].

Unfractionated heparin (UFH) is an antithrombotic agent which can be given IV or SC. At a dose of 5,000 IU SC two to three times daily, it can be used for thromboembolism prophylaxis. Therapeutic UFH may be used for patients with mechanical heart valves, pulmonary embolism, and acute coronary syndromes. Dosing is largely empirical, with different centers often using different dosing regimens. Most regimens require a bolus intravenous dose followed by a maintenance dose of 1,000–1,500 IU/h by continuous intravenous infusion, with a target activated partial thromboplastin time (APTT) ratio between 1.5 and 2.5 compared with the arithmetic mean of the normal range [21, 22] (or the laboratory reference range). It is well documented that achieving a target APTT ratio within the first 24 h is difficult, because levels vary considerably, even when measured every 4 h [23]. UFH does not cross the placenta and therefore has no fetal side-effects. Maternal side-effects include heparin-induced thrombocytopenia (HIT) in 1–3 % of patients [24–26] and osteoporosis (rare in short-term use and at low dose, but a 10 % or greater decrease in bone density was reported in around one-third of women; and a symptomatic vertebral fracture rate of 2.2 % at therapeutic dose, in 4 of 184 women for whom the dosage of heparin ranged from 15,000 to 30,000 (mean 24,500) IU per 24 hours, and the duration of treatment ranged from 7 to 27 (mean 17) weeks) [27, 28].

Low molecular weight heparin (LMWH) has replaced UFH as the anticoagulant of choice for the majority of prothrombotic conditions during pregnancy [29]. Its use in patients with mechanical valves in pregnancy, however, remains contentious, with reports of high rates of thromboembolic complications in this group [30, 31]. It is administered SC and does not cross the placenta; there are therefore no adverse fetal effects. It has a better side-effect profile than UFH, with substantially less HIT<0.1 % [22, 24, 32] and osteoporosis (<0.1 %) [33, 34], has a longer half-life than UFH (3–6 h after SC injection), and has a more predictable anticoagulant effect. LMWH is eliminated by the kidneys. In the presence of renal insufficiency, the half-life is prolonged and dose adjustment is needed [35]. Prophylactic dose LMWH (LMWH-P) is administered once daily (the dose varies between different preparations), whereas high prophylactic (LMWH-HP) and therapeutic doses (LMWH-T) have twice daily (12 hourly) dosing regimens (see Tables 7.2 and 7.3). For the treatment and prevention of deep vein thrombosis and pulmonary embolism, routine anti-Xa monitoring is not recommended except in specific situations including at the extremes of body weight (<50 or >90 kg) or if there is renal insufficiency [22]. If used in patients with mechanical heart valves, however, anti-Xa must be measured every 1–2 weeks (peak levels at 3–5 h post-dose depending on the preparation) with regular dose adjustment to maintain anti-Xa levels between 1.0 and 1.2 IU/mL [36].

Table 7.2 Indications and recommended regimens for anticoagulation in pregnancy

Cardiac lesion	Thromboprophylactic agent during pregnancy	Dose
Mitral stenosis (mild)/SR	Aspirin	75 mg od
Mitral stenosis (>mild)/SR	LMWH	P/HP/T
LV dilatation EF<40 %	LMWH	P/HP/T
LV dilatation EF>50 %	Aspirin	75 mg od
Persistent AF	LMWH	HP/T
Paroxysmal AF	LMWH	HP/T
LVNC EF>50 %	Aspirin	75 mg od
LVNC EF<40 %	LMWH	P/HP
Severe LA dilatation (>×cm^2)	LMWH	P/HP
Fontan (any)	LMWH	HP/T
Unrepaired ASD/PFO	Aspirin	75 mg od
Unrepaired ASD/PFO with a history of stroke	LMWH	HP/T
>Mild Ebstein's	LMWH	P/HP
ARVC RVEF<40 %	LMWH	P/HP
Prosthetic heart valves	LMWH ± Aspirin	HI

LMWH low molecular weight heparin, *P* prophylactic dose, *HP* high prophylactic dose, *T* therapeutic ("treatment" dose), *HI* high intensity, *EF* ejection fraction, *SR* sinus rhythm, *AF* atrial fibrillation, *LA* left atrium, *LVNC* left ventricular non-compaction, *ASD* atrial septal defect, *PFO* persistent foramen ovale, *ARVC* Arrhythmogenic Right Ventricular Cardiomyopathy, *RVEF* right ventricular ejection fraction.

7.4 Maternal Heart Disease Associated with Increased Thromboembolic Risk

For simplicity heart disease will be categorized as acquired, inherited, or congenital. The focus will be on those conditions associated with increased thromboembolic risk, rather than an exhaustive list of all cardiac disorders.

7.4.1 Acquired Heart Disease

7.4.1.1 Valvular Heart Disease
Native Obstructive Valvular Disease
There are two main valve lesions associated with increased thromboembolic risk, both in the pregnant and nonpregnant state, namely, mitral steno-sis (usually rheumatic [RHD]) and tricuspid stenosis (rare and due to RHD or abnormality of valve leaflets or its apparatus). Mitral stenosis (MS) is more common, but it is now rare in the developed world (0.02 % prevalence [37]), whereas in some parts of the developing world, the incidence is much higher (0.2–0.5 % in rural India and parts of Arabia) [38, 39]. There has been a resurgence of RHD in some areas of the UK where there are large immigrant communities, and some UK centers report that around 10–15 % of maternal heart disease is rheumatic in origin [40].

Rheumatic mitral valve disease may cause valvar stenosis (MS) or regurgitation (MR). As a consequence of these valve lesions, the left atrium dilates which leads to a high incidence of atrial arrhythmias (flutter [AFL] and/or fibrillation [AF]). Most women with more than mild mitral or tricuspid stenosis will be anticoagulated with warfarin or another vitamin K antagonist (target INR 2.5 (range 2.0–3.0)) even if in sinus rhythm, due to the presence of sluggish intra-atrial blood flow and the risk of atrial arrhythmia. Too often the first presentation of mitral stenosis is cerebral thromboembolism associated with new onset of AF. If there is persistent AF or a prior history of paroxysmal atrial fibrillation or flutter (PAF/PAFL), this is also an indication for anticoagulation with warfarin, irrespective of the degree of valve obstruction. If there is only mild stenosis (MVA>1.6 cm^2) and mild left atrial (LA) dilatation (<3.9 cm or 20 cm^2) and no prior history of arrhythmia, aspirin alone is used for thromboprophylaxis. During pregnancy, patients previously on warfarin are converted to LMWH-T, while those previously taking aspirin are commenced on prophylactic dose LMWH.

Other acquired obstructive valve lesions such as aortic stenosis (AS) are not associated with an increased risk of thrombus formation per se, as there is a high velocity of blood flow across the valve. Thromboembolism risk assessment in AS should, however, take into account the degree of valvar calcification/thickening and left ventricular size and function. In the presence of a heavily calcified valve or significant LV dilatation (LV end-diastolic diameter >6.2 cm or >3.8 cm/m^2) [41] and or dysfunction (EF <40 %), there may be an increased thromboembolic risk, and treatment with aspirin or LMWH should be considered during pregnancy.

Regurgitant Valve Lesions

The most common regurgitant valve lesions are mitral (MR) and aortic regurgitation (AR).

The common causes of MR are valve leaflet prolapse, myxomatous degeneration, annular dilatation, or following infective endocarditis. Irrespective of etiology, when important MR is present, it causes left atrial dilatation, and there is a risk of atrial arrhythmias, which is an indication for thromboprophylaxis (see Table 7.2).

AR frequently occurs in the context of aortic root dilatation secondary to aortopathy and connective tissue disease such as Marfan syndrome or bicuspid aortic valve (BAV), but endocarditis is also a common cause. Thromboprophylaxis is rarely indicated in those with aortopathy because the assessment of risk versus benefits of treatment must take into account the increased risk of aortic dissection in this patient group.

Ischemic Heart Disease (IHD)

The number of women with IHD in pregnancy is increasing due to advancing maternal age and increasing risk factors for IHD in younger people. It is therefore not surprising that pregnant women with acute coronary syndromes including myocardial infarction, coronary dissection, and long-term sequelae of IHD now account for the largest number of maternal cardiac deaths in the UK, a trend likely to continue [42]. Women with a prior history of IHD and prior coronary intervention are treated with dual antiplatelet therapy (aspirin and clopidogrel) for 4 weeks if a bare metal stent is deployed [43, 44] and 12 months for a drug-eluting stent [45, 46]. Aspirin 75 mg od is safe in pregnancy, but there is only anecdotal evidence for the safety of clopidogrel in pregnancy. However, when assessing the risks versus benefits of stopping clopidogrel, it must be borne in mind that stent thrombosis may be a fatal event and continuation of therapy is usually indicated.

Prosthetic Heart Valves

Prosthetic valves may be tissue/bioprosthetic (homografts/xenografts/pericardial) or mechanical (metal). Mechanical valves are highly thrombogenic and require anticoagulation with warfarin to prevent valve thrombosis [47]; bioprosthetic valves, on the other hand, do not require formal anticoagulation with warfarin.

The European Society of Cardiology (ESC) offers guidance on target INR levels for different types of metallic prostheses and patient-related factors influencing thromboembolic risk in the nonpregnant state, as follows [49]:

Prostheses

Low thromboembolic risk prostheses include Carbomedics (aortic position), Medtronic Hall, and St. Jude Medical. Medium thromboembolic risk prostheses are Bjork-Shiley and other bileaflet valves, and high thromboembolic risk prostheses are Lillehei-Kaster, Omniscience, and Starr-Edwards valves.

Patient-Related Factors

Mitral, tricuspid, or pulmonary valve replacement; previous history of thromboembolism; atrial fibrillation; left atrial diameter > 50 mm; left atrial spontaneous echo contrast; mitral stenosis of any degree; LVEF < 35 %; and hypercoagulable states such as pregnancy. If more than one patient-related risk factor is present, the INR target is increased to a higher value.

Recommended INR Levels

Low-risk prosthesis and < or = 1 patient risk factor: INR target 2.5, >1 risk factor: target INR 3.0

Medium-risk prosthesis and < or = 1 patient risk factor: INR target 3.0; >1 risk factor: target INR 3.5

High-risk prosthesis and < or = 1 patient risk factor: INR target 3.5; >1 risk factor: target INR 4.0.

The American Heart Association/American College of Cardiology (AHA/ACC) guidelines, on the other hand, recommend a target INR of 3.0, regardless of valve type and patient risk, with additional low-dose aspirin if this is felt necessary [47].

The British Committee for Standards in Haematology (BCSH) guidelines recommend that the target INR should be raised from 2.5 to 3.0 and 3.0 to 3.5 in the low risk and medium risk groups, respectively, if there are any patient risk factors for thrombosis, namely: mitral, tricuspid or pulmonary position; previous arterial thromboembolism; atrial fibrillation; left atrium diameter >50 mm; mitral stenosis of any degree; left ventricular ejection fraction <35 %; left atrial dense spontaneous echo contrast [48].

The main problem with anticoagulation for mechanical valves during pregnancy is that there is no ideal anticoagulant which is both safe and effective for both mother and fetus. Warfarin therapy throughout pregnancy results in the lowest observed rate of thromboembolism (3.9 %). However, vitamin K antagonist use is associated with fetal and neurodevelopmental problems [50, 18]. In these women, the rate of thromboembolism with UFH is high at 25 % if used throughout pregnancy and 9 % if used for the first trimester [51]. Therapeutic dose LMWH is an attractive alternative to warfarin and UFH. However, in the HIP-CAT study, which compared enoxaparin with sequential UFH and warfarin in pregnant women with mechanical valves, 2/7 women receiving therapeutic dose enoxaparin 1mg/kg 12-hourly developed fatal valve thrombosis [51]. James et al found an overall thromboembolism rate of 22 % and a maternal mortality of 4 %. Another study [30] found an overall incidence of valve thrombosis of 8.6 % (7/81) and an overall thromboembolism rate of 12.4 % (10/81). Notably, 9 of these 10 patients received a fixed dose of LMWH, and in 2 of these a low fixed dose was used. Among 51 pregnancies where anti-Xa levels were monitored, only one patient was reported to have had thromboembolism. A more recent study [53] reported that compliance with therapeutic dose enoxaparin and aspirin is associated with a low risk of valve thrombosis: 5 thromboembolism events in 34 pregnancies treated with enoxaparin, with non-compliance or sub-therapeutic anti-Xa levels contributory in each case of thromboembolism. However [52] the authors reported fatal valve thrombosis despite therapeutic anti-Xa levels in 1 of 23 pregnancies and other adverse cardiac events in 22 % (5/23). Women must therefore be counseled of the pros and cons, regarding the choice of anticoagulant and anticoagulant regimen, in order to make an informed decision about which treatment regimen to use during pregnancy.

There is no consensus between cardiac societies on the optimal regimen, and current guidelines (ESC, AHA and the ACCP [49, 47, 24]) offer different advice. In practice most cardiologists consider three possible treatment regimens:

1. Warfarin throughout pregnancy, if the dose is <5 mg od, until week 36, then conversion to UFH or LMWH in preparation for delivery planning.
2. Stop warfarin before week 6 and convert to adjusted therapeutic dose UFH or LMWH for weeks 6–12. Then resume warfarin until week 36 when UFH or LMWH is restarted in preparation for delivery.
3. Stop warfarin before week 6 and convert to adjusted high intensity LMWH, and continue LMWH for duration of pregnancy until the time of delivery [36, 53].

If UFH or LMWH is used at any stage of pregnancy, the APTT (UFH) or anti-Xa (LMWH) must be monitored. For UFH administered by continuous intravenous infusion, the APTT ratio is measured within 4 h of starting treatment and thereafter every 6 h or after every dose adjustment, aiming for an APTT ratio which is 1.5–2.5 times that of normal controls [54] (or the laboratory reference range). If LMWH is used, the anti-Xa is measured every 1–2 weeks. The ACCP guidelines (2012) advise that if LMWH is used, doses are adjusted to achieve 'the manufacturer's peak anti-Xa LMWH 4 h post-SC injection' (that is, approximately 1.0 IU/mL). As detailed above, therapeutic dose LMWH can be associated with thromboembolic events. We reported that high intensity adjusted LMWH, aiming for a peak level (4 hours post-dose) of 1.0–1.2 IU/mL is associated with absence of thromboembolism unless levels of LMWH are subtherapeutic [36] (for suggested LMWH doses, see Table 7.3; in patients with prosthetic heart valves, considerable increases in LMWH doses may be needed during pregnancy, with a mean increase of >50% reported by Quinn et al. [36]). Low-dose aspirin may be added in women who are at particularly high risk of thrombosis, for example, those with atrial fibrillation.

In our practice, patients have a planned delivery at around 37–38 weeks gestation. A written delivery plan is formulated by the multidisciplinary team, which includes peripartum anticoagulation management and anaesthetic options. For a vaginal delivery, patients are admitted for induction of labour (IOL), taking the last dose of LMWH (dalteparin 100 units/kg or equivalent) on the morning (or the evening in primigravidae) of the day prior to the day of IOL. In women also receiving low-dose aspirin, this is stopped one week prior to elective delivery. The timeline for completion of delivery is 36 hours and if unsuccessful a Caesarean section (CS) should be performed.

Table 7.3 Weight-adjusted dosing regimens for LMWH

Weight (kg)	Enoxaparin	Dalteparin	Tinzaparin (75 U/kg od)
P dose			
<50	20 mg od	2,500 U od	3,500 U od
50–90	40 mg od	5,000 U od	4,500 U od
91–130	60 mg od	7,500 U od	7,000 U od
131–170	80 mg od	10,000 U od	9,000 U od
>170	0.6 mg/kg od	75 U/kg od	75 U/kg od
HP dose	40 mg bd	5,000 U bd	4,500 U bd
T dose	1 mg/kg bd antenatally 1.5 mg/kg od postnatally	100 U/kg bd or 200 U/kg od postnatally	175 U/kg od (ante- and postnatally)

If the creatinine clearance is <30 mL/min (<20 mL/min for tinzaparin), the LMWH dose should be reduced accordingly
Doses above as per RCOG guidelines for prevention of VTE in pregnancy [29] and the Heart Disease and Pregnancy – study group statement (http://www.rcog.org.uk/womens-health/clinical-guidance/heart-disease-and-pregnancy-study-group-statement)

For elective CS, no LMWH should be administered for 24 hours prior to admission, allowing use of regional anaesthesia. Postdelivery, the management of LMWH is along the lines detailed in Chapter 4, aiming to start warfarin on day 4 postdelivery.

Tissue valves generally do not require anticoagulation, unless there is concomitant atrial arrhythmia, poor ventricular function, or significant chamber dilatation. Depending on thromboembolic risk assessment, low-dose aspirin may also be given.

Acquired Dilated Cardiomyopathies (ADCM)

There are many causes of acquired DCM. In the younger age group, the most common causes are viral myocarditis, toxins, drugs, and pregnancy-associated cardiomyopathy which will be discussed in more detail below. Irrespective of the etiology, if there is only mild residual impairment of LV function, a subsequent pregnancy may precipitate a decline in function, and regular echo surveillance is advisable (monthly in our service). In the presence of severe LV or RV dilatation, there is blood stasis within the chamber, in addition to reduced endothelial antithrombotic properties and increased platelet adhesion [55–57]. There is no clear consensus as to whether patients with DCM and low LV ejection fraction (<40 %) should receive thromboprophylaxis in

the absence of other prothrombotic risk factors, but many are treated with warfarin, especially if there is spontaneous echo contrast on transthoracic echo cardiography (TTE) [58, 59]. During pregnancy, those with DCM and poor function (EF<40 %) will be given LMWH, although the majority with this degree of LV impairment will have been advised against pregnancy as they represent a high-risk group with important maternal morbidity and mortality [60]. For those with DCM and an EF>40 %, LMWH or aspirin 75 mg od should be considered.

Peripartum Cardiomyopathy (PPCM)

PPCM is defined as an idiopthic cardiomyopathy preseting with heart failure secondary to LV systolic dysfunction towards the end of pregnancy or in the months following delivery where no other cause is found. Patients may present acutely in pulmonary edema or may develop progressive signs and symptoms of congestive cardiac failure. There is important morbidity and mortality from thromboembolic complications [61], and women with a new diagnosis of PPCM should be treated with LMWH during pregnancy and converted to warfarin postpartum. Around 50 % have recovery of LV function over a timeframe of ~6 months and during this time they remain should warfarinized [62]. If LV function recovers, warfarin can be stopped. For subsequent pregnancies, a recurrence risk of up to 50 % is quoted, especially if there is persistent LV dysfunction following the index pregnancy [63]. If there is persistent LV dysfunction with EF<50 %, pregnancy is inadvisable, but some patients will accept risk and become pregnant and they should be considered for treatment with LMWH. If LV function is normal, aspirin should be considered.

7.4.1.2 Inherited Heart Diseases
Familial Dilated Cardiomyopathy (FDCM)

In FDCM, both the right and left ventricles are dilated and dysfunctional. Approximately 25 % of DCM cases have a familial etiology. The most common inheritance pattern is autosomal dominant but an X-linked inheritance is also reported. Atrial arrhythmias and atrial dilatation are common, and warfarin anticoagulation is often needed (target INR of 2.5, range 2–3). In pregnancy warfarin is converted to LMWH.

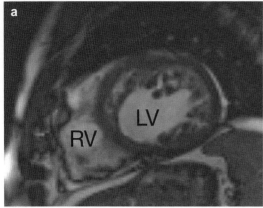 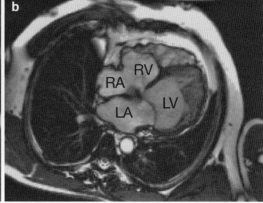

Fig. 7.1 Magnetic resonance images of left ventricular non-compaction (*LVNC*). (**a**) Short axis view with increased trabeculations and recesses in the anterior, lateral, and inferior wall. (**b**) Four-chamber view showing the distribution of non-compacted myocardium in both *LV* and *RV* toward the apex. *RA* right atrium, *RV* right ventricle, *LA* left atrium, *LV* left ventricle (Images courtesy Dr. Andrew Flett, The Heart Hospital, UCLH)

Left Ventricular Non-compaction (LVNC)

LVNC is characterized by excessive trabeculation and recesses within the left ventricular myocardium (Fig. 7.1). The natural history of this disorder is poorly defined, but some develop progressive dilatation and LV dysfunction. If the LV is non-dilated, patients are given aspirin thromboprophylaxis, but in the presence of LV dysfunction and or dilatation, warfarin is used to reduce thromboembolic risk. During pregnancy, those taking warfarin are converted to LMWH, while all others are treated with aspirin.

Familial Hypertrophic Cardiomyopathy (FHCM)

FHCM is the most common form of inherited cardiomyopathy with an incidence of 1 in 500. It is inherited in a mostly autosomal dominant pattern. It is characterized by asymmetrical hypertrophy predominantly of the left ventricle and occasionally the right ventricle. The distribution of hypertrophy can vary, but basal septal hypertrophy is common, and this may cause left ventricular outflow tract obstruction (LVOTO). The myocardium is abnormal in structure and there is systolic and diastolic dysfunction. Diastolic (relaxation) abnormalities cause an elevation in LV filling pressure, which in turn leads to left atrial dilatation and atrial arrhythmias (30 % affected). The presence of LVH per se does not increase thromboembolic risk, but if there is a history of atrial arrhythmias, patients are anticoagulated with warfarin, which is converted to LMWH during pregnancy.

Arrhythmogenic Right Ventricular Cardiomyopathy (ARVC)

ARVC is a rare inherited cardiomyopathy characterized by right ventricular (RV) dilatation, malignant ventricular arrhythmias (ventricular tachycardia [VT] or ventricular fibrillation [VF]), and sudden cardiac death (SCD). Atrial arrhythmias are less common. Many patients have implantable defibrillators in situ for primary or secondary prevention of SCD. Over time there is progressive remodeling and dilatation of the RV, and RV dysfunction is common. In the presence of RV dilatation and paroxysmal VT/VF, patients require anticoagulation with warfarin, which is converted to LMWH during pregnancy.

7.4.1.3 Congenital Heart Disease
Unrepaired Atrial Septal Defect (ASD)

ASDs are the most common congenital abnormality, accounting for ~10 % of all congenital defects. Although the majority are diagnosed and repaired in infancy or childhood, some are newly detected in adulthood, especially during pregnancy. The most common defect is the ostium secundum ASD, which represents 75 % of all ASDs. Other defects including the ostium primum defect and sinus venosus defect are less common. In the presence of any type

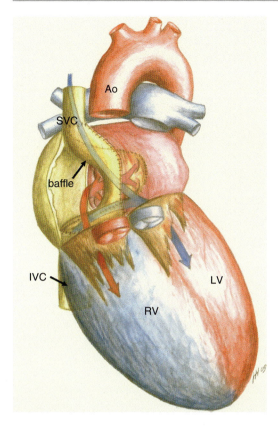

Fig. 7.2 Transposition of the great arteries (TGA), status post Mustard operation: systemic venous return is directed across to the left atrium, then subpulmonary left ventricle and the pulmonary artery. Pulmonary venous return is into the right atrium, then systemic right ventricle, then aorta. *RV* right ventricle, *LV* left ventricle, *IVC* inferior vena cava, *SVC* superior vena cava, *Ao* aorta (Image courtesy Dr. JPM Hamer, The Netherlands)

of ASD, there is a left-to-right shunt at atrial level, which causes volume overload of the right heart, leading to right atrial and right ventricular dilatation. Atrial arrhythmias are therefore common. During pregnancy, if there is no history of atrial arrhythmias, patients are given aspirin, but if there is a prior history of atrial arrhythmias, they will be anticoagulated with LMWH.

Atrioventricular Septal Defects (AVSDs)
The majority of adults with AVSD will have been diagnosed and surgically repaired in infancy or childhood. Residual problems in adulthood include left AV valve (LAVV) regurgitation and atrial arrhythmias. If arrhythmias are persistent or paroxysmal, patients are anti-

coagulated with warfarin and converted to LMWH during pregnancy.

Mustard or Senning Repair of Transposition of the Great Arteries (TGA)
The Mustard and Senning operations for TGA physiologically correct blood flow by complex intra-atrial baffling, whereby deoxygenated caval blood is directed across the interatrial septum (IAS), through the mitral valve into the left ventricle and via the pulmonary artery to the lungs, and oxygenated pulmonary venous blood is diverted across the IAS, through the tricuspid valve into the right ventricle (RV) and into the aorta (Fig. 7.2). Although blood flow is physiologically corrected, the anatomy remains uncorrected, and the right ventricle is the systemic/subarterial ventricle (SRV). As a consequence, the RV dilates and hypertrophies and over time becomes dysfunctional. Atrial arrhythmias are also common. Patients with SRV impairment (EF < 50 %) are advised that pregnancy is high risk and SRV function may deteriorate. Those with only mild impairment (EF > 50 %) who embark on pregnancy are given aspirin thromboprophylaxis, unless there is a history of ARR whereby LMWH is indicated. Any patients taking warfarin prior to pregnancy will be converted to LMWH during pregnancy.

Congenitally Corrected TGA (CCTGA)
The anatomy of this rare lesion is such that the left atrium connects to a morphological RV via a tricuspid valve and the right atrium connects to the LV via a mitral valve (Fig. 7.3). There is often a VSD or pulmonary stenosis (PS), and patients with this more complex form of anatomy will often have undergone surgery in childhood to close the VSD and relieve the PS. Late complications include SRV dysfunction, atrial arrhythmias, and complete heart bock. The indication for anticoagulation is the same as for patients with the Mustard/Senning repairs.

Ebstein's Anomaly
In Ebstein's anomaly the tricuspid valve is displaced caudally toward the RV apex. This causes atrialization of the RV, reducing the functional size of the RV cavity (Fig. 7.4). The majority have a PFO or small ASD. Accessory electrophysiological pathways are common,

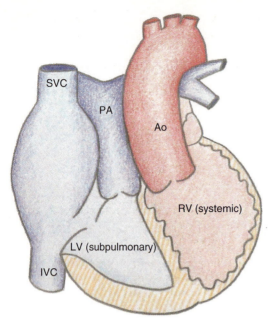

Fig. 7.3 Congenitally corrected TGA (CCTGA): systemic venous return via *IVC* and *SVC* into the right atrium, then subpulmonary left ventricle, then pulmonary artery. Pulmonary venous return via left atrium, systemic right ventricle to aorta. *TGA* transposition of the great arteries, *RV* right ventricle, *LV* left ventricle, *IVC* inferior vena cava, *SVC* superior vena cava, *Ao* aorta, *PA* pulmonary artery (Image courtesy Dr. Raquel Prieto, Centro de Salud Salvador Pau, Valencia, Spain)

leading to a high prevalence of ARR and supraventricular tachycardia (SVT). In its mildest form there is near-normal RV volume and function and only mild tricuspid regurgitation (TR), but with more severe TV displacement, the functional RV is small and severely restrictive, which leads to right heart failure and severe TR with cyanosis (right-to-left shunting across the PFO/ASD). The indication for anticoagulation in this heterogeneous group of patients must be considered on an individual case-by-case basis. Those with atrial arrhythmias and severe atrialization of the RV will be anticoagulated with warfarin and converted to LMWH during pregnancy.

The Fontan Circulation

The Fontan operation is a palliative surgery for those born with complex congenital heart disease and in whom a biventricular repair is not possible. Since the original Fontan operation, there have been many modifications, but all represent a form of right heart bypass, whereby caval blood is diverted directly into the pulmonary arteries, negating the need for a subpulmonary ventricle. The total cavopulmonary connection (TCPC) is now the preferred palliation (Fig. 7.5). Although

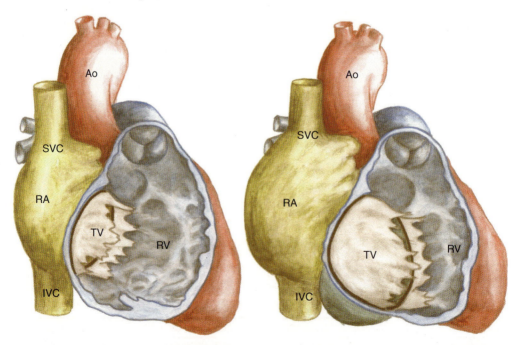

Fig. 7.4 Normal heart (*left*) versus Ebstein's anomaly (*right*): the tricuspid valve is displaced apically, resulting in a dilated right atrium and a small right ventricle. *RA* right atrium, *TV* tricuspid valve, *RV* right ventricle, *Ao* aorta, *SVC* superior vena cava, *IVC* inferior vena cava (Image courtesy Dr. JPM Hamer, The Netherlands)

the Fontan circulation is a single ventricle circulation, unlike those born with a single ventricle, there is separation of the systemic venous and arterial circulations, and oxygen saturations are therefore normal. In the Fontan circulation, blood flow into the pulmonary artery (PA) is passive, assisted by spontaneous respiration and negative intrathoracic pressure. Blood flow is therefore sluggish, and when coupled with the coagulation

abnormalities inherent to Fontan patients (increased platelet activation, impaired endothelial function, acquired protein C deficiency), there is a high risk of thromboembolic complications [64, 65] (Figs. 7.6 and 7.7). Studies have shown around 20 % incidence of asymptomatic PE in Fontan patients [66, 67]. The majority of patients with a Fontan circulation and/or severe RA dilatation are anticoagulated with warfarin, which is converted to LMWH during pregnancy. The remainder take aspirin, but during pregnancy all Fontan patients should be treated with LMWH.

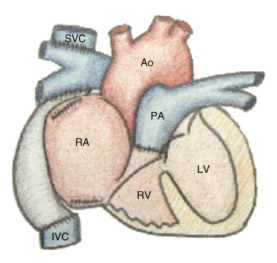

Fig. 7.5 Tricuspid atresia and status post Fontan operation (*TCPC* total cavopulmonary connection): the *SVC* is connected to the *PA* (bidirectional Glenn Shunt), and the *IVC* is connected to the *PA* via an extracardiac conduit. A functionally univentricular heart. *RV* right ventricle, *LV* left ventricle, *IVC* inferior vena cava, *SVC* superior vena cava, *Ao* aorta, *PA* pulmonary artery (Image courtesy Dr. Raquel Prieto, Centro de Salud Salvador Pau, Valencia, Spain)

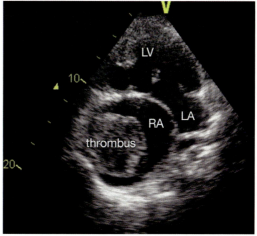

Fig. 7.6 Transthoracic echo image showing thrombus within the right atrium in a patient with APC Fontan circulation. *RA* right atrium, *LA* left atrium, *LV* left ventricle (Image courtesy Justin O'Leary, The Heart Hospital, UCLH)

Fig. 7.7 Transthoracic echo image showing thrombus attached to internal cardiac defibrillator (ICD) lead prolapsing through the tricuspid valve into the RV in a patient with hypertrophic cardiomyopathy. *RA* right atrium, *RV* right ventricle, *LA* left atrium, *LV* left ventricle (Image courtesy Ruth Brooks, The Heart Hospital, UCLH)

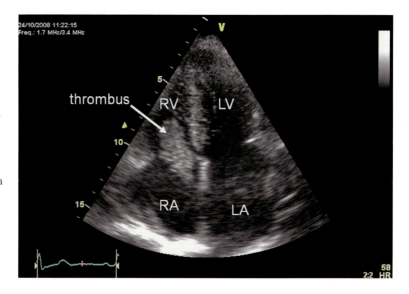

Eisenmenger Syndrome (ES)

ES is a syndrome characterized by cyanosis, pulmonary hypertension, and a right-to-left shunt at atrial, ventricular, or great vessel level. The most common causes of ES are VSD, PDA, and AVSD [68]. The initial left-to-right shunt and consequent increased pulmonary blood flow cause remodeling of the pulmonary microvasculature with subsequent increase in pulmonary vascular resistance (PVR). The elevated PVR causes secondary RV hypertension and reversal of the shunt. Right-to-left shunting of deoxygenated blood causes cyanosis and secondary polycythemia which leads to a multitude of hematological abnormalities including erythrocytosis, hyperviscosity, and iron deficiency [69]. There is both a prothrombotic (increased fibrinogen levels in the presence of reduced fibrinolytic activity) and bleeding tendency (thrombocytopenia secondary to reduced platelet production, increased activation, and increased destruction) [70, 71]. Up to a third of patients have evidence of pulmonary thromboemboli [72, 73], and around 20 % will have hemoptysis secondary to bronchial collaterals [74]. There is therefore no consensus as to whether these patients should be routinely anticoagulated, although warfarin treatment is indicated if there has been a proven thrombotic event. Pregnancy in ES is associated with a 30–50 % maternal mortality, and women are therefore advised against pregnancy [75, 76]. Fetal complications are also common, and the live-birth rate is closely associated with maternal oxygen saturation, such that if maternal resting O_2 saturation is <85 %, the chance of a live birth is ~12 % but if >90 % the live-birth rate is ~92 % [77]. If a woman with ES embarks on pregnancy, she will require anticoagulation with LMWH.

Conclusion

Thromboembolism is a major risk for women with heart disease embarking on pregnancy. While thromboembolic events are seen in 1 in 1,000 to 1 in 2,000 normal pregnancies [78, 79], the ZAHARA review of pregnancy outcomes in ~2,500 women with congenital heart disease concluded that thromboembolic risk in this group is 50 times higher than that of the normal pregnant population [80]. The CARPREG study also found that thromboembolic events were a major cause of morbidity and mortality within a similar pregnant population. Assessment of thromboembolic risk in any woman with heart disease embarking on pregnancy is therefore essential. Currently, however, there are no good data or guidelines specific to this patient group, with the exception of patients with mechanical valves. Clearly guidelines are needed, but until they are available, clinical practice and experience provide some insight into how to reduce thromboembolic risk in women with heart disease during pregnancy.

From our own institutional experience of managing over 500 pregnancies in women with heart disease, 90 women have received thromboprophylaxis. Their underlying cardiac lesions are shown in Fig. 7.8. There have been a total of five thromboembolic complications. Three thromboembolic events were in women prescribed thromboprophylaxis (aspirin [1], LMWH [2]) and 2 were in patients on nil therapy. There was one major thromboembolic event of mechanical valve thrombosis in a young woman with a Bjork-Shiley mitral prosthesis anticoagulated with LMWH. She had a genetic prothrombotic tendency (heterozygosity for the G20210A prothrombin gene mutation) and had subtherapeutic anti-Xa levels as a result of suboptimal anti-Xa monitoring due to geographical remoteness. She presented at 24 weeks with acute pulmonary edema. Of the other two events on treatment, a patient with HOCM and an ICD in situ developed a large thrombus on the ICD lead at 24 weeks' gestation. She had been noncompliant with aspirin therapy and was found to be heterozygous for factor V Leiden. On further questioning she reported a family history of VTE, a sibling having had a prior PE. The other patient with a TCPC Fontan presented with a pulmonary embolism at 20 weeks' gestation. She had been noncompliant with LMWH therapy. Two thromboembolic events were in women on no VTE prophylaxis. One patient with anthracycline cardiomyopathy and near-normal LV function pre-pregnancy had a spontaneous pregnancy loss at 24 weeks' gestation and was found to have poor LV function and LV thrombus at review 2 weeks later. The second patient had moderate to severe valvar aortic stenosis and

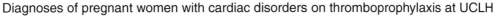

Diagnoses of pregnant women with cardiac disorders on thromboprophylaxis at UCLH

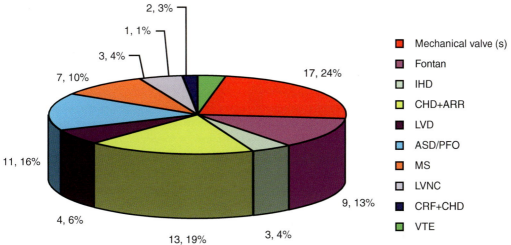

Fig. 7.8 Diagnoses of pregnant women with cardiac disorders on thromboprophylaxis at UCLH. *IHD* ischemic heart disease, *ARR* atrial arrhythmia, *LVD* left ventricular dysfunction, *ASD* atrial septal defect, *PFO* persistent foramen ovale, *MS* mitral stenosis, *LVNC* left ventricular non-compaction, *CRF* chronic renal failure, *VTE* venous thromboembolism (Chart courtesy Ruth Brooks, The Heart Hospital, UCLH)

48 h post vaginal delivery had a left-sided CVA. This clinical experience provides several learning points.

Learning Points

- If LMWH is used for mechanical valves in pregnancy, it must be monitored meticulously every 1–2 weeks and the dose up-titrated promptly to maintain target anti-Xa levels.
- Any patient at risk of a deterioration in ventricular function during pregnancy should be considered for LMWH thromboprophylaxis.
- Inherited or acquired thrombophilias should be excluded in those with a past or family history of VTE.
- Calcified valves pose a thromboembolic risk and patients with these should be considered for thromboprophylaxis.
- Patient compliance with any treatment regimen is of paramount importance, and thromboembolic risk and its prevention needs to be highlighted and reiterated at clinic review.

Acknowledgements The authors would like to thank Ruth Brooks, cardiac specialist nurse for the maternal cardiology service at the Heart Hospital, for her input.

References

1. Arafeh JM, Baird SM. Cardiac disease in pregnancy. Crit Care Nurs Q. 2006;29:32–52.
2. Lewis G, editor. The Confidential Enquiry into Maternal and Child Health (CEMACH). Saving mothers' lives: reviewing maternal deaths to make motherhood safer – 2003–2005. The seventh report on confidential enquiries into maternal deaths in the United Kingdom. London: CEMACH; 2007.
3. Siu SC, Sermer M, Colman JM, Alvarez AN, Mercier LA, Morton BC, Kells CM, Bergin ML, Kiess MC, Marcotte F, Taylor DA, Gordon EP, Spears JC, Tam JW, Amankwah KS, Smallhorn JF, Farine D, Sorensen S, Cardiac Disease in Pregnancy (CARPREG) Investigators. Prospective multicenter study of pregnancy outcomes in women with heart disease. Circulation. 2001;104(5):515–21.
4. Siu SC, Sermer M, Harrison DA, Grigoriadis E, Liu G, Sorensen S, Smallhorn JF, Farine D, Amankwah KS, Spears JC, Colman JM. Risk and predictors for pregnancy-related complications in women with heart disease. Circulation. 1997;96:2789–94.
5. Walker F. In: Steer PJ, Gatzoulis MA, Baker P, editors. Antenatal care of women with cardiac disease: a cardiologists perspective. Heart disease and pregnancy. London: RCOG Press; 2006.
6. Klinzing P, Markert UR, Liesaus K, Peiker G. Case report: successful pregnancy and delivery after myocardial infarction and essential thrombocythemia treated with clopidrogel. Clin Exp Obstet Gynecol. 2001;28:215–6.

7. Cuthill JA, Young S, Greer IA, Oldroyd K. Anaesthetic considerations in a parturient with critical coronary artery disease and a drug-eluting stent presenting for caesarean section. Int J Obstet Anesth. 2005;14:167–71.

8. Taguchi K. Pregnancy in patients with a prosthetic heart valve. Surg Gynecol Obstet. 1977;145:2068.

9. Nassar AH, Hobeika EM, Abd Essamad HM, Taher A, Khalil AM, Usta IM. Pregnancy outcome in women with prosthetic heart valves. Am J Obstet Gynecol. 2004;191:1009–13.

10. Blickstein D, Blickstein I. The risk of fetal loss associated with Warfarin anticoagulation. Int J Gynaecol Obstet. 2002;78:221–5.

11. Srivastava AK, Gupta AK, Singh AV, Husain T. Effect of oral anticoagulant during pregnancy with prosthetic heart valve. Asian Cardiovasc Thorac Ann. 2002;10:306–9.

12. Hall JG. Embryopathy associated with oral anticoagulant therapy. Birth Defects. 1965;12:133–40.

13. Iturbe-Alessio I, Fonseca MC, Mutchinik O, Santos MA, Zajarias A, Salazar E. Risks of anticoagulant therapy in pregnant women with artificial heart valves. N Engl J Med. 1986;315:1390–3.

14. Sadler L, McCowan L, White H, Stewart A, Bracken M, North R. Pregnancy outcomes and cardiac complications in women with mechanical, bioprosthetic and homograft valves. BJOG. 2000;107:245–53.

15. Meschengieser SS, Fondevila CG, Santarelli MT, Lazzari MA. Anticoagulation in pregnant women with mechanical heart valve prostheses. Heart. 1999; 82:23–6.

16. Chen WW, Chan CS, Lee PK, Wang RY, Wong VC. Pregnancy in patients with prosthetic heart valves: an experience with 45 pregnancies. Q J Med. 1982;51: 358–65.

17. Hall JAG, Paul RM, Wilson KM. Maternal and fetal sequelae of anticoagulation during pregnancy. Am J Med. 1980;68:122–40.

18. Wesseling J, Van Driel D, Heymans HSA, Rosendaal FR, Geven-Boere LM, Smrkovsky M, Touwen BCL, Sauer PJJ Van der Veer E. Coumarins during pregnancy: Long-term effects on growth and development of school-age children. Thrombosis and Haemostasis. 2001;85(4):609–13.

19. Hung L, Rahimtoola SH. Prosthetic heart valves and pregnancy. Circulation. 2003;107:1240–6.

20. Cotrufo M, De Feo M, De Santo LS, Romano G, Della Corte A, Renzulli A, Gallo C. Risk of warfarin during pregnancy with mechanical valve prostheses. Obstet Gynecol. 2002;99:35–40.

21. Eikelboom JW, Hirsh J. Monitoring unfractionated heparin with the aPTT: time for a fresh look. Thromb Haemost. 2006;96(5):547–52.

22. Thromboembolic disease in pregnancy and the puerperium: Acute management. Royal College of Obstetricians and Gynaecologists. Green-top guideline no.37b, February 2007. Reviewed 2010. London: RCOG.

23. Schaefer DC, Hufnagle J, Williams L. Rapid heparin anticoagulation: use of a weight-based nomogram. Am Fam Physician. 1996;54:2517–21.

24. Bates SM, Greer IA, Middeldorp S, Veenstra DL, Prabulos A-M, Vandvik PO. VTE, Thrombophilia, Antithrombotic Therapy, and Pregnancy: Antithrombotic Therapy and Prevention of Thrombosis, 9th ed: American College of Chest Physicians Evidence-Based Clinical Practice Guidelines. Chest February 2012 141(2): e691S–36.

25. Warkentin TE, Levine MN, Hirsh J, Horsewood P, Roberts RS, Gent M, Kelton JG. Heparin-induced thrombocytopenia in patients treated with low-molecular-weight-heparin or unfractionated heparin. NEJM. 1995;332:1330–6.

26. Girolami B, Prandoni P, Stefani PM, Tanduo C, Sabbion P, Eichler P, Ramon R, Baggio G, Fabris F, Girolami A. The incidence of heparin-induced thrombocytopenia in hospitalized medical patients treated with subcutaneous unfractionated heparin: a prospective cohort study. Blood. 2003;101:2955–9.

27. Barbour LA, Kick SD, Steiner JF, LoVerde ME, Heddleston LN, Lear JL, Baron AE, Barton PL. A prospective study of heparin-induced osteoporosis in pregnancy using bone densitometry. Am J Obstet Gynecol. 1994;170:862–9.

28. Dahlman, TC. Osteoporotic fractures and the recurrence of thromboembolism during pregnancy and the puerperium in 184 women undergoing thromboprophylaxis with heparin. American Journal of Obstetrics and Gynecology. 1993;168(4):1265–70.

29. Royal College of Obstetricians and Gynaecologists. Green-top guideline no. 37a. Thrombosis and embolism during pregnancy and the puerperium, Reducing the risk. London. Royal College of Obstetricians and Gynaecologists; 2009.

30. Oran B, Lee-Parritz A, Ansell J. Low molecular weight heparin for the prophylaxis of thromboembolism in women with prosthetic mechanical heart valves during pregnancy. Thromb Haemost. 2004;92:747–51.

31. James AH, Brancazio LR, Gehrig TR, Wang A, Ortel TL. Low-molecular-weight heparin for thromboprophylaxis in pregnant women with mechanical heart valves. J Matern Fetal Neonatal Med. 2006; 19:543–9.

32. Bazzan M, Donvito V. Low molecular weight heparin during pregnancy. Thromb Res. 2001;101:V175–86.

33. Sanson BJ, Lensing AW, Prins MH, Ginsberg JS, Barkagan ZS, Lavenne-Pardonge E, Brenner B, Dulitzky M, Nielsen JD, Boda Z, Turi S, Mac Gillavry MR, Hamulyak K, Theunissen IM, Hunt BJ, Buller HR. Safety of low-molecular-weight heparin in pregnancy: a systematic review. Thromb Haemost. 1999; 81:668–72. .

34. Greer IA, Nelson-Piercy C. Low-molecular-weight heparins for thromboprophylaxis and treatment of venous thromboembolism in pregnancy: a systematic review of safety and efficacy. Blood. 2005;106:401–7.

35. Hirsh J, Bauer KA, Donati MB, Gould M, Samama MM, Weitz JI, American College of Chest Physicians. Parenteral anticoagulants: American College of Chest Physicians Evidence-Based Clinical Practice Guidelines (8th Edition). Chest. 2008;133 Suppl 6:141S–59.

36. Quinn J, Von Klemperer K, Brooks R, Peebles D, Walker F, Cohen H. Use of high intensity adjusted

dose low molecular weight heparin in women with mechanical heart valves during pregnancy: a single-center experience. Haematologica. 2009;94:1608–12.

37. Nkomo VT, Gardin JM, Skelton TN, Gottdiener JS, Scott CG, Enriquez-Sarano M. Burden of valvular heart diseases: a population-based study. Lancet. 2006;368(9540):1005–11.

38. Vijaykumar M, Narula J, Reddy KS. Incidence of rheumatic fever and prevalence of rheumatic heart disease in India. Int J Cardiol. 1994;43:221–8.

39. Agarwal AK. Rheumatic fever and rheumatic heart disease in Arabia. Int J Cardiol. 1994;43:221–8.

40. Personal communication with Dr. Lorna Swan, consultant cardiologist, Royal Brompton Hospital, London, and Dr. Sara Thorne, consultant cardiologist, University Hospital Birmingham, Birmingham. 2010.

41. British Society of Echocardiography guidelines for chamber quantification. www.bsecho.org.

42. Curry R, Swan L, Steer PJ. Cardiac disease in pregnancy. Curr Opin Obstet Gynecol. 2009;21:508–13.

43. Leon MB, Baim DS, Popma JJ, Gordon PC, Cutlip DE, Ho KK, Giambartolomei A, Diver DJ, Lasorda DM, Williams DO, Pocock SJ, Kuntz RE. A clinical trial comparing three antithrombotic-drug regimens after coronary-artery stenting. Stent Anticoagulation Restenosis Study Investigators. N Engl J Med. 1998; 339:1665–71.

44. Urban P, Macaya C, Rupprecht HJ, Kiemeneij F, Emanuelsson H, Fontanelli A, Pieper M, Wesseling T, Sagnard L. Randomized evaluation of anticoagulation versus antiplatelet therapy after coronary stent implantation in high-risk patients: the multicenter aspirin and ticlopidine trial after intracoronary stenting (MATTIS). Circulation. 1998;98(20):2126–32.

45. Brener SJ, Steinhubl SR, Berger PB, Brennan DM, Topol EJ, for the CREDO Investigators. Prolonged dual antiplatelet therapy after percutaneous coronary intervention reduces ischemic events without affecting the need for repeat revascularization: insights from the CREDO trial. J Invasive Cardiol. 2007;19:287–90.

46. Galla JM, Lincoff AM. The role of clopidogrel in the management of ischemic heart disease. Curr Opin Cardiol. 2007;22:273–9.

47. Bonow RO, Carabello BA, Chatterjee K, de Leon Jr AC, Faxon DP, Freed MD, Gaasch WH, Lytle BW, Nishimura RA, O'Gara PT, O'Rourke RA, Otto CM, Shah PM, Shanewise JS, American College of Cardiology/American Heart Association Task Force on Practice Guidelines. 2008 focused update incorporated into the ACC/AHA 2006 guidelines for the management of patients with valvular heart disease: a report of the American College of Cardiology/ American Heart Association Task Force on Practice Guidelines (Writing Committee to revise the 1998 guidelines for the management of patients with valvular heart disease). Endorsed by the Society of Cardiovascular Anesthesiologists, Society for Cardiovascular Angiography and Interventions, and Society of Thoracic Surgeons. J Am Coll Cardiol. 2008;52:e1–142.

48. Keeling, D, Davidson, S, Watson, H and British Comm Standards, H. The management of heparin-induced thrombocytopenia. British Journal of Haematology. 2006;133(3):259–69

49. Vahanian A, Baumgartner H, Bax J, Butchart E, Dion R, Filippatos G, Flachskampf F, Hall R, Iung B, Kasprzak J, Nataf P, Tornos P, Torracca L, Wenink A, Task Force on the Management of Valvular Hearth Disease of the European Society of Cardiology; ESC Committee for Practice Guidelines. Guidelines on the management of valvular heart disease: The Task Force on the Management of Valvular Heart Disease of the European Society of Cardiology. Eur Heart J. 2007; 28:230–68.

50. Chan WS, Anand S and Ginsberg JS. Anticoagulation of pregnant women with mechanical heart valves - A systematic review of the literature. Archives of Internal Medicine. 2000;160(2):191–6.

51. Ginsberg JS, Chan WS, Bates SM, Kaatz S. Anticoagulation of pregnant women with mechanical heart valves. Arch Intern Med. 2003;163:694–8.

52. Yinon Y, Siu SC, Warshafsky C, Maxwell C, McLeod A, Colman JM, Sermer M, Silversides CK. Use of low molecular weight heparin in pregnant women with mechanical heart valves. Am J Cardiol. 2009;104(9):1259–63.

53. McLintock C, McCowan LM, North RA. Maternal complications and pregnancy outcome in women with mechanical prosthetic heart valves treated with enoxaparin. BJOG. 2009;116(12):1585–92.

54. Raschke R, Gollihare B, Peirce J. The effectiveness of implementing the weight-based heparin nomogram as a practice guideline. Arch Intern Med. 1996;156:1645–9.

55. Elkayam U, Khan S, Mehboob A, Ahsan N. Impaired endothelium-mediated vasodilation in heart failure: clinical evidence and the potential for therapy. J Card Fail. 2002;8:15–20.

56. Ahnert AM, Freudenberger RS. What do we know about anticoagulation in patients with heart failure? Curr Opin Cardiol. 2008;23:228–32.

57. Chong AY, Freestone B, Patel J, Lim HS, Hughes E, Blann AD, Lip GY. Endothelial activation, dysfunction, and damage in congestive heart failure and the relation to brain natriuretic peptide and outcomes. Am J Cardiol. 2006;97:671–5.

58. Abdo AS, Kemp R, Barham J, Geraci SA. Dilated cardiomyopathy and role of antithrombotic therapy. Am J Med Sci. 2010;339(6):557–60.

59. Cleland JG, Findlay I, Jafri S, Sutton G, Falk R, Bulpitt C, Prentice C, Ford I, Trainer A, Poole-Wilson PA. The Warfarin/Aspirin Study in Heart failure (WASH): a randomized trial comparing antithrombotic strategies for patients with heart failure. Am Heart J. 2004;148:157–64.

60. Grewal J, Siu SC, Ross HJ, Mason J, Balint OH, Sermer M, Colman JM, Silversides CK. Pregnancy outcomes in women with dilated cardiomyopathy. J Am Coll Cardiol. 2009;55:45–52.

61. Sliwa K, Fett J, Elkayam U. Peripartum cardiomyopathy. Lancet. 2006;368:687–93.

62. Sutton MS, Cole P, Plappert M, Saltzman D, Goldhaber S. Effects of subsequent pregnancy on left

ventricular function in peripartum cardiomyopathy. Am Heart J. 1991;121(6 Pt 1):1776–8.

63. Elkayam U, Tummala PP, Rao K, Akhter MW, Karaalp IS, Wani OR, Hameed A, Gviazda I, Shotan A. Maternal and fetal outcomes of subsequent pregnancies in women with peripartum cardiomyopathy. N Engl J Med. 2001;344(21):1567–71.

64. Kajimoto H, Nakazawa M, Murasaki K, Hagiwara N, Nakanishi T. Increased P-selectin expression on platelets and decreased plasma thrombomodulin in Fontan patients. Circ J. 2009;73:1705–10.

65. Odegard KC, McGowan Jr FX, Zurakowski D, Dinardo JA, Castro RA, del Nido PJ, Laussen PC. Procoagulant and anticoagulant factor abnormalities following the Fontan procedure: increased factor VIII may predispose to thrombosis. J Thorac Cardiovasc Surg. 2003;125:1260–7.

66. Varma C, Warr MR, Hendler AL, Paul NS, Webb GD, Therrien J. Prevalence of "silent" pulmonary emboli in adults after the Fontan operation. J Am Coll Cardiol. 2003;41:2252–8.

67. Monagle P, Cochrane A, McCrindle B, Benson L, Williams W, Andrew M. Thromboembolic complications after Fontan procedures – the role of prophylactic anticoagulation. J Thorac Cardiovasc Surg. 1998; 115:493–8.

68. Wood P. Pulmonary hypertension with special reference to the vasoconstrictive factor. Br Heart J. 1958;20:557–70.

69. Perloff JK, Rosove MH, Child JS, Wright GB. Adults with cyanotic congenital heart disease: hematologic management. Ann Intern Med. 1988;109:406–13.

70. Lill MC, Perloff JC, Child JS. Pathogenesis of thrombocytopenia in cyanotic congenital heart disease. Am J Cardiol. 2006;98(2):254–8.

71. Huber K, Beckmann R, Frank H, Kneussl M, Mlczoch J, Binder BR. Fibrinogen, t-PA, and PAI-1 plasma levels in patients with pulmonary hypertension. Am J Respir Crit Care Med. 1994;150:929–33.

72. Diller GP, Gatzoulis MA. Pulmonary vascular disease in adults with congenital heart disease. Circulation. 2007;115:1039–50.

73. Broberg CS, Ujita M, Prasad S, Li W, Rubens M, Bax BE, Davidson SJ, Bouzas B, Gibbs JS, Burman J, Gatzoulis MA. Pulmonary arterial thrombosis in eisenmenger syndrome is associated with biventricular dysfunction and decreased pulmonary flow velocity. J Am Coll Cardiol. 2007;50:634–42.

74. Daliento L, Somerville J, Presbitero P, Menti L, Brach-Prever S, Rizzoli G, Stone S. Eisenmenger syndrome. Factors relating to deterioration and death. Eur Heart J. 1998;19:1845–55.

75. Warnes CA. Pregnancy and pulmonary hypertension. Int J Cardiol. 2004;97 Suppl 1:11–3.

76. Bédard E, Dimopoulos K, Gatzoulis MA. Has there been any progress made on pregnancy outcomes among women with pulmonary arterial hypertension? Eur Heart J. 2009;30:256–65.

77. Presbitero P, Somerville J, Stone S, Aruta E, Spiegelhalter D, Rabajoli F. Pregnancy in cyanotic congenital heart disease. Outcome of mother and fetus. Circulation. 1994;89(6):2673–6.

78. Toglia MR, Weg JG. Venous thromboembolism during pregnancy. N Engl J Med. 1996;335:108–14.

79. Greer IA. Thrombosis in pregnancy: maternal and fetal issues. Lancet. 1999;353:1258–65.

80. Drenthen W, Pieper PG, Roos-Hesselink JW, van Lottum WA, Voors AA, Mulder BJ, van Dijk AP, Vliegen HW, Yap SC, Moons P, Ebels T, van Veldhuisen DJ, ZAHARA Investigators. Outcome of pregnancy in women with congenital heart disease: a literature review. J Am Coll Cardiol. 2007;49(24): 2303–11.

Inherited Bleeding Disorders in Pregnancy: von Willebrand Disease, Factor XI Deficiency, and Hemophilia A and B Carriers

8

Christine A. Lee and Rezan A. Kadir

Abstract

Obstetric management of women with von Willebrand Disease (VWD) and FXI deficiency, and carriers of hemophilia A and B, requires a multidisciplinary team approach with obstetricians, midwives, hematologists, anesthetists, and neonatologists. This chapter discusses these disorders with particular emphasis on their management during pregnancy, delivery and postpartum. Diagnostic (carrier) testing before becoming pregnant in order to allow appropriate preconception counselling and timely provision of prenatal diagnosis, especially in those who could potentially carry a severely affected baby, are also addressed.

8.1 von Willebrand Disease

8.1.1 History

In a classic paper published in 1926, Erik von Willebrand described 66 members of a bleeder family in the Aland Islands. It was noted that whereas 16 of 35 women had the trait, it was only present in 7 of 31 men, and therefore von Willebrand suggested that "the trait seemed espe-

cially to be seen among women…in the female bleeders, the diathesis becomes manifest both in a milder and graver form…Among the females five deaths have occurred." The index Hjordis, who had presented with epistaxis, later died at the onset of her fourth menstrual period, but her own mother produced 12 siblings and her deliveries were normal without heavy bleeding. However, the maternal grandmother had bled to death in childbirth. It is likely that this represented Type 1 and Type 3 von Willebrand Disease (VWD) in the mother and maternal grandmother, respectively [1] (Fig. 8.1).

8.1.2 Inheritance and Clinical Picture

A large epidemiological study conducted in a young normal population in Italy in 1987 showed a prevalence of VWD of 1 % or 1 in 100 [2]. In a study in which the United States Nationwide Inpatient Sample (NIS) for the years 2000–2003 was queried

C.A. Lee, MA, MD, DSc, FRCP, FRCPath (✉)
University of London, London, UK
Oxford Haemophilia and Thrombosis Centre,
Department of Haematology,
Churchill Hospital, Oxford OX3 7LJ, UK
e-mail: profcalee@hotmail.com

R.A. Kadir, MD, FRCS, FRCOG
Department of Obstetrics and Gynaecology,
Royal Free Hospital, Hampstead, London
NW3 2QG, UK
e-mail: rezan.abdul-kadir@royalfree.nhs.uk

H. Cohen, P. O'Brien (eds.), *Disorders of Thrombosis and Hemostasis in Pregnancy*,
DOI 10.1007/978-1-4471-4411-3_8, © Springer-Verlag London 2012

Fig. 8.1 A bleeder family from Føglø in the Aland archipelago (From von Willebrand [1])

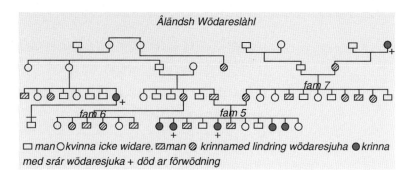

Âländsh Wödareslàhl

☐ *man* ○ *kvinna icke widare.* ⊠ *man* ⊘ *krinnamed lindring wödaresjuha* ● *krinna med srár wödaresjuka* + *död ar förwödning*

fam 7

fam 6   *fam 5*

for pregnancy-related discharges, women with a diagnosis of VWD were compared with women without VWD; the frequency of a diagnosis of VWD among women giving birth was 0.024 % or 1 in 4,000 [3]. A study of symptomatic patients at hemostasis centers found an incidence of 0.002–0.01 % or 1 in 10,000 [4].

There are explanations for some of these discrepancies – the level of VWF in a young population tends to be lower, and it has been found that the level of VWF increases by 15 % each decade [5]. National Indicator set data are derived from discharge summaries, and there is a strong possibility of errors in coding toward underdiagnosis. Furthermore, many patients remain undiagnosed or are seen outside hemostasis centers, particularly in the USA [3]. It has also been pointed out that the wide spectrum of clinical and laboratory manifestations and the lack of strong penetrance mean that making the diagnosis can be very difficult [6].

Thus, VWD is the most common inherited bleeding disorder, and a low von Willebrand factor (VWF) may be found with a frequency of 1 % in young women [2].

8.1.3   Classification of VWD

von Willebrand disease has been classified into three main types [7].

Type 1 is a quantitative deficiency of VWF with a mild to moderate VWF level, 15–50 IU/dL, and normal VWF multimer structure. It occurs in approximately 85 % of cases.

Type 2 is a qualitative deficiency occurring in 15 % of cases and is further subdivided – type 2A, loss of high- and intermediate-weight multimers; type 2B, loss of high molecular weight multimers

and often associated with thrombocytopenia; and type 2M, normal VWF multimers and poor binding to platelets. Type 2N VWD involves a mutation in the VWF protein which leads to decreased binding of FVIII with resultant FVIII deficiency, and is often misdiagnosed as hemophilia A.

Type 3 is a severe quantitative deficiency with undetectable VWF protein. It is rare, occurring at a frequency of one in a million in the UK population. However, in those populations where first cousin marriage is practised, it is more common [10].

8.1.4   Prepregnancy Counseling

Type 1 and 2 von Willebrand disease is inherited as an autosomal dominant condition with variable inheritance; therefore for type 1 and 2 VWD, there is a 50 % risk of a mother transmitting VWD to her child. However, type 3 VWD is an autosomal recessive disorder, and an affected individual is either homozygote or compound heterozygote. Thus, when a child with type 3 VWD has already been born in a family, the risk of a subsequent child being affected is 25 %. This is common in first cousin marriages; the parents may request antenatal diagnosis, but this should be planned in advance to allow the causative mutation to be identified [11].

8.1.5   Antenatal management

The physiological response to pregnancy is an increase in FVIII and VWF; thus, most women with VWD do not bleed excessively during pregnancy (Fig. 8.2) [12, 13].

Most women with type 1 VWD achieve levels in the normal nonpregnant range by the third

Fig. 8.2 Levels of FVIIIC, VWF:Ag, and VWF:AC during pregnancy (From Kadir et al. [12])

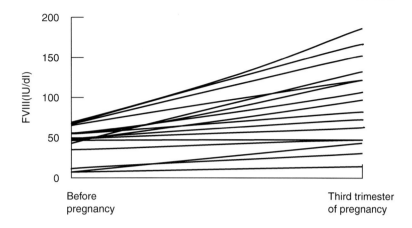

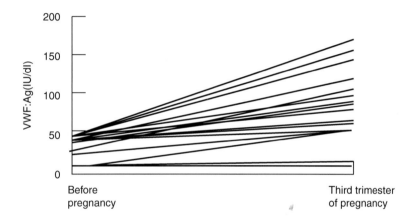

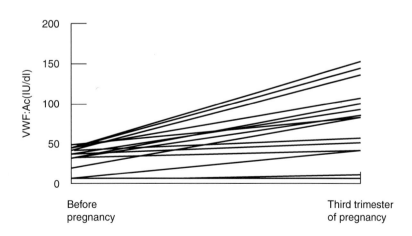

trimester [12]. In a series of 24 pregnancies in 24 women with VWD studied retrospectively, it was found that the FVIIIC and VWF:Ag rose above baseline levels by 1.5 times in most cases. However, some women who are severely affected with type 1 VWD may fail to achieve normal

VWF levels by the third trimester, and a baseline level of <15 IU/dL was predictive of a third trimester level <50 IU/dL [14].

In type 2 VWD, although FVIII and VWF:Ag levels increase, there is minimal or no increase in VWF:AC levels [14]. In type 2N VWD, the FVIII level remains low because of impaired binding by VWF. In type 2B VWD, thrombocytopenia may worsen in pregnancy because the increase in intermediate multimers induces platelet aggregation [15].

There is little or no increase of VWF in type 3 VWD [16, 12].

Regular monitoring of VWF:Ag and VWF:AC together with FVIIIC is recommended at booking, 28 and 34 weeks 'gestation, and prior to invasive procedures [11]. The platelet count should be monitored in those with type 2B VWD [15]. If the VWF:AC does not reach 50 IU/dL by the third trimester, prophylaxis with clotting factor concentrate to cover delivery should be considered [17, 11].

8.1.6 Miscarriage

The spontaneous miscarriage rate has been reported as 14 % [18]. In a review of 84 pregnancies in women with VWD during the years 1980–1996, it was found that 33 % presented with vaginal bleeding during the first trimester and there was an overall spontaneous miscarriage rate of 21 % [12]. A miscarriage rate of 21 % was reported in another study of pregnant women with VWD [19]. Thus, although women with VWD have a higher rate of bleeding during the first trimester, there is not an increased rate of miscarriage.

Spontaneous miscarriage or elective termination in women with VWD is associated with an increased risk of bleeding complications [19, 12, 15]. In one study, transfusion was required for bleeding in association with 10 % of spontaneous miscarriages or elective abortions, and intermittent bleeding occurred for 2 weeks after miscarriage in 30 % of cases [12]. Most miscarriages occur during the first trimester before the VWF:AC has increased substantially [14]. It is therefore recommended that women with VWD who present with spontaneous miscarriage or who elect for

termination of pregnancy should have the VWF:AC measured and prophylactic treatment given if the VWF:AC is <50 IU/dL [11].

8.1.7 Treatment

8.1.7.1 DDAVP

The use of DDAVP in pregnancy remains controversial. A survey in the USA showed that 50 % and 30 % of hematologists used intravenous and intranasal DDAVP, respectively, for postpartum hemorrhage (PPH) in type 1 VWD but 31 % considered pregnancy as a contraindication [20]. There are reports of the use of DDAVP to cover chorionic villus sampling or amniocentesis [21], to cover 52 deliveries and 20 Caesarean sections in women with a low third trimester VWF [22], and to cover mothers with VWD after cutting the cord [23].

The evidence suggests that DDAVP is not contraindicated in uncomplicated pregnancy.

8.1.7.2 Clotting Factor Concentrate Containing VWF

Virally inactive plasma-derived concentrate containing VWF is the treatment of choice for those women who are unresponsive to DDAVP. If the FVIIIC and/or VWF:AC is <50 IU/dL, a prophylactic infusion should be started at the onset of labor and a VWF:AC >50 IU/dL maintained for at least 3 days post vaginal delivery and 5 days post-Caesarean section [11]. In type 2N VWD, recombinant FVIII has been successfully used [24]. In type 3 VWD, concentrate is always required to cover delivery because the VWF level does not increase in pregnancy [79].

8.1.8 Regional Analgesia and Anesthesia

Several case reports have described women with VWD who received epidural anaesthesia without bleeding complications [76, 77, 78].

In a series, eight women with VWD received regional anesthesia during labour and delivery without bleeding complications and only one woman received prophylactic therapy as the clotting factor levels were >50 IU dL^{-1} in the other cases [80]. Epidural anesthesia may be considered for use in the majority of women with type 1 VWD whose levels have risen to >50 IU dL^{-1}. However, the decision on its use needs to be made jointly by an experienced anesthetist, obstetrician and hematologist after considerations are given to hemostatic concerns such as the degree of correction of the plasma FVIII:C and VWF levels, possible degree of residual platelet impairment, possible rate of postpartum decline of VWF and the consequent risks of bleeding/spinal hematoma. The risks of an epidural or spinal anesthetic for Caesarean section should be balanced against the risk of a general anesthetic. In all cases the epidural should be inserted by an experienced anesthetist. Epidural anesthesia is generally not recommended for use in type 2 or 3 VWD [81].

8.1.9   Postpartum management

There is an increased risk of both primary (>500 mL blood loss in the first 24 h after delivery) and secondary (excessive bleeding from 24 h to 6 weeks postpartum) PPH in women with VWD. This is due to a fall in VWF and FVIIIC postnatally [13] (Fig. 8.3). Three series including 51 women and 92 deliveries showed a primary PPH rate of 16–29 % and a secondary PPH rate of 20–29 % [12, 14, 25]. All women with VWD should therefore be advised to have active management of the third stage of labor; this involves administration of an oxytocic drug with the birth

of the baby, early cord clamping, and controlled cord traction. The VWF level should be checked postdelivery particularly in those with a low predelivery baseline. The risk of PPH is higher in types 2 and 3 VWD, and in these women, the VWF should be maintained >50 IU/dL for at least 3 days post vaginal delivery or 5 days post-Caesarean section. The fall in VWF postdelivery can be very variable – there are anecdotal reports of a fall from 41 to 9 IU/dL over the course of a week [14] and a fall of 50 % within 24 h of delivery [26]. One study found that the average time of presentation of secondary PPH in women with VWD is 16 days postdelivery [27] and therefore there is a need for observation and possibly prophylaxis for several weeks postpartum. Prolonged and/or intermittent secondary PPH has also been reported in VWD [12, 14]. In a recent study, the duration of lochia was significantly longer in women with VWD compared to those with no bleeding disorders [28].

8.2   Factor XI Deficiency

8.2.1   Inheritance and Clinical Picture

The management of pregnancy and delivery for women with Factor XI (FXI) deficiency is difficult because the bleeding tendency is so unpredictable. This deficiency was first described in 1953 [29] and was termed hemophilia C. Although the inheritance was initially thought to be autosomal dominant [30], a study in 1961 showed autosomal recessive inheritance [31]. Factor XI deficiency

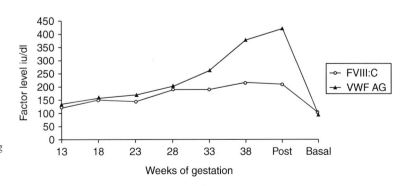

Fig. 8.3 The levels of FVIII and VWF:Ag during pregnancy and postdelivery (From Stirling et al. [13])

was found to be very common in Jews where the frequency of the heterozygous state among Ashkenazi Jews was found to be 8 % [32].

Individuals with severe FXI deficiency, FXI below 15–20 IU/dL, are at risk of bleeding with surgery and trauma, but some individuals with this severe deficiency do not have a bleeding tendency [33]. The bleeding may be inconsistent within a particular family and is not related to the factor level, in contrast to hemophilias A and B [34, 35]. Studies of the relationship of the FXIC level and the bleeding tendency have also shown that individuals with a level between 50 and 70 IU/dL may have a bleeding tendency [34] (Fig. 8.4). Thus, it is important to take a good bleeding history and to test for additional coexisting abnormalities of VWF and platelet function [36].

8.2.2 Treatment of FXI Deficiency

Comprehensive guidelines on treatment are available [37, 38].

8.2.2.1 Fresh Frozen Plasma (FFP)
FFP was the mainstay of treatment until FXI plasma-derived concentrate became available. This was used in Rosenthal's original patients [29]. FFP has been made safer with respect to possible viral transmission either by pooled solvent detergent treated plasma or single donor units treated with methylene blue [38]. However, in the UK, there remains a concern about possible transmission of abnormal prions following the large epidemic of BSE in cattle and ingestion by potential plasma donors [39].

8.2.2.2 Plasma-Derived FXI Concentrate
A plasma-derived FXI concentrate derived from German plasma is available in the UK [38]. However, there have been concerns about potential thrombogenicity [40], therefore the dose used should not raise the plasma level above 70 IU/dL, and the maximum dose should be 30 IU/dL. The use of FXI concentrate should be limited to those with severe deficiency (<20 IU/dL) or in mild deficiency (20–70 IU/dL) where there is a clear history of bleeding [38].

8.2.2.3 Tranexamic Acid
Tranexamic acid alone has been demonstrated to be sufficient to cover dental extractions in people with severe FXI deficiency [8]. It can be used in those with milder FXI deficiency (20–70 IU/dL) where bleeding is difficult to predict. However, tranexamic acid should not be used concurrently with FXI concentrate because of the potential thrombotic risk [38].

8.2.2.4 Recombinant Factor VIIa
Recombinant VIIa (rVIIa) has been used to cover surgery in FXI deficiency in order to overcome the potential risk of transfusion-transmitted infection. The dose used was 90 mcg/kg intravenously 2

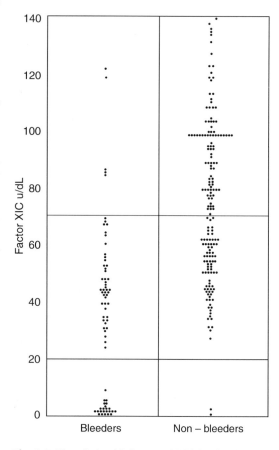

Fig. 8.4 The relationship between FXIC level and bleeding tendency. Pooled data from two UK studies [34, 35] – 249 individuals from 54 families transmitting factor XI deficiency. Of 128 heterozygotes, 45 (35 %) are bleeders. The *upper horizontal line* defines the lower limit of the normal range, and the lower line cut-off between severe and partial deficiency (From Bolton-Maggs [33])

hourly for the first 24 h, and 4 hourly for the second 24 h [41]. Low doses (30 mcg/kg) have recently been used and shown to effectively induce hemostasis in patients with FXI deficiency undergoing surgery [42]. Due to the unpredictable length of labor and short half-life of rFVIIa, its use is not practical to cover labor, but it has been used successfully to cover elective Caesarean section.

8.2.3   Genetic Counseling and Prenatal Diagnosis

Prenatal diagnosis should be offered to patients where there is a risk of severe deficiency [11]. A partner of a female with FXI deficiency should be offered screening with a FXIC assay.

There are a large number of different mutations [43, 44]. Thus, prenatal diagnosis may be difficult although Ashkenazi Jewish individuals exhibit two common mutations: type II, a stop codon in exon 5, and type III, a missense mutation in exon 9 leading to reduced expression of FXI.

8.2.4   Antenatal Management

Factor XI levels usually remain constant during pregnancy [45, 12, 46]. A study in London followed 61 pregnancies in 30 women, two with severe deficiency (FXI 2–8 IU/dL) and 28 with partial deficiency (FXI median 51 IU/dL, range 34–65 IU/dL). The median (range) prepregnancy and third trimester FXI levels were 55 (34–65) and 54 (37–75) IU/dL, respectively, in women with a partial deficiency, and 2 and 8 and 4 and 13 IU/dL in the two women with severe deficiency. Overall, the FXI levels did not change significantly during pregnancy ($p = 0.09$) [45]. Routine monitoring of FXI levels should ideally be carried out at booking, 28 and 34 weeks. The rate of miscarriage does not seem to be increased in these women [46], but they may be at increased risk of hemorrhage following miscarriage or termination of pregnancy, especially if there is a bleeding history [12, 46]. Therefore, consideration of prophylaxis with FXI concentrate or virally inactivated FFP should be given to those with severe FXI deficiency or a bleeding history for invasive procedures, such as CVS or amniocentesis, and termination of pregnancy. Probable "nonbleeders" can be managed expectantly, with treatment available [11].

8.2.5   Intrapartum Management

The risk of PPH can be reduced by active management of the third stage of labor and prophylactic use of FFP or FXI concentrate [47, 48, 12, 49]. In severe deficiency (FXI < 20 IU/dL), regardless of mode of delivery, we recommend FXI concentrate in a dose such that peak levels do not exceed 70 IU/dL (NR 70–150 IU/dL) or, if unavailable, FFP is given at the onset of labor, prior to induction or Caesarean section. For women with partial deficiency and a bleeding history, or no previous hemostatic challenge, tranexamic acid 1G 6–8 hourly intravenously during labor and orally postdelivery for 3 days is recommended. A "wait and watch" policy is advised for those with partial deficiency and no bleeding history despite hemostatic challenge [11]. The decision to give prophylactic cover for Caesarean section in women with partial deficiency should be individualized and dependent on bleeding history and type of anesthetic or analgesia [45, 50, 11].

8.2.6   Regional Analgesia and Anesthesia

Epidural anesthesia has been carried out in FXI-deficient women without complication [48, 12, 46]. A total of 60 women with inherited bleeding disorders have been identified in the English literature describing the use of regional block during labor and delivery, and there were no reported complications [45, 50]. If epidural is necessary, it should be covered with FXI concentrate – FFP contains a variable quantity of FXI and is not recommended [11]. Consideration can be given to the use of rFVIIa [52].

8.2.7 Postpartum Management

Women with FXI deficiency are at increased risk of postpartum hemorrhage [34, 12, 46]. A recent series documented obstetric outcome in 61 pregnancies in 30 women with FXI deficiency over 10 years (1997–2006) [46]. The rate of PPH was 11 % for both primary and secondary PPH but only 3 of the 10 PPH occurred after prophylaxis with factor XI concentrate or tranexamic acid was given – clearly prophylactic hemostatic support reduces PPH as the rate of primary PPH and secondary PPH has previously been reported as 16 % and 24 %, respectively, in untreated patients (Fig. 8.5; [45, 50, 12]). Prophylactic tranexamic acid in a dose of 1G 6 hourly should be considered for 3 days post vaginal delivery partum or 5 days following Caesarean section. Since the

half-life of FXI is 52 h [52], subsequent doses of FXI concentrate are rarely needed [11].

8.3 Hemophilia A and Hemophilia B

8.3.1 Inheritance

Hemophilia A and B are sex-linked recessive disorders with an incidence in male births of 1 in 5,000 and 1 in 30,000, respectively. The daughter of a male with hemophilia is an obligate carrier, and a carrier has a 50 % chance of passing the gene defect to her children – there is a 50 % chance of having an affected son and a 50 % chance of having a daughter who is a carrier (Fig. 8.6). Carriers may have a reduced clotting

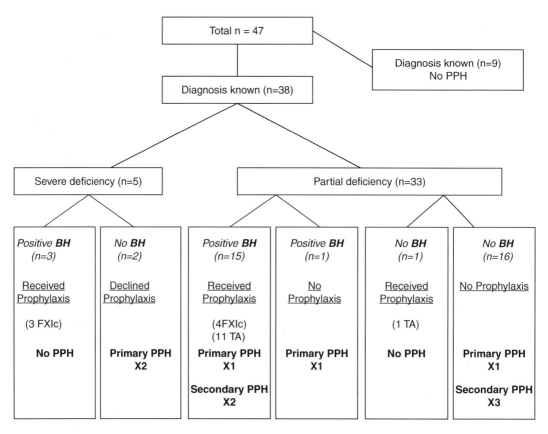

Fig. 8.5 The use of intrapartum prophylaxis and postpartum hemorrhage in women with FXI deficiency (From Chi et al. [44]). BH = bleeding history. TA = tranexamic acid

factor level but a wide range of values, 22–116 IU/dL, has been reported [53] because of the phenomenon of lyonization where there is random inactivation of one of the two X chromosomes [54]. Where there is extreme lyonization, the clotting factor level may be very low with an increased risk of bleeding. However, there is also an increased bleeding risk at mildly reduced clotting factor levels [55]. Management of carriers of hemophilia requires a multidisciplinary approach, and ideally they should be managed in a combined clinic with both expertise and facilities to provide a management plan [56].

8.3.2   Genetic Counseling and Carrier Detection

The purpose of genetic counseling is to provide the potential carrier and her parents or partner with the information required to reach a decision about carrier testing and prenatal diagnosis and to provide support during the process [57]. Genetic counseling for hemophilia includes discussion of the medical condition – the inheritance and treatment, personal and relationship concerns related to hemophilia, and beliefs and wishes of the person discussing possible inheritance, as well as others who might be affected [57]. A framework for genetic service provision has been provided as a guideline by the UK Haemophilia Centre Doctors' Organisation (UKHCDO) [58] (Table 8.1). The first step in carrier diagnosis is the family tree – the daughter of a man with hemophilia is an obligate carrier and her sons have a 50 % chance of having hemophilia and her daughters have a 50 % chance of being a carrier (Fig. 8.6). Within a family where an index patient with hemophilia has been identified, there may be many females at risk of being carriers. However, newly diagnosed cases of hemophilia may be sporadic – one study reported this as being 50 % of newly diagnosed cases [59]. However, in a mother of a sporadic case of hemophilia, there is the possibility of mosaicism – a mixture of normal and mutation-carrying cells. Carriership should be established before pregnancy and before prenatal diagnosis.

8.3.3   Testing the Carrier Status of Healthy Girls

There has been a review of the testing of healthy children for recessively inherited conditions [60]. The United Nations Convention on the Rights of the Child has declared that any action or decision affecting this group should be in their "best interests" [61]. The World Health Organization (WHO) has proposed that the reason for genetically testing children was to improve their medical care [62]. The British Medical Association (BMA) has presented a more flexible approach which suggests that the dynamics within the family should be taken into account when consider-

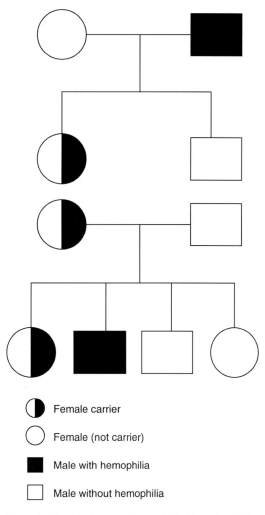

○) Female carrier

○ Female (not carrier)

■ Male with hemophilia

□ Male without hemophilia

Fig. 8.6 The inheritance of hemophilia (From Lee [56])

Table 8.1 Counseling and consent for genetic testing in hemophilia

Establish that hemophilia is present in the family and determine its type and severity
Establish family pedigree(tree) to identify possible or definite (obligate) carriers
Provide a full explanation of the potential clinical effects of being a hemophilia carrier or affected male
Provide a full explanation of mode of inheritance of hemophilia
Discuss the rationale for identifying the genetic defect in patients with hemophilia
Outline the means by which carrier status is assessed
Discuss what is involved in genetic testing: sample collection, transfer/storage of data, research projects on stored material, insurance issues, and risk of error
If appropriate, advise on the techniques for prenatal testing
Provide an opportunity to ask questions
Provide an opportunity for the individual being consulted to present her understanding of the information that has been discussed
Provide patient information sheet and an opportunity for follow-up appointment

From Lee [56]

ing carrier testing of children [9]. A systematic review of guidelines and position papers has found that, although there were some exceptions, there was general agreement to wait until children can give informed consent for themselves [9].

In a study considering "the attitudes towards and beliefs about genetic testing in the hemophilia community," female carriers and family members thought testing was necessary for adolescent girls to determine carrier status [60].

Women who are hemophilia carriers may have a low level of FVIII or IX, and it is therefore recommended that the respective clotting factor is measured in young obligate carriers [58]. The ethical debate is redundant in this situation.

8.3.4 Genetic Diagnosis

It is now possible to perform genetic diagnosis for the specific mutation causing hemophilia in a family. In severe hemophilia A, approximately

50 % of families carry an inversion of intron 22 which is a rearrangement of the long arm of the X chromosome [63]. In this situation, it may be possible to establish carriership without knowledge of the mutation in the index member of the family. For most potential carriers, it is necessary to know the mutation in the index family member, and mutations for hemophilia A are listed on the HAMSTeRS database (http://europium.csc.mrc.ac.uk). In hemophilia B, almost all families have a unique mutation, and in the UK most of these are identified [64].

8.3.5 Reproductive Options

The options possible for families known to be at risk of transmitting an inherited bleeding disorder include:
- Conceiving naturally, having prenatal diagnosis (PND), and the option of terminating an affected fetus
- Taking the risk and consequences of having an affected child
- Not having a child
- Adoption
- Assisted conception with egg donation
- Assisted conception with preimplantation diagnosis (PGD)

The decision will be influenced by ethnic and cultural issues, the severity of hemophilia in the family, and the personal and family experience of the disorder [65].

8.3.6 Prenatal Diagnosis

The noninvasive determination of fetal sex is now often possible in the first trimester through the analysis of free fetal DNA in the maternal circulation and/or ultrasound examination of the fetal genital tubercle [66]. This means that invasive prenatal diagnostic tests can usually be avoided in female pregnancies. Chorionic villus sampling (CVS) is the most widely used method in the prenatal diagnosis of hemophilia. It is important to arrange prophylactic treatment with clotting factor concentrate if the clotting factor level is <50 IU/dL. Since invasive testing may cause feto-maternal hemorrhage, anti-D should be given to Rhesus D-negative mothers. CVS is performed between 11 and 14 weeks' gestation under ultrasound guidance to obtain a sample of placenta for genetic analysis. It is associated with a 1–2 % risk of miscarriage [67]. CVS should not be performed before 10 weeks' gestation because of the risk of fetal limb deformity [68, 69]. Amniocentesis can also be used for PND – this is usually performed between 15 and 18 weeks of gestation. Fetal cells within the amniotic fluid can be sexed by in situ hybridization (FISH), and/or DNA can be extracted for PCR-based linkage analysis or mutation detection [70]. Cordocentesis or percutaneous umbilical cord sampling can be performed to measure the FVIII or FIX – this is considered if the causative mutation in the family is unknown. There is a 1–2 % risk of fetal loss [71] and probably increased if the fetus has a bleeding tendency, so this is not commonly performed.

Preimplantation Genetic Diagnosis (PGD) uses in vitro fertilization (IVF) to create embryos. One or two cells from each fertilized embryo are tested for the specific genetic diagnosis, and unaffected embryos are identified for transfer to the uterus. In hemophilia the technique was initially used for diagnosis of fetal sex, but there are reports of specific diagnosis [72]. However, IVF is expensive, invasive and stressful, and the success rate is lower than for spontaneous conception [73].

8.3.7 Management of Pregnancy

The FVIII levels increase in carriers of hemophilia A during pregnancy, and most carriers will have a normal FVIII level (>50 IU/dL) at term. In contrast, FIX levels do not change during pregnancy [74]. Clotting factor levels should be checked at booking, 28 and 34 weeks, and prophylaxis should be given to cover invasive procedures when the level is <50 IU/dL [11].

8.3.8 Management of Delivery

For women with low factor levels, intravenous access should be established, the third stage of labor should be actively managed, and prophylactic treatment should be given to cover labor and delivery when the clotting factor level is <50 IU/dL. Invasive intrapartum monitoring techniques, such as fetal scalp blood sampling and application of a fetal scalp electrode, should be avoided. The risk factors for cranial bleeding in affected newborns include prolonged labor and instrumental delivery, particularly vacuum (ventouse) extraction, which can cause cephalhematoma, or the use of high or rotational forceps. Potentially difficult instrumental delivery (high or rotational forceps) should be avoided because of the risk of intracranial bleeding in an affected baby, and there should be a low threshold for early recourse to Caesarean section. However, instrumental delivery is not completely contraindicated; there are some situations where an easy "lift-out" forceps delivery may be safer for an affected baby than a difficult Caesarean delivery of a head deeply impacted in the pelvis. It is important that a cord plasma sample is obtained to measure FVIII or FIX levels in order to make or exclude a diagnosis of hemophilia.

After birth, IM injections for the baby should be avoided until the results of the cord blood factor levels are known (results should be requested urgently). The first dose of vitamin K should therefore be given orally. Circumcision should not be performed unless and until factor levels in the baby have been shown to be normal. These factor levels should be rechecked when the baby is 2–3 months old in order to establish its true status.

8.3.9 Regional Analgesia and Anesthesia

The management plan should be made in consultation with the anesthetist prior to labor. The use of regional blockade is of some concern because of the potential risk of epidural or spinal hemorrhage and hematoma. However, provided the clotting factor level is >50 IU/dL, regional block is not contraindicated and has been shown to be safe [50]. It is important to check clotting factor levels prior to removal of the epidural catheter because the pregnancy-induced rise in FVIII is reversed after delivery.

8.3.10 Postpartum Management

The incidence of primary and secondary PPH has been reported as 22 and 11 %, respectively [75] compared to 5–8 and 0.8 % in the general population (in whom routine prophylactic oxytocics are used). Therefore, the factor level should ideally be checked after delivery, and it should be maintained at >50 IU/dL. Tranexamic acid can be used to treat heavy lochia, if necessary [70].

Learning Points
- Obstetric management of women with VWD and FXI deficiency and carriers of hemophilia requires a multidisciplinary team approach with obstetricians, midwives, hematologists, anesthetists, and neonatologists.
- Women in families with such inherited bleeding disorders should undergo diagnostic (carrier) testing before becoming pregnant in order to allow appropriate preconception counseling and timely provision of prenatal diagnosis, especially in those who could potentially carry a severely affected baby.
- Women with VWD and FXI deficiency and carriers of hemophilia are at risk of postpartum hemorrhage, especially those with low factor (>50 iu/dL) levels at term. Appropriate hemostatic cover, based on the mother's factor level, her bleeding tendency, and mode of

delivery, minimizes the risk, and the third stage of labor should be actively managed.
- Regional block is not contraindicated in these women provided the clotting defects have normalized during pregnancy or been corrected by replacement therapy. The decision should be made on an individual basis prior to labor after careful evaluation of the potential risks and benefits.
- Affected newborns are also at risk of bleeding during the process of birth. Cranial bleeding, including cephalhematoma and intracranial hemorrhage, is the most common and serious site. Thus, very prolonged labor and difficult instrumental delivery, in particular vacuum extraction, should be avoided, and delivery achieved by the least traumatic method with early recourse to Caesarean section.
- Umbilical cord blood should be taken at birth to measure factor levels in the baby. IM injections and surgical procedures, including circumcision, should be avoided until the levels are known to be normal.

Case Study 1
A 23-year-old Caucasian woman registered with our hemophilia center with severe type 1 VWD (VWF:Ag = 5 IU/dL, VWF:Ac = 4 IU/dL, FVIII = 10 IU/dL at diagnosis) reported pregnant at 5 weeks' gestation in her first pregnancy. She was from a traveler family and decided against medical advice to travel to Italy with her husband during pregnancy due to her worries about infection with swine flu in the UK. She did not have regular antenatal care in Italy and had repeated episodes of mild to moderate vaginal bleeding during pregnancy that was managed with tranexamic acid (TA). At 32 weeks' gestation, she had a significant antepartum hemorrhage and required factor replacement therapy. After discharge form hospital in Italy, she returned to London and reported to our center. The scan showed

normal fetal well-being and a posterior high placenta. Her factor levels were unchanged from prepregnancy, and her bleeding was minimal. We managed her with TA 1 g 6 hourly with the plan to give factor replacement if the bleeding increased.

For delivery, it was planned to continue TA and start factor replacement with the first sign of labor, aiming to maintain her VWF and FVIII above 50 IU/dL for at least 2 weeks. She presented in spontaneous labor at 39 weeks of gestation and during labor was managed according to the plan. She progressed well, did not require epidural analgesia, and delivered a girl by vaginal delivery with the aid of an episiotomy.

The third stage of labor was actively managed, and she also received misoprostol 600 mcg rectally prophylactically after delivery of the placenta. Her episiotomy was sutured without any complications. She required twice daily factor replacement. On day 3 postpartum, her TA was stopped, and her factor replacement was reduced to once daily by the on-call team, contrary to the plan of management provided by the joint hemophilia/obstetric team, due to concerns of an increased risk of thrombosis.

On day 4, she had an episode of severe secondary PPH, requiring a 4-unit red cell transfusion, uterine balloon insertion, and vaginal packing. Her factor levels had dropped to 28 IU/dL. TA and twice daily factor replacement were restarted. She recovered well and was discharged home on day 7 on TA and once daily factor replacement. Her hemoglobin was 9.5 g/dL and she was given iron therapy. Three weeks after delivery, her lochia had reduced but remained moderate. Factor replacement was reduced to twice weekly until 5 weeks postdelivery. A combined oral contraceptive pill was then started and her factor replacement stopped. She continued taking TA 1 g 6 hourly until her lochia had completely stopped.

On review at 8 weeks, she had stopped bleeding, and her hemoglobin had risen to 10.9 g/dL. Her daughter was progressing well. Her cord blood factor level was borderline. It was advised that mild VWD could not be excluded and that repeat testing would be organized at a later stage and to inform the center if there was any concern regarding bleeding in her daughter.

Case Study 2

A 30-year-old carrier of hemophilia A was in her first pregnancy. Free fetal DNA testing at 10 weeks' gestation showed a male fetus. The mother declined CVS and was aware that there was a 50 % chance of her son being affected. Her prepregnancy FVIII level was 38 IU/dL. The pregnancy progressed without any complication, and her third trimester FVIII level normalized, rising to 140 IU/dL. She was therefore advised that there would be no need for hemostatic cover for labor and delivery, including for regional block.

She did not go into spontaneous labor by 42 weeks of gestation, so her cervix was assessed by ultrasound scan and reported to be 3.8 cm long and closed. The woman was counseled about induction of labor and the high chance of prolonged labor and operative delivery when the cervix is >3 cm long in a primip at the start of induction. She was aware that her unborn son had a 50 % chance of being affected, thus very prolonged labor and, in particular, difficult operative delivery needed to be avoided to avoid the risk of cranial bleeding. Following this counseling, the mother opted for an elective Caesarean section. This was performed under combined spinal/epidural block without any complications. Her estimated blood loss during delivery was 400 mL. Cord blood confirmed her son to be affected with severe hemophilia A.

References

1. von Willebrand EA. Hereditar pseudohenofili. Finska lakarsallskapets Handl. 1926;67:7–112.
2. Rodeghiero F, Castaman G, Dini E. Epidemiological investigation of the prevalence of von Willebrand's disease. Blood. 1987;69:454–9.
3. James AH, Jamison MG. Bleeding events and other complications during pregnancy and childbirth in women with von Willebrand disease. J Thromb Haemost. 2007;5:1165–9.
4. Sadler JE, Mannucci PM, Berntorp E, Bochkov N, Meyer D, Peake I, Rodeghiero F, Srivastava A. Impact, diagnosis and treatment of von Willebrand disease. Thromb Haemost. 2000 Aug;84(2):160–74.
5. Kadir RA, Economides DL, Sabin CA, Pollard D, Lee CA. Variations in coagulation factors in women: effects of age, ethnicity, menstrual cycle and combined oral contraceptive. Thromb Haemost. 1999;82: 1456–61.
6. Rodgiero F, Castaman G. von Willebrand Disease: epidemiology. In: Lee CA, Berntorp EE, Hoots WK, editors. Textbook of hemophilia. 2nd ed. London: Wiley-Blackwell; 2010. p. 286–93.
7. Sadler JE, Budde U, Eikenboom JC, Favaloro EJ, Hill FG, Holmberg L, Ingerslev J, Lee CA, Lillicrap D, Mannucci PM, Mazurier C, Meyer D, Nichols WL, Nishino M, Peake IR, Rodeghiero F, Schneppenheim R, Ruggeri ZM, Srivastava A, Montgomery RR, Federici AB; Working Party on von Willebrand Disease Classification. Update on the pathophysiology and classification of von Willebrand disease: a report of the Subcommittee on von Willebrand Factor. J Thromb Haemost. 2006 Oct;4(10):2103–14.
8. Berliner S, Horowitz I, Martinowitz U, Brenner B, Seligsohn U. Dental surgery in patients with severe factor XI deficiency without plasma replacement. Blood Coagul Fibrinolysis. 1992;3:465–74.
9. BMA. Consent, rights and choices in health care for children and young people. London: BMJ Books; 2001.
10. Lak M, Peyvandi F, Mannucci PM. Clinical manifestations and complications of childbirth and replacement therapy in 385 Iranian patients with type 3 von Willebrand disease. Br J Haematol. 2000;4:1236–9.
11. Lee CA, Chi C, Pavord SR, Bolton-Maggs PHB, Pollard D, Hinchcliffe-Wood A, Kadir RA. The obstetric and gynaecological management of women with inherited bleeding disorders – review with guidelines produced by a taskforce of UK Haemophilia Centre Doctors' Organisation. Haemophilia. 2006;12:301–36.
12. Kadir RA, Lee CA, Sabin CA, Pollard D, Economides DL. Pregnancy in women with von Willebrand's disease or factor XI deficiency. BJOG. 1998;105:314–21.
13. Stirling Y, Woolf L, North WR, Seghatchian MJ, Meade TW. Haemostasis in normal pregnancy. Thromb Haemost. 1984;52:176–82.
14. Ramsahoye BH, Davies SV, Dasani H, Pearson JF. Obstetric management in von Willebrand's disease: a report of 24 pregnancies and a review of the literature. Haemophilia 1995;1:140–144.
15. Rick ME, Williams SB, Sacher RA, McKeown LP. Thrombocytopenia associated with pregnancy in a patient with type IIB von Willebrand disease. Blood. 1987;69:786–9.
16. Caliezi C, Tsakiris DA, Behringer H, Kuhne T, Marbet GA. Two consecutive pregnancies and deliveries in a patient with von Willebrand's disease type 3. Haemophilia. 1998;4:845–9.
17. James AH, Kouides PA, Kadir RA, et al. von Willebrand disease and other bleeding disorders in women: consensus on diagnosis and management from an international panel. Am J Obstet Gynecol. 2009;201:12.e1–8.
18. Steer C, Campbell S, Davies M, Mason B, Collins W. Spontaneous abortion rates after natural and assisted conception. BMJ. 1989;299:1317–8.
19. Foster PA. The reproductive health of women with von Willebrand disease unresponsive to DDAVP: the results of an international survey. On behalf of the subcommittee on VWF of the SSC of the ISTH. Thromb Haemost. 1995;74:784–90.
20. Cohen AJ, Kessler CM, Ewenstein BM. Management of von Willebrand disease: a survey on the current clinical practice from the haemophilia centres of North America. Haemophilia. 2001;7:235–41.
21. Mannucci PM. How I treat patients with von Willebrand disease. Blood. 2001;97:1915–9.
22. Sanchez-Luceros A, Meschengieser SS, Turdo K, et al. Evaluation of desmopressin during pregnancy in women with low plasmatic von Willebrand factor level and bleeding history. Thromb Res. 2007;120:387–90.
23. Castaman G, Tosetto A, Rodeghiero F. Pregnancy and delivery in women with von Willebrand disease and different von Willebrand factor mutations. Abstract As-Mo-029 XXII congress ISTH, Boston, 2009.
24. Dennis MW, Clough V, Toh CH.Unexpected presentation of type 2N von Willebrand disease in pregnancy. Haemophilia. 2000 Nov;6(6):696–7.
25. Greer IA, Lowe GD, Walker JJ, Forbes CC. Haemorrhagic problems in obstetrics and gynaecology in patients with congenital coagulopathies. BJOG. 1991; 98:909–18.
26. Hanna W, McCarroll D, McDonald T, et al. Variant von Willebrand disease and pregnancy. Blood. 1981; 58:873–9.
27. Roque H, Funai E, Lockwood CJ. von Willebrand disease and pregnancy. J Matern Fetal Med. 2000;9: 257–66.
28. Chi C, Bapir M, Lee CA, Kadir RA. Puerperal loss (lochia) in women with or without inherited bleeding disorders. Am J Obstet Gynecol. 2010;203(1):56.e1–5.
29. Rosenthal RL, Dreskin OH, Rosenthal N. New hemophilia-like disease caused by deficiency of a third plasma thromboplastin factor. Proc Soc Exp Biol Med. 1953;82:171–4.

30. Seligsohn U, Bolton-Maggs PH. Factor XI deficiency. In: Lee CA, Berntorp EE, Hoots WK, editors. Textbook of hemophilia. 2nd ed. London: Wiley-Blackwell; 2010. p. 355–61.
31. Rapaport SI, Proctor RR, Patch NJ, Yettra M. The role of inheritance of PTA deficiency: evidence for the existence of major PTA deficiency and minor PTA deficiency. Blood. 1961;18:149–65.
32. Seligsohn U. Factor XI deficiency. Thromb Haemost. 1993;70:68–71.
33. Bolton-Maggs PHB. Factor XI deficiency. In: Lee CA, editor. Bailliere's clinical haematology: haemophilia. London: Bailliere Tindall; 1996. p. 356–67.
34. Bolton-Maggs PH, Young Wan-Yin B, McCraw AH, Slack J, Kernoff PB. Inheritance and bleeding in factor XI deficiency. Br J Haematol. 1988;69:521–8.
35. Bolton-Maggs PH, Patterson DA, Wensley RT, Tuddenham EG. Definition of bleeding tendency in factor-XI deficient kindred's – a clinical and laboratory study. Thromb Haemost. 1995;73:194–202.
36. Bolton-Maggs PHB. The management of factor XI deficiency. Haemophilia. 1998;4:683–8.
37. Bolton-Maggs PH, Perry DJ, Chalmers EA, Parapia LA, Wilde JT, Williams MD. The rare coagulation disorders – review with guidelines for management from the UK Doctors' Organisation. Haemophilia. 2004;10:593–628.
38. Keeling D, Tait C, Makris M. Guideline on the selection and use of therapeutic products to treat haemophilia and other hereditary bleeding disorders. Haemophilia. 2008;14:671–84.
39. Peden A, Fairfoul G, Lowrie S, McCardle L, Head MW, Love S, Ward HJT, Cousens SN, Keeling D, Millar CM, Hill FGH, Ironside JW. Variant CJD infection in the spleen of an asymptomatic adult patient with haemophilia. Haemophilia. 2010; 16:296–304.
40. Bolton-Maggs PH, Colvin BT, Satchi BT, Lee CA, Lucas GS. Thrombogenic potential of factor XI concentrate. Lancet. 1994 Sep 10;344(8924):748–9.
41. O'Connell NM, Riddell AF, Pascoe G, Perry DJ, Lee CA. Recombinant factor VIIa to prevent surgical bleeding in factor XI deficiency. Haemophilia. 2008; 14:775–81.
42. Kenet G, Lubetsky A, Luboshitz J, Ravid B, Tamarin I, Varon D, Martinowitz U. Lower doses of rFVIIa therapy are safe and effective for surgical interventions in patients with severe FXI deficiency and inhibitors. Haemophilia. 2009;15(5):1065–73. Epub 2009 May 26.
43. Seligsohn U. Factor XI deficiency in humans. J Thromb Haemost. 2009 Jul;7 Suppl 1:84–7.
44. O'Connell NM. Factor XI deficiency. Semin Hematol. 2004;41:76–81.
45. Chi C, Kulkarni A, Lee CA, Kadir RA. The obstetric experience of women with factor XI deficiency. Acta Obstet Gynecol. 2009;1:1–6.
46. Myers B, Pavord S, Kean L, Hill M, Dolan G. Pregnancy outcome in factor XI deficiency: incidence of miscarriage, antenatal and postnatal haemorrhage in 33 women with FXI deficiency. BJOG. 2007;114:643–6.
47. Collins P, Goldman E, Lilley P, Pasi KJ, Lee CA, et al. Clinical experience of factor XI deficiency: the role of fresh frozen plasma and factor XI concentrate. Haemophilia. 1995;1:227–31.
48. David AL, Paterson-Brown S, Letsky EA. Factor XI deficiency presenting in pregnancy: diagnosis and management. BJOG. 2002;109:840–3.
49. Mavromatidis G, Dinas K, Delkos D, Goutzioulis F, Vosnakis C, Hatzipantelis E. Uneventful caesarean delivery with administration of factor XI concentrate in a patient with severe factor XI deficiency. Int J Hematol. 2007;86:222–4.
50. Chi C, Lee CA, England A, Hingorani J, Paintsil J, Kadir RA. Obstetric analgesia and anaesthesia in women with inherited bleeding disorders. Thromb Haemost. 2009;101:1104–11.
51. O'Connell NM, Riddell AF, Pascoe G, Perry DJ, Lee CA. Recombinant factor VIIa to prevent surgical bleeding in factor XI deficiency. Haemophilia. 2008 Jul;14(4):775–81.
52. Bolton-Maggs PH, Wensley RT, Kernoff PB, et al. Production and therapeutic use of a factor XI concentrate from plasma. Thromb Haemost. 1992;67:314–9.
53. Rizza CR, Rhymes IL, Austen DE, Kernoff PB, Aroni SA. Detection of carriers of haemophilia: a 'blind' study. Br J Haematol. 1975;30:447–56.
54. Lyon MF. Chromatin and gene action in the mammalian X-chromosome. Am J Hum Genet. 1962;14:135–48.
55. Plug I, Mauser-Bunschoten EP, Brocker-Vriends AH, van Amstel HK, van der Bom JG, van Diemen-Homan JE, Willemse J, Rosendaal FR. Bleeding in carriers of haemophilia. Blood. 2008;111:1811–5.
56. Lee CA, Chi C, Shiltagh N, Pollard D, Griffioen A, Dunn N, Kadir RA. Review of a multidisciplinary clinic for women with inherited bleeding disorders. Haemophilia. 2009;15:359–60.
57. Miller R. Genetic counselling for haemophilia. WFH treatment monograph 2002; No 25 World Federation of haemophilia www.wfh.org.
58. Ludlam CA, Pasi KJ, Bolton-Maggs P, Collins P, Cumming AM, Dolan G. A framework for genetic service provision for haemophilia and other inherited bleeding disorders. Haemophilia. 2005;11:145–63.
59. Ljund R, Petrini P, Nilsson IM. Diagnostic symptoms of severe and moderate haemophilia A and B – a survey of 140 cases. Acta Paediatr Scand. 1990;79:196–200.
60. Dunn NF, Miller R, Griffioen A, Lee CA. Carrier testing in haemophilia A and B: adult carriers and their partners experiences and their views on the testing of young females. Haemophilia. 2008;14:584–92.
61. United Nations Convention on the Rights of the Child 20. Xi. 1989: TS 44: Cm 1976 http://www.un.org/Docs/journal/asp/ws.asp?m=A/RES/44/25.
62. World Health Organisation. Proposed international guidelines on ethical issues in medical genetics and genetic services. Geneva: World Health Organisation; 1998. p. 1998.

63. Antonarakis S, Rossiter JP, Young M, Horst J, de Moerloose P, Sommer SS, Ketterling RP, et al. Factor VIII gene inversions in severe hemophilia A: results of an international consortium study. Blood. 1995;86:2206–12.

64. Giannelli F, Green PM, Somner S. Haemophilia B (sixth edition); a database of point mutations and short editions and deletions. Nucleic Acids Res. 1996;24:103–18.

65. Kadir RA, Sabin C, Gouldman E, Pollard D, Lee C, Economides DL. Reproductive experience and attitude of carriers of haemophilia. Haemophilia. 2000;6:33–40.

66. Chi C, Hyett JA, Finning KM, Lee CA, Kadir RA. Non-invasive first trimester determination of fetal gender: a new approach for prenatal diagnosis of haemophilia. BJOG. 2006;113:239–42.

67. Mujezinovic F, Alfirevic Z. Procedure-related complications of amniocentesis and chorionic villous sampling: a systematic review. Obstet Gynecol. 2007;110: 687–94.

68. Firth HV, Boyd PA, Chamberlain PF, et al. Analysis of limb reduction defects in babies exposed to chorionic villus sampling. Lancet. 1994;343:1069–71.

69. RCOG. Amniocentesis and chorionic villus sampling. Green-top Guideline No. 8. London; RCOG: 2005.

70. Kadir RA, Lee CA. Obstetrics and gynaecology: haemophilia. In: Lee CA, Berntorp EE, Hoots WK, editors. Textbook of hemophilia. 2nd ed. London: Wiley-Blackwell; 2010. p. 355–61.

71. Buscaglia M, Ghisoni L, Bellotti M, et al. Percutaneous umbilical blood sampling: indication changes and procedure loss rate in a nine years' experience. Fetal Diagn Ther. 1996;11:106–13.

72. Michaelides K, Tuddenham EG, Turner C, Lavender B, Lavery SA. Live birth following the first mutation specific pre-implantation genetic diagnosis. Thromb Haemost. 2006;95:373–9.

73. Human Fertilization and Embryology Authority. HFEA guide to infertility and directory of clinics 2005/6. London: Human Fertilisation and Embryology Authority; 2006.

74. Chi C, Lee CA, Shiltagh N, Khan A, Pollard D, Kadir RA. Pregnancy in carriers of haemophilia. Haemophilia. 2008;14:56–64.

75. Kadir RA, Economides DL, Braithwaite J, Goldman E, Lee CA. The obstetric experience of carriers of haemophilia. BJOG. 1997;104:803–10.

76. Caliezi C, Tsakiris DA, Behringer H, Kuhne T, Marbet GA; Jones BP, Bell EA, Maroof M. Epidural labor analgesia in a parturient with von Willebrand's disease type IIA and severe preeclampsia. Anesthesiology 1999;90:1219–1220.

77. Milaskiewicz RM, Holdcroft A, Letsky E. Epidural anaesthesia and von Willebrand's disease. Anaesthesia 1990;45:462–464.

78. Cohen S, Daitch JS, Amar D, Goldiner PL. Epidural analgesia for labor and delivery in a patient with von Willebrand's disease. Reg Anesth 1989;14:95–97.

79. Caliezi C, Tsakiris DA, Behringer H, Kühne T, Marbet GA. Two consecutive pregnancies and deliveries in a patient with von Willebrand's disease type 3. Haemophilia 1998;4(6):845–849.

80. Kadir RA, Lee CA, Sabin CA, Pollard D, Economides DL. Pregnancy in women with von Willebrand's disease or factor XI deficiency. Br J Obstet Gynaecol 1998;105:314–32.

81. Pasi KJ, Collins PW, Keeling DM et al. Management of von Willebrand disease: a guideline from the UK Haemophilia Centre Doctors' Organization. Haemophilia 2004;10:218–231.

Inherited Bleeding Disorders in Pregnancy: Rare Coagulation Factor Defects

9

Flora Peyvandi, Marzia Menegatti, and Simona Maria Siboni

Abstract

Inherited deficiencies of plasma proteins involved in blood coagulation generally lead to lifelong bleeding disorders. Rare bleeding disorders (RBDs), discussed in this chapter, represent 3–5 % of all the inherited coagulation deficiencies, with prevalence ranging from approximately 1:500,000 to 1:2,000,000 in the general population. Patients affected by bleeding disorders present a wide spectrum of clinical symptoms that vary from a mild or moderate bleeding tendency to significant episodes. Women with inherited bleeding disorders are particularly disadvantaged since, in addition to suffering from general bleeding symptoms, they are also at risk of bleeding complications from regular haemostatic challenges during menstruation, pregnancy and childbirth. Moreover, such disorders pose important problems for affected women due to their reduced quality of life caused by limitations in activities and work, and alteration of their reproductive life. Management of these women is difficult because of considerable inter-individual variation. Furthermore, reliable information on clinical management is scarce, with only a few long-term prospective studies of large cohorts providing evidence to guide diagnosis and treatment.

9.1 Introduction

Inherited deficiencies of plasma proteins involved in blood coagulation generally lead to lifelong bleeding disorders, whose severity is directly pro-

F. Peyvandi, MD, PhD (✉) • M. Menegatti, PhD
S.M. Siboni, MD
A. Bianchi Bonomi Hemophilia and Thrombosis Center,
Fondazione IRCCS Cá Granda Ospedale Maggiore
Policlinico, and Dipartimento di Fisiopatologia
Medico-Chirurgica e dei Trapianti, Università degli Studi
di Milano and Luigi Villa Foundation,
Milan, Italy
e-mail: flora.peyvandi@unimi.it; f.payvandi@ucl.ac.uk

portional to the degree of factor deficiency (less factor/more severe bleeding tendency). Hemophilia A and B are the most frequently inherited bleeding disorders and, together with von Willebrand disease (VWD), a defect of primary hemostasis associated with a secondary defect in coagulation factor VIII (FVIII), comprise 95–97 % of all the inherited deficiencies of coagulation factors. The remaining defects, named rare bleeding disorders (RBDs) represent 3–5 % of all the inherited coagulation deficiencies, with their prevalence ranging from approximately 1:500,000 to 1:2,000,000 in the general population [1]. The RBDs include the

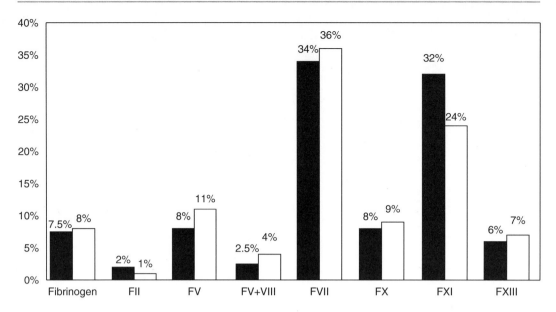

Fig. 9.1 Prevalence of RBDs according to WFH 2008 survey (*closed bars*) and EN-RBD (www.rbdd.eu) (*open bars*)

inherited deficiencies of fibrinogen, factor (F) II, FV, FV+FVIII, FVII, FX, FXI, and FXIII. They are usually transmitted as autosomal recessive traits, meaning that women represent about half of the affected patients. The prevalence of homozygous or double heterozygous patients, who generally carry the most severe form of the disease, is usually low in the general population [2]. However, in countries where consanguineous marriages are practiced such as Africa, India, and the Middle East, the number of affected patients seems 8–10-fold higher, representing a significant burden for public health, with greater demand for diagnosis and treatment [3]. Recent immigration from these countries to Europe has also increased the demand for diagnosis and treatment in this region of the world.

Information on the worldwide prevalence of RBDs can be derived from the data collected by the European Network of RBDs (EN-RBD: www.rbdd.eu) [4] and the World Federation of Hemophilia (WFH) global survey, showing that FVII and FXI deficiencies are the most prevalent RBDs representing 34 and 32 % of the total number of affected patients respectively, followed by the deficiencies of fibrinogen, FV and FX (7.5–8 %), FXIII (6 %), the rarest disorders being FII, and FV+FVIII deficiencies (2–2.5 %) (Fig. 9.1).

Due to the rarity of RBDs, the available information on their clinical severity, including symptoms, laboratory measurements, and type of treatment, are still limited, because only a few centers follow and manage a significant number of patients. Accordingly, scientific reports are usually limited to small groups of patients or even single cases. Even the most reliable registries designed to gather detailed information are limited to single aspects of the disease (clinical or therapeutic) or to the analysis of a single RBD.

The management of patients during bleeding episodes remains a challenge due to the scant availability of specific evidence-based guidelines for treatment of RBDs patients and the limited availability of specific factor concentrates. The lack of adequate information on several aspects of RBDs makes it very difficult to prepare evidence-based guidelines for the diagnosis and treatment of affected patients.

9.2 Classification of RBDs

Most RBDs are expressed phenotypically as a parallel reduction of plasma factors measured by functional assays and immunoassays (so-called type I deficiencies). Qualitative defects, characterized by normal, slightly reduced, or increased levels of factor antigen contrasting with much lower or undetectable functional activity (type II), are less frequent [2]. Regarding fibrinogen and prothrombin deficiency, quantitative defects are expressed by afibrinogenemia (as <10 mg/dL) or hypofibrinogenemia (10–50 mg/dL) and hypoprothrombinemia respectively (total absence of prothrombin is not compatible with life and no patient with <5 % of prothrombin level has been reported [5]). Qualitative defects are expressed by dysfibrinogenemia and dysprothrombinemia.

9.3   Clinical Symptoms

Patients affected by RBDs present with a wide spectrum of clinical symptoms that vary from a mild or moderate bleeding tendency to significant bleeding episodes and with different patterns among RBDs. Mucosal tract bleeding is the most frequently reported type of symptom, whereas spontaneous life-threatening manifestations such as central nervous system (CNS), gastrointestinal (GI), and musculoskeletal bleeding are relatively more frequent in patients with some specific deficiencies such as afibrinogenemia, severe FX or FXIII deficiency [2, 6–13]. A sign reported to be common to all RBDs is the occurrence of excessive bleeding at the time of surgical procedures [2, 6–13].

Women affected by RBDs are particularly disadvantaged because in addition to suffering from these bleeding symptoms, they may also experience excessive monthly bleeding associated with menstruation. Menorrhagia, defined as blood loss of more than 80 mL per menstruation, is reported to be one of the most important symptoms in women affected with RBDs [14, 15]. Menstruation may be a source of inconvenience to women in general but is significantly more problematic for women affected with coagulation disorders who have excessive blood loss, which can have a major impact on their quality of life and employment. Many women do not go out at all during their periods, avoiding activities such as working, taking part in sports, traveling, and studying. Menorrhagia is not the only gynecological problem that women with RBDs are more likely to

experience, they are also at risk of increased bleeding in conditions such as hemorrhagic ovarian cysts, endometriosis, endometrial hyperplasia, polyps, and fibroids [14].

Pregnancy and childbirth, two important stages in the life of a woman, pose particular clinical challenges in women with RBDs, since information about these issues are very scarce and limited to just a few case reports. Pregnancy is accompanied by increased concentrations of fibrinogen, FVII, FVIII, FX, and von Willebrand factor, particularly marked in the third trimester [16–20]. At variance, FII, FV, FIX, and FXIII are relatively unchanged [16]. The active, unbound form of free protein S is decreased during pregnancy secondary to increased levels of its binding protein, the complement component C4b [19, 21]. Plasminogen activator inhibitor type 1 (PAI-1) levels are increased [22]. All of these changes contribute to the hypercoagulable state of pregnancy and, in women with RBDs, contribute to improved hemostasis. Despite improved hemostasis, however, women with factor deficiencies do not achieve the same factor levels as those of women without factor deficiencies [14], increasing the possibility of pregnancy loss or bleeding complications, especially if the defect is severe.

Detailed information about the pregnancy, pregnancy complication, and the management of women with RBDs is limited and often, apart from FXI deficiency [23, 24] (addressed in detail in Chapter 8), derived from small series or case reports. For FV + FVIII deficiency, no data have been reported in relation to pregnancy; the obstetric experience of women with FV deficiency could probably serve as a guide. In this chapter, a summary of the information currently available on complications of pregnancy in women with RBDs are reported.

9.3.1   Miscarriages

Miscarriage is common in the general population, with at least 12–13.5 % of recognized pregnancies resulting in spontaneous miscarriage [25, 26]. An increased risk of miscarriage and placental abruption resulting in recurrent fetal loss or premature delivery among women with afibrinogenemia [7, 27, 28] or FXIII deficiency [29, 30] has been reported. A study of the Scientific and Standardization Committee of the International Society on Thrombosis and Haemostasis (ISTH) reported a high incidence of spontaneous miscarriage (38 %) and also stillbirth in 15 women with 64 reported pregnancies fulfilling the criteria of familial dysfibrinogenemia and thrombosis not due to other causes [31]. It is generally believed that women with bleeding disorders are protected from miscarriage by the hypercoagulable state of pregnancy, but whether women with bleeding disorders other than familial dysfibrinogenaemia have an increased risk of miscarriage is unclear. Only two reports describe miscarriages: the first a case report of miscarriages in four out of eight pregnancies in a hypoprothrombinemic woman [32]; and the second, excessive bleeding after two early pregnancy losses in a series including ten pregnancies in four women affected with FVII deficiency [33]. Similarly, Kumar and Mehta reported four pregnancies in a woman with FX severe deficiency [34]: two pregnancies resulted in preterm labor and birth at 21 and 25 weeks' gestation (both babies died in the neonatal period). The mother was treated early in two subsequent pregnancies with regular FX replacement, and she delivered healthy babies at 34 and 32 gestational weeks of gestation. Whilst, prophylactic factor replacement therapy seemed to improve pregnancy outcome in this patient, other case reports have described successful term pregnancies in women with severe FX deficiency without antenatal prophylaxis [35, 36]. Further studies are needed to confirm whether inherited bleeding disorders, other than deficiency of fibrinogen or FXIII, are associated with a higher rate of miscarriage.

9.3.2   Bleeding During Pregnancy

Pregnancy is not contraindicated in patients with rare bleeding disorders but requires a multidisciplinary approach for their management of the affected women. As previously discussed, pregnancy is accompanied by increased concentrations of fibrinogen, FVII, FVIII, FX, and von Willebrand factor, while FII, FV, and FIX are relatively unchanged, making women with RBDs at risk of bleeding during pregnancy. There are no previous suitable studies based on adequate sample size confirming or refuting these data. An investigation by Siboni et al. which collected information on bleeding at the time of menarche, and bleeding during pregnancy and the postpartum period in 35 women affected with RBDs and 114 controls recorded that bleeding during pregnancy occurred in 21% of patients vs 6% of controls, however, this difference was not statistically significant $P=0.11$) [37].

However, bleeding during pregnancy is a symptom reported in women with afibrinogenemia and severe FX deficiency [28, 34, 38]. Six successful pregnancies were achieved by afibrinogenemic women receiving fibrinogen replacement therapy throughout pregnancy. Vaginal bleeding began at around 5 weeks' gestation in cases where replacement therapy was not commenced [39].

9.3.3   Postpartum Hemorrhage (PPH)

PPH can be an anticipated problem in women with bleeding disorders. At the end of a normal pregnancy, an estimated 10–15 % of a woman's blood volume, or at least 750 mL/min, is lost through the uterus within the first few weeks after birth [40]. Normally after delivery of the baby and placenta, the uterine musculature or myometrium contracts around the uterine vasculature and the vasculature constricts in order to prevent exsanguination. Retained placental fragments and lacerations of the reproductive tract may also cause heavy bleeding, but the single most important cause of PPH is uterine atony [41]. Despite the critical role of uterine contractility in controlling postpartum blood loss, women with bleeding disorders are at an increased risk of PPH. There are multiple case reports and several case series documenting the incidence of PPH in women with bleeding disorders [23, 34, 42–44], but there are limited data that compare women with bleeding disorders and controls.

PPH was found to be the most common obstetric complication occurring in 45 % (14/31 deliveries) among ten patients affected with hypofibrinogenemia [45], while a high incidence of postpartum thrombosis was noted among dysfibrinogenemic women (7/15, 47 %) [31]. PPH was also reported in 13 (76 %) of 17 deliveries among nine women with FV deficiency [46], who appear to be at increased risk of developing this complication (especially women with low FV activity levels). Although at a lower rate, PPH was also reported in patients with FVII [47], FX [48], and FXI deficiencies [23]. Particularly interesting is the latter report of a large study of 164 pregnancies in 62 women with FXI deficiency (levels <17 IU dL) showing that 69 % of the women never experienced PPH during 93 deliveries without any prophylactic cover. The authors therefore argued that prophylactic treatment is not mandatory for these women, especially with vaginal delivery (however, excessive bleeding at delivery did occur in around 20 % of deliveries not covered by fresh frozen plasma (FFP)). The incidence of PPH in women with FXIII deficiency is not known. Successful pregnancy in women with FXIII subunit A deficiency is generally achieved only with replacement therapy throughout pregnancy and at delivery [49]. No data are published on the rate of PPH in women affected with FII deficiency.

Among all women, the median duration of bleeding after delivery is 21–27 days [50, 51], but coagulation factors, elevated during pregnancy, return to baseline within 14–21 days [52]. Therefore, there is a period of time, 2–3 weeks after delivery, when coagulation factors have returned to prepregnancy levels but women are still bleeding. Women with bleeding disorders are particularly vulnerable to delayed or 'secondary' PPH during this same period of time. The implication is that women with bleeding disorders may require prophylaxis and/or close observation for several weeks after birth.

9.4 Laboratory Diagnosis

9.4.1 Phenotype Analysis

The combined performance of the screening coagulation tests, the prothrombin time (PT) and activated partial thromboplastin time (aPTT), is usually applied to identify RBDs of clinically significant severity, but not FXIII deficiency. A prolonged aPTT with a normal PT is suggestive

of FXI deficiency (after exclusion of FVIII, FIX, and FXII deficiencies). The reverse pattern (normal aPTT and prolonged PT) is typical of FVII deficiency, whereas the prolongation of both tests directs further analysis towards possible deficiencies of FX, FV, prothrombin, or fibrinogen. This paradigm is not valid for RBDs due to combined deficiencies, which prolong both the PT and the aPTT. The sensitivity of the PT and aPTT to the presence of clotting factor deficiencies is dependent on the test system employed [53, 54]. Specific assays of factor coagulant activity are necessary when the degree of prolongation of the global tests suggests the presence of clinically significant deficiencies. Factor antigen assays are not strictly necessary for diagnosis and treatment but are necessary to distinguish type I from type II deficiencies. However, these data are important in deficiency of fibrinogen or FII deficiency, where a normal antigen level associated with reduced activity (dysfibrinogenemia and dysprothrombinemia) is associated with higher risk of thrombosis.

The standard laboratory clotting tests (PT, aPTT, fibrinogen level, platelet counts, bleeding time) are normal in FXIII deficiency. The diagnosis of FXIII deficiency is established by the demonstration of increased clot solubility in 5 M urea, dilute monochloroacetic acid, or acetic acid.

However, the method is not quantitative and is difficult to standardize. The sensitivity of these assays mainly depends on the fibrinogen level, on the reagents used to trigger the coagulation of the plasma (thrombin and/or Ca^{2+}), on specific features of the solubilizing agent, and on the concentration of FXIII. In a UK NEQAS study, 15 combinations of these variables were used among participant laboratories [55], and the clot solubility test could detect only very severe FXIII deficiency (where the FXIII activity in the patient's plasma was significantly <5 %). If clot solubility in these reagents is found, a mixing study (FXIII activity determination on a mixture of patient and normal plasma) is needed to exclude the presence of a FXIII inhibitor. In the presence of neutralizing antibody, FXIII present in normal plasma will be inhibited. Factor XIII activity may also be determined quantitatively by measuring the incorporation of fluorescent or radioactive amines into proteins [56]. Specific ELISA tests have been developed to establish FXIII-A and FXIII-B antigen levels [57].

These tests can be ordered by a gynecologist or the family physician, or alternatively, the woman may be referred directly to a hematologist. However, interpretation of abnormal or borderline results usually requires referral to a hematology (or an internal medicine) consultant. These assays are routinely available in many coagulation laboratories in Europe and North America but are seldom carried out, so that proficiency and standardization may be limited.

9.4.2 Molecular Diagnosis

RBDs are usually due to DNA defects in genes encoding the corresponding coagulation factors [2]. Exceptions are the combined deficiencies of coagulation FV and FVIII and of vitamin-K-dependent proteins (FII, FVII, FIX, and FX) caused, respectively, by mutations in genes encoding proteins involved in the FV and FVIII intracellular transport mechanism and in genes that encode enzymes involved in posttranslational modifications and in vitamin K metabolism [58–61].

The identification of gene defects in patients with RBDs could represent the basis on which to carry out prenatal diagnosis in families that already have one affected child with a severe bleeding history. Molecular characterization and subsequent prenatal diagnosis gain importance particularly in developing countries, where patients with these deficiencies rarely survive beyond childhood and where management is still largely inadequate; therefore, prenatal diagnosis is an important option for the prevention of the birth of children affected by RBDs and severe bleeding manifestations, particularly in region with low economic resources.

9.5 Therapeutic Management

Based on the observations detailed above, regular replacement therapy throughout pregnancy in order to maintain a minimum activity level is recommended in women with afibrinogenemia and should be commenced as soon as possible in

pregnancy to reduce the probability of early fetal loss in women with deficiency of fibrinogen [39, 62, 63]. In these women, treatment should also be continued during labor and delivery to minimize the risk of bleeding complications. Thrombotic events have also been reported in patients with inherited afibrinogenemia [7] so the risks of bleeding and thrombosis should be considered and balanced during pregnancy. Management of women with hypofibrinogenemia should follow similar lines depending on the fibrinogen level, individual bleeding tendency, and family history, as well as previous obstetric history [64]. Thrombotic events during the puerperium have also been reported among women with afibrinogenemia and hypofibrinogenemia [65], and here again the potential for thrombosis associated with replacement therapy must be carefully evaluated and balanced against the risk of bleeding. The management of pregnancy in women with dysfibrinogenemia needs to be individualized, taking into account the fibrinogen level and personal and family history of bleeding and thrombosis [62]. No specific treatment is required in asymptomatic women.

Based on very limited available data, it is difficult to make recommendations for the obstetric management of women with prothrombin, FV, and FV + FVIII deficiencies. It is unknown whether or not prophylactic replacement therapy is required or not during pregnancy. However, women with prothrombin and FV deficiency particularly those with low levels appear to be at increased risk of PPH. Therefore, careful management of labor and the immediate postpartum period is necessary. Regarding women with FV + FVIII deficiency, the obstetric experience of women with FV deficiency and carriers of hemophilia could probably serve as a useful guide.

A significant rise in the FVII level is observed during pregnancy in women with mild/moderate forms of FVII deficiency (heterozygotes) [33], but not in women with severe deficiency [44, 47, 66]. Therefore, in women with mild/moderate deficiency, in whom the FVII level may normalize at term, replacement therapy may not be required for labor and delivery. However, this decision should again be individualized and should take into account the mother's bleeding tendency. Women with severe deficiency or a positive bleeding history are more likely to be at risk of PPH; hence, prophylactic treatment is required for women with low FVII coagulant activity levels at term and/or a significant bleeding history [42, 47, 67, 68].

In women with FX deficiency, replacement therapy should be considered if bleeding occurs or if the patient is undergoing an invasive procedure. Women with severe deficiency and a history of adverse pregnancy outcome may benefit from replacement therapy during a subsequent pregnancy [62]. Replacement therapy is also required to cover labor and delivery in these women to minimize the risk of bleeding complications [69, 70].

Treatment is not mandatory for women with FXI (addressed in detail in Chapter 8) deficiency, especially with vaginal delivery [23]; however, due to the unpredictable bleeding tendency in FXI deficiency, especially during surgery, the decision whether or not to give prophylaxis during labor and delivery needs to be individualized and must take into consideration the FXI level, personal/family bleeding history, and mode of delivery. In FXIII deficiency replacement therapy should be commenced as early as possible in pregnancy to prevent fetal loss [71, 72]; the treatment should also be continued during labor and delivery to minimize the risk of bleeding complications. Higher FXIII levels may be required for delivery [73]. Table 9.1 provides some recommendations on the treatment during pregnancy/delivery and surgery based on previous published reviews [62, 74, 75].

9.6 Multidisciplinary Clinics

Women with an inherited coagulation defect are ideally managed in a multidisciplinary clinics with a gynaecologist/obstetrician, haematologist and, when relevant, an anaesthetist. However, at the present time, few such clinics exist and these women are usually managed suboptimally in separate gynaecology and/or haematology clinics. The ideal multidisciplinary team would have an even broader representation of expertise and would include a haemostasis clinician, a laboratory hematologist, an obstetrician-gynecologist, an anesthetist, a family physician, a social worker, a pharmacist, and a biomedical scientist.

Case Series 1 [33]
Four different cases are described:

A patient who had FVII deficiency with a baseline level of 7 IU/dL had a total of three pregnancies. Two term vaginal deliveries were uneventful and the third pregnancy resulted in a miscarriage requiring surgical evacuation. There was excessive intraoperative blood loss during the procedure, but not requiring blood transfusion.

A patient who had FVII deficiency with a baseline factor level of 22 IU/dL had a surgical termination in the first trimester. This was associated with major intraoperative hemorrhage requiring transfusion of multiple blood components.

A patient who had FVII deficiency and a baseline factor level of 30 IU/dL had two pregnancies with FVII levels at term of 62 and 60 IU/dL, respectively. She had two cesarean sections covered with prophylactic recombinant activated FVII (rFVIIa) treatment to cover delivery. One was complicated by excessive blood loss (1,400 mL) not requiring blood transfusion.

A patient who had FVII deficiency and a baseline factor level of 49 IU/dL had four pregnancies: three full-term vaginal deliveries and one cesarean section, all without replacement therapy and without hemorrhage.

Case Report 2 [36]
A 30-year-old nulliparous woman was referred for investigation of an irregular menstrual cycle.

On clinical examination, a 20-week normal pregnancy was diagnosed. She gave a history of a congenital FX deficiency diagnosed at 6 years of age when she presented with an unexplained and unspecified bleeding tendency. Laboratory measurements showed FX activity coagulant level less than 2–3 % of normal and a trace of FX antigen

Table 9.1 Available recommendation for treatment during pregnancy/delivery and surgery on the basis of previous published literature

Deficient factor	Pregnancy/delivery		Surgery (cesarean section)	
	Minimum level	Treatment	Minimum level	Treatment
Afibrinogenemia	100 mg/dL	Successful pregnancy in afibrinogenemia is difficult without fibrinogen replacement therapy No strong data to support routine post-partum fibrinogen prophylaxis beyond the first 1–2 days	100 mg/dL	Fibrinogen concentrates (20/30 mg/kg) Cryoprecipitate (1 single donor unit/10 kg)
Hypofibrinogenemia		Should be individualized taking into account fibrinogen level, individual bleeding tendency and family history, as well as previous obstetric history		
Dysfibrinogenemia		As for hypofibrinogenemia. The potential for thrombosis in this disease must be carefully evaluated and balanced against the risk of bleeding		
Prothrombin	25 %	No data	20–40 %	SD-treated plasma (15–20 mL/kg) PCC (20–30 IU/kg)
Factor V	15–25 %	SD-treated plasma (15–20 mL/kg, until after delivery)	25 %	SD-treated plasma (15–20 mL/kg)
Factors V + VIII	15–25 % FV; 50 % FVIII	FV levels in pregnancy do not change, whereas FVIII levels rise throughout the pregnancy. Therefore, any possible bleeding is likely to be dependent on the FV level	25 % FV; 50 % FVIII	As for FV
Factor VII	15–20 %	Not required during pregnancy, unless there is a bleeding history with previous pregnancies If FVII < 20 %, peripartum prophylaxis should be considered	10–15 %	FVII concentrates (30–40 mL/kg) monitoring FVII levels and clinical response rFVIIa (15–30 ug/kg every 4–6 h)
Factor X	10–20 %	In severe FX deficiency and history of adverse pregnancy outcome replacement therapy to cover pregnancy, labor and delivery (up to 3 days) is indicated	10–20 %	SD-treated plasma (10–20 mL/kg) PCC (20–30 IU/kg)
Factor XI	15–20 %	FXI levels 15–70 IU/dL: with bleeding history, tranexamic acid up to 3 days (first dose during labor) FXI levels <15 IU/dL replacement therapy should be considered at the onset of labor, only if patient has bleeding history, but it is not mandatory and should be reserved for patients who develop excessive hemorrhages	15–20 %	FXI concentrate at low-dose treatment (10 IU/kg) for FXI deficiency (<10 IU/L)
Factor XIII	3–10 %	FXIII concentrates: it is recommended that regular therapy is commenced as early as possible in pregnancy to prevent bleeding and pregnancy loss Factor replacement should be given at delivery to maintain FXIII levels >20 %	5–10 %	Cryoprecipitate (1 single donor unit/10 kg) SD-treated plasma (15–20 mL/kg) FXIII concentrates (10–20 IU/kg)

As modified from [1, 74, 75]

SD solvent detergent, *PCC* prothrombin complex concentrate, *rFVIIa* recombinant-activated FVII level. Both parents were heterozygous with activity and antigen levels around 50 % of normal. The patient received several blood transfusions during her lifetime, and in 1990, she tested positive for the hepatitis C virus. In the previous decade, however, no therapy had been required apart from contraceptive treatment for menorrhagia. No therapy was necessary during pregnancy since she did not have any bleeding symptom. A multidisciplinary meeting was held in collaboration with pediatricians and anesthetists in order to decide on the mode of delivery Cesarean section at the 38 weeks was scheduled because of the potential risk of cranial and/or abdominal hemorrhage in the newborn as a consequence of vaginal delivery. From 30 weeks of gestational she had weekly clinical examination and ultrasound scans for fetal growth and placental function in view of the risk of preterm labor reported in the literature.

At weeks of gestation, cesarean section was performed, and, to prevent hemorrhage, she was treated with intravenous prothrombin complex concentrate (PCC; which contains factor II, IX, and X +/- factor VII): 1,000 IU was started one hour before the delivery. A normal prothrombin time was rapidly attained, and a healthy male baby was delivered. Following cesarean delivery, 500 IU infusions of prothrombin complex concentrate were administered 12 hourly for 3 days. The day after the therapy was stopped, factor X quickly fell to 7 % of normal. In order to prevent PPH, the patient was started on oral progestogen.

Learning Points
- In women who have a personal or a family history of bleeding, further investigation should be considered.
- Inherited bleeding disorders should be considered in the differential diagnosis of all women presenting with menorrhagia or other gynecological bleeding complications.

- Pregnancy is accompanied by increased concentrations of fibrinogen, FVII, FVIII, FX, and von Willebrand factor, while FII, FV, and FIX are relatively unchanged. Despite improved hemostasis, however, women with coagulation factor deficiencies may not achieve the same factor levels as those of women without factor deficiencies.
- Miscarriage is common in the general population, with at least 12–13.5 % of recognized pregnancies resulting in spontaneous miscarriage. An increased risk of miscarriage and placental abruption resulting in fetal loss or preterm delivery is reported in women with deficiency of fibrinogen or FXIII.
- Women affected with RBDs may still bleed during the first 2–3 weeks after delivery, when coagulation factors return to prepregnancy levels. Women with bleeding disorders are particularly vulnerable to delayed or secondary PPH during this period. The implication is that women with bleeding disorders may require prophylaxis and/or close observation for several weeks after delivery.

References

1. Mannucci PM, Duga S, Peyvandi F. Recessively inherited coagulation disorders. Blood. 2004;104:1243–52.
2. Tuddenham EGD, Cooper DN. The molecular genetics of haemostasis and its inherited disorders. Oxford: Oxford Medical Publications; 1994 (Oxford Monography on Medical Genetics No. 25).
3. Peyvandi F, Palla R, Menegatti M, Mannucci PM. Introduction: rare bleeding disorders: general aspects of clinical features, diagnosis, and management. Semin Thromb Hemost. 2009;35:349–55.
4. Peyvandi F, Palla R, Menegatti M. European Registry of Rare Bleeding Disorders. Hematology Education: the education programme for the annual congress of the European Hematology Association 2010;4:43.
5. Sun WY, Witte DP, Degen JL, et al. Prothrombin deficiency results in embryonic and neonatal lethality in mice. Proc Natl Acad Sci USA. 1998;95: 7597–602.
6. Lak M, Sharifian R, Peyvandi F, Mannucci PM. Symptoms of inherited factor V deficiency in 35 Iranian patients. Br J Haematol. 1998;103:1067–9.
7. Lak M, Keihani M, Elahi F, et al. Bleeding and thrombosis in 55 patients with inherited afibrinogenaemia. Br J Haematol. 1999;107:204–6.

8. Lak M, Peyvandi F, Ali Sharifian A, et al. Pattern of symptoms in 93 Iranian patients with severe factor XIII deficiency. J Thromb Haemost. 2003;1:1852–3.

9. Peyvandi F, Mannucci PM, Asti D, et al. Clinical manifestations in 28 Italian and Iranian patients with severe factor VII deficiency. Haemophilia. 1997;3:242–6.

10. Peyvandi F, Mannucci PM, Lak M, et al. Congenital factor X deficiency: spectrum of bleeding symptoms in 32 Iranian patients. Br J Haematol. 1998;102: 626–8.

11. Peyvandi F, Tuddenham EG, Akhtari AM, et al. Bleeding symptoms in 27 Iranian patients with the combined deficiency of factor V and factor VIII. Br J Haematol. 1998;100:773–6.

12. Peyvandi F, Lak M, Mannucci PM. Factor XI deficiency in Iranians: its clinical manifestations in comparison with those of classic hemophilia. Haematologica. 2002;87:512–4.

13. Acharya SS, Coughlin A, Dimichele DM. Rare Bleeding Disorder Registry: deficiencies of factors II, V, VII, X, XIII, fibrinogen and dysfibrinogenemias. J Thromb Haemost. 2004;2:248–56.

14. James AH. More than menorrhagia: a review of the obstetric and gynaecological manifestations of bleeding disorders. Haemophilia. 2005;11:295–307.

15. Kadir RA, Economides DL, Sabin CA, et al. Frequency of inherited bleeding disorders in women with menorrhagia. Lancet. 1998;351:485–9.

16. Stirling Y, Woolf L, North WR, et al. Haemostasis in normal pregnancy. Thromb Haemost. 1984;52:176–82.

17. Sanchez-Luceros A, Meschengieser SS, Marchese C, et al. Factor VIII and von Willebrand factor changes during normal pregnancy and puerperium. Blood Coagul Fibrinolysis. 2003;14:647–51.

18. Wickstrom K, Edelstam G, Lowbeer CH, et al. Reference intervals for plasma levels of fibronectin, von Willebrand factor, free protein S and antithrombin during third-trimester pregnancy. Scand J Clin Lab Invest. 2004;64:31–40.

19. Bremme KA. Haemostatic changes in pregnancy. Best Pract Res Clin Haematol. 2003;16:153–68.

20. Hellgren M, Blomback M. Studies on blood coagulation and fibrinolysis in pregnancy, during delivery and in the puerperium. Normal condition. Gynecol Obstet Invest. 1981;12:141–54.

21. Bremme K, Ostlund E, Almqvist I, et al. Enhanced thrombin generation and fibrinolytic activity in normal pregnancy and the puerperium. Obstet Gynecol. 1992;80:132–7.

22. Sie P, Caron C, Azam J, et al. Reassessment of von Willebrand factor (VWF), VWF propeptide, factor VIII:C and plasminogen activator inhibitors 1 and 2 during normal pregnancy. Br J Haematol. 2003;121: 897–903.

23. Salomon O, Steinberg DM, Tamarin I, et al. Plasma replacement therapy during labor is not mandatory for women with severe factor XI deficiency. Blood Coagul Fibrinolysis. 2005;16:37–41.

24. Myers B, Pavord S, Kean L, et al. Pregnancy outcome in Factor XI deficiency: incidence of miscarriage, antenatal and postnatal haemorrhage in 33 women with Factor XI deficiency. BJOG. 2007;114:643–6.

25. Everett C. Incidence and outcome of bleeding before the 20th week of pregnancy: prospective study from general practice. BMJ. 1997;315:32–4.

26. Nybo Andersen AM, Wohlfahrt J, Christens P, et al. Maternal age and fetal loss: population based register linkage study. BMJ. 2000;320:1708–12.

27. Evron S, Anteby SO, Brzezinsky A, et al. Congenital afibrinogenemia and recurrent early abortion: a case report. Eur J Obstet Gynecol Reprod Biol. 1985;19:307–11.

28. Kobayashi T, Kanayama N, Tokunaga N, et al. Prenatal and peripartum management of congenital afibrinogenaemia. Br J Haematol. 2000;109:364–6.

29. Inbal A, Kenet G. Pregnancy and surgical procedures in patients with factor XIII deficiency. Biomed Prog. 2003;16:69–71.

30. Burrows RF, Ray JG, Burrows EA. Bleeding risk and reproductive capacity among patients with factor XIII deficiency: a case presentation and review of the literature. Obstet Gynecol Surv. 2000;55:103–8.

31. Haverkate F, Samama M. Familial dysfibrinogenemia and thrombophilia. Report on a study of the SSC Subcommittee on Fibrinogen. Thromb Haemost. 1995;73:151–61.

32. Catanzarite VA, Novotny WF, Cousins LM, Schneider JM. Pregnancies in a patient with congenital absence of prothrombin activity: case report. Am J Perinatol. 1997;14:135–8.

33. Kulkarni AA, Lee CA, Kadir RA. Pregnancy in women with congenital factor VII deficiency. Haemophilia. 2006;12:413–6.

34. Kumar M, Mehta P. Congenital coagulopathies and pregnancy: report of four pregnancies in a factor X-deficient woman. Am J Hematol. 1994;46:241–4.

35. Larrain C. Congenital blood coagulation factor X deficiency. Successful result of the use prothrombin concentrated complex in the control of caesarean section hemorrhage in 2 pregnancies. Rev Med Chil. 1994;122:1178–83.

36. Romagnolo C, Burati S, Ciaffoni S, et al. Severe factor X deficiency in pregnancy: case report and review of the literature. Haemophilia. 2004;10:665–8.

37. Siboni SM, Spreafico M, Calò L, Maino A, Santagostino E, Federici AB, Peyvandi F. Gynaecological and obstetrical problems in women with different bleeding disorders. Haemophilia. 2009;15:1291–9.

38. Greer IA, Lowe GD, Walker JJ, Forbes CD. Haemorrhagic problems in obstetrics and gynaecology in patients with congenital coagulopathies. Br J Obstet Gynaecol. 1991;98:909–18.

39. Inamoto Y, Terao T. First report of case of congenital afibrinogenemia with successful delivery. Am J Obstet Gynecol. 1985;153:803–4.

40. Ross M. Placental and fetal physiology. In: Gabbe S, Niebyl J, Simpson J, editors. Obstetrics: normal and problem pregnancies. New York: Churchill Livingstone; 2002. p. 37–62.

41. Benedetti T. Obstetrical hemorrhage. In: Gabbe S, Niebyl J, Simpson J, editors. Obstetrics: normal and

problem pregnancies. New York: Churchill Livingstone; 2002. p. 503–38.

42. Fadel HE, Krauss JS. Factor VII deficiency and pregnancy. Obstet Gynecol. 1989;73:453–4.

43. Strickland DM, Galey WT, Hauth JC. Hypofibrinogenemia as a cause of delayed postpartum hemorrhage. Am J Obstet Gynecol. 1982;143:230–1.

44. Robertson LE, Wasserstrum N, Banez E, et al. Hereditary factor VII deficiency in pregnancy: peripartum treatment with factor VII concentrate. Am J Hematol. 1992;40:38–41.

45. Goodwin TM. Congenital hypofibrinogenemia in pregnancy. Obstet Gynecol Surv. 1989;44:157–61.

46. Noia G, De Carolis S, De Stefano V, et al. Factor V deficiency in pregnancy complicated by Rh immunization and placenta previa. A case report and review of the literature. Acta Obstet Gynecol Scand. 1997;76:890–2.

47. Rizk DE, Castella A, Shaheen H, Deb P. Factor VII deficiency detected in pregnancy: a case report. Am J Perinatol. 1999;16:223–6.

48. Girolami A, Lazzarin M, Scarpa R, Brunetti A. Further studies on the abnormal factor X (factor X Friuli) coagulation disorder: a report of another family. Blood. 1971;37:534–41.

49. Ichinose A, Asahina T, Kobayashi T. Congenital blood coagulation factor XIII deficiency and perinatal management. Curr Drug Targets. 2005;6:541–9.

50. Edwards A, Ellwood DA. Ultrasonographic evaluation of the postpartum uterus. Ultrasound Obstet Gynecol. 2000;16:640–3.

51. Visness CM, Kennedy KI, Ramos R. The duration and character of postpartum bleeding among breast-feeding women. Obstet Gynecol. 1997;89:159–63.

52. Dahlman T, Hellgren M, Blombäck M. Changes in blood coagulation and fibrinolysis in the normal puerperium. Gynecol Obstet Invest. 1985;20:37–44.

53. Lawrie AS, Kitchen S, Purdy G, et al. Assessment of actin FS and actin FSL sensitivity to specific clotting factor deficiencies. Clin Lab Haematol. 1998;20:179–86.

54. Turi DC, Peerschke EI. Sensitivity of three activated partial thromboplastin time reagents to coagulation factor deficiencies. Am J Clin Pathol. 1986;85:43–9.

55. Jennings I, Kitchen S, Woods TAL, Preston FE. Problems relating to the laboratory diagnosis of factor XIII deficiency: a UK NEQAS study. J Thromb Haemost. 2003;1:2603–8.

56. Fickenscher K, Aab A, Stuber W. A Photometric assay for blood coagulation factor XIII. Thromb Haemost. 1991;65:535–40.

57. Katona E, Haramura G, Karpati L, et al. A simple, quick one-step ELISA assay for the determination of complex plasma factor XIII (A2B2). Thromb Haemost. 2000;83:268–73.

58. Nichols WC, Seligsohn U, Zivelin A, et al. Mutations in the ER-Golgi intermediate compartment protein ERGIC-53 cause combined deficiency of coagulation factors V and VIII. Cell. 1998;93:61–70.

59. Zhang B, Cunningham MA, Nichols WC, et al. Bleeding due to disruption of a cargo-specific ER-to-Golgi transport complex. Nat Genet. 2003;34:220–5.

60. Mousallem M, Spronk HM, Sacy R, et al. Congenital combined deficiencies of all vitamin K-dependent coagulation factors. Thromb Haemost. 2001;86:1334–6.

61. Rost S, Fregin A, Ivaskevicius V, et al. Mutations in VKORC1 cause warfarin resistance and multiple coagulation factor deficiency type 2. Nature. 2004;427:537–41.

62. Bolton-Maggs PH, Perry DJ, Chalmers EA, et al. The rare coagulation disorders – review with guidelines for management from the United Kingdom Haemophilia Centre Doctors' Organisation. Haemophilia. 2004;10:593–628.

63. Trehan AK, Fergusson IL. Congenital afibrinogenaemia and successful pregnancy outcome (Case report). Br J Obstet Gynaecol. 1991;98:722–4.

64. Frenkel E, Duksin C, Herman A, Sherman DJ. Congenital hypofibrinogenemia in pregnancy: report of two cases and review of the literature. Obstet Gynecol Surv. 2004;59:775–9.

65. Dupuy E, Soria C, Molho P, et al. Embolized ischemic lesions of toes in an afibrinogenemic patient: possible relevance to in vivo circulating thrombin. Thromb Res. 2001;102:211–9.

66. Braun MW, Triplett DA. Case report: factor VII deficiency in an obstetrical patient. J Indiana State Med Assoc. 1979;72:900–2.

67. Eskandari N, Feldman N, Greenspoon JS. Factor VII deficiency in pregnancy treated with recombinant factor VIIa. Obstet Gynecol. 2002;99:935–7.

68. Jimenez-Yuste V, Villar A, Morado M, et al. Continuous infusion of recombinant activated factor VII during caesarean section delivery in a patient with congenital factor VII deficiency. Haemophilia. 2000;6:588–90.

69. Konje JC, Murphy P, de Chazal R, et al. Severe factor X deficiency and successful pregnancy. Br J Obstet Gynaecol. 1994;101:910–1.

70. Bofill JA, Young RA, Perry Jr KG. Successful pregnancy in a woman with severe factor X deficiency. Obstet Gynecol. 1996;88:723.

71. Rodeghiero F, Castaman GC, Di Bona E, et al. Successful pregnancy in a woman with congenital factor XIII deficiency treated with substitutive therapy. Report of a second case. Blut. 1987;55:45–8.

72. Kobayashi T, Terao T, Kojima T, et al. Congenital factor XIII deficiency with treatment of factor XIII concentrate and normal vaginal delivery. Gynecol Obstet Invest. 1990;29:235–8.

73. Asahina T, Kobayashi T, Takeuchi K, Kanayama N. Congenital blood coagulation factor XIII deficiency and successful deliveries: a review of the literature. Obstet Gynecol Surv. 2007;62:255–60.

74. Kadir R, Chi C, Bolton-Maggs P. Pregnancy and rare bleeding disorders. Haemophilia. 2009;15:990–1005.

75. Todd T, Perry DJ. A review of long-term prophylaxis in the rare inherited coagulation factor deficiencies. Haemophilia. 2010;16:569–83.

Inherited Bleeding Disorders in Pregnancy: Platelet Defects

10

Andrew D. Mumford and Amanda Clark

Abstract

Platelet function disorders (PFDs) include the severe bleeding disorders Glanzmann thrombasthenia (GT) and Bernard Soulier syndrome (BSS), and a heterogenous group of other non-severe phenotype platelet defects. GT and BSS confer significant risk of ante-partum and post-partum bleeding and may be complicated by alloimmunisation against platelet antigens, potentially causing maternal platelet refractoriness and fetal alloimmune thrombocytopenia. This chapter reviews the prevalence of bleeding in GT and BSS, and in non-severe PFDs. We describe the available therapies to prevent or treat obstetric bleeding in women with PFD and summarise current management strategies.

10.1 Introduction

Platelets are anuclear cellular components of blood that are a critical component of primary hemostasis and support the activation of plasma coagulation factors to enable fibrin clot formation. Platelets also have pro-inflammatory and pro-proliferative activities and mediate vascular disorders such as atherothrombosis. In pregnancy, platelets are essential to maintain adequate hemostasis at delivery and contribute to the pathogenesis of vascular disorders such as preeclampsia and other microangiopathic coagulopathies.

Disorders of platelet number may give rise to significant maternal and fetal morbidity because of bleeding, and this group of disorders are described elsewhere in this volume. Similar morbidity may arise from platelet function disorders (PFDs) which include rare heritable disorders such as Glanzmann thrombasthenia (GT) and Bernard-Soulier syndrome (BSS) which may be associated with severe bleeding in pregnancy. This group also includes non-severe PFDs which are heterogeneous and common disorders that may also be associated with adverse pregnancy outcomes. The non-severe PFDs often present significant difficulties in diagnosis and management.

This chapter provides a description of the expected changes in platelet function in normal and abnormal pregnancies and summarizes the key diagnostic features of the major platelet

A.D. Mumford, PhD, FRCPath (✉)
Bristol Heart Institute, University of Bristol,
Level 7 Bristol Royal Infirmary, Bristol BS2 8HW, UK
e-mail: a.mumford@bristol.ac.uk

A. Clark, FRCPath
Bristol Haemophilia Centre, University Hospitals
NHS Foundation Trust,
Bristol, BS2 8ED, UK

H. Cohen, P. O'Brien (eds.), *Disorders of Thrombosis and Hemostasis in Pregnancy*,
DOI 10.1007/978-1-4471-4411-3_10, © Springer-Verlag London 2012

function disorders. A systematic review is presented of the worldwide experience of pregnancy in women with severe GT and BSS and non-severe PFDs and includes consensus guidance for optimum management.

10.2   Changes in Platelet Function in Normal Pregnancy

Platelet aggregation and ATP secretion in response to activating agonists have been shown to increase in women during normal pregnancy compared to nonpregnant controls [1–3]. This difference was most evident in the third trimester, but by 6–12 weeks after delivery, platelets from the pregnant and nonpregnant groups were indistinguishable [1, 2]. Increased platelet surface expression of the lysosome marker CD63 also increased during normal pregnancy both in non-stimulated and agonist-stimulated platelets [4, 5]. Similarly, the plasma concentrations of the soluble platelet activation markers β-thromboglobulin and soluble CD40 ligand increased during normal pregnancy [5, 6] suggesting an increase in basal activation of platelets in vivo. However, alternative markers of platelet activation, such as platelet binding of fibrinogen or other markers of the open-conformation $\alpha_{IIb}\beta_3$ integrin, were shown not to increase in non-stimulated platelets during normal pregnancy [3, 5]. There was also no increase in the platelet surface expression of P-selectin which is a marker of platelet α-granule secretion [7, 8]. Other smaller studies have shown decreased platelet surface expression of P-selectin in response to agonist stimulation during pregnancy and lower plasma concentrations of β-thromboglobulin [9, 10].

Interpretation of these observational data is hampered by the limited sample sizes of the individual studies and by difficulties in standardization of platelet function assays between laboratories. However, taken together, these data suggest that normal pregnancy is associated with increased platelet responsiveness to activating stimuli but not necessarily an increase in basal platelet activation in vivo. This increase in responsiveness has been linked mechanistically to suppression of the cAMP pathway which normally inhibits plate-

let activation [3, 11], increased thromboxane A_2 synthesis [3], and increased mobilization of cytoplasmic Ca^{2+} [3] which have been observed consistently in platelets during normal pregnancy. The initiating stimulus for these changes is unknown.

10.3   Changes in Platelet Function in Abnormal Pregnancy

Pregnancy complicated by preeclampsia has been associated with increased expression of P-selectin and CD63 on non-stimulated and ADP-stimulated platelets compared to normotensive pregnancy controls [5, 8, 12]. Plasma concentrations of P-selectin [13] and soluble CD40 ligand [10, 14] also markedly increased supporting the notion that preeclampsia is associated with pathological platelet activation in vivo. In apparent conflict with this, platelets obtained from pregnant women with preeclampsia showed reduced aggregation responses to activating agonists compared to normotensive pregnancy controls [15, 16]. However, this apparent loss of function *ex vivo* may be a consequence of increased in vivo activation because of depletion or downregulation of activating receptors and signaling pathways. A similar phenomenon may be observed in other disorders such as the myeloproliferative disorders in which there is also increased platelet activation in vivo. Evidence for platelet activation in vivo during non-proteinuric hypertension during pregnancy is less compelling and contradictory [17].

10.4   Spectrum of Platelet Function Disorders

The heritable PFDs may be subclassified according to clinical severity into groups that comprise *severe GT and BSS* in which there are frequent or severe bleeding episodes and *non-severe PFDs* in which abnormal bleeding usually only follows trauma or surgery. Within the non-severe PFD group are some uncommon GT and BSS variants (e.g., type II GT, Bolzano BSS variant) in which bleeding is usually mild (Table 10.1).

Table 10.1 Classification of platelet function disorders

Severe phenotype platelet function disorders
Severe Glanzmann thrombasthenia
Severe Bernard-Soulier syndrome
Non-severe phenotype disorders
Defects in platelet aggregation or adhesion
Rare Glanzmann thrombasthenia variants (type II)
Rare Bernard-Soulier syndrome variants
Some "heterozygous" Bernard-Soulier syndrome variants
Defects of platelet receptors
Deficiency of receptors ADP ($P2Y_{12}$), thromboxane A_2, collagen (GPVI)
Defects in signal transduction
Thromboxane synthesis defect ("aspirin-like" defect)
G-protein activation defect
Ca^{2+} mobilization defect
Integrin $\alpha_{IIb}\beta_3$ activation defect
Protein phosphorylation defects (e.g., protein kinase-θ defect)
Phosphatidylinositol metabolism defects (e.g., phospholipase C deficiency)
Defects in platelet secretion
Isolated δ-storage pool disease
Combined αδ-storage pool disease
α-granule deficiency (e.g., Grey platelet syndrome)
Syndromic secretion defects (e.g., Hermansky-Pudlak syndrome)
Quebec platelet disorder
Miscellaneous disorders
Platelet procoagulant function disorder (Scott syndrome)

Modified from [24]

10.4.1 Severe Glanzmann Thrombasthenia

Severe GT is a rare autosomal recessive disorder caused by a quantitative deficiency of the platelet glycoprotein (GP) IIb-IIIa ($\alpha_{IIb}\beta_3$ integrin) which is the major platelet receptor of fibrinogen and other macromolecular adhesive proteins. Absence of functional GPIIb-IIIa therefore results in a major defect in platelet-platelet aggregation and markedly impaired primary hemostasis [18]. Laboratory analysis of platelets shows markedly reduced or absent aggregation responses to all agonists except ristocetin. Flow cytometry shows markedly reduced or absent surface expression of GPIIb (CD41) and GPIIIa (CD61) [19]. The platelet count and morphology are normal. Affected individuals are homozygous or compound heterozygous for deleterious mutations in *ITGA2B* and *ITGB3* which encode GPIIb and GPIIIa, respectively [20].

Fetal intracranial hemorrhage before or during delivery is rare in severe GT. However, most affected children present before the age of 5 years with purpura, petechiae, or abnormal bruising [21]. Abnormal mucocutaneous bleeding persists through childhood, and gingival bleeding and severe epistaxis are common [21]. Menorrhagia is frequently severe in GT, and life-threatening bleeding has been reported at the menarche [22]. Other prominent symptoms include bleeding from the gastrointestinal and urinary tracts, prolonged surgical and traumatic bleeding, and oral bleeding after exfoliation of deciduous teeth [21].

10.4.2 Severe Bernard-Soulier Syndrome

Severe BSS is an autosomal recessive disorder caused by a quantitative deficiency of the platelet glycoprotein GPIb-IX-V complex. This complex is the major platelet receptor for von Willebrand factor (VWF) and mediates platelet adhesion to collagen in primary hemostasis. The GPIb-IX-V complex also facilitates platelet activation by thrombin and regulates pro-platelet formation by megakaryocytes. BSS patients therefore have defective platelet adhesion but also thrombocytopenia with large circulating platelets [23].

Laboratory analysis of platelets in severe BSS shows failure of agglutination with ristocetin but normal aggregation with other activating agonists. Flow cytometry shows markedly reduced or absent platelet surface expression of the GPIb-IX-V complex. The platelet count is usually reduced and the mean platelet volume increased, but these features are highly variable among affected individuals [19, 24]. Severe BSS is associated with homozygous or compound heterozygous mutations in *GPIBA*, *GPIBB,* or *GP9* which encode components of GPIb and GPIX [25].

Severe BSS usually presents in early life with abnormal mucocutaneous or traumatic bleeding that is more severe than expected from the degree of thrombocytopenia. However, the clinical bleeding phenotype in BSS is variable. Some individuals with a marked deficiency of GPIb-IX-V present later in childhood or in early adulthood with abnormal bleeding after trauma or surgery or with prolonged bleeding at menarche [26].

10.4.3 Non-severe Platelet Function Disorders

Non-severe PFDs include some rare GT or BSS variants in which there is partial loss of glycoprotein function rather than absence of expression. Mild bleeding may also arise in some individuals who are "carriers" of severe BSS and who are heterozygous for mutations affecting GPIb-IX-V [27]. Otherwise, the non-severe PFDs comprise a heterogeneous group of defects of platelet surface receptors, signal transduction, and secretion pathway proteins [24, 28, 29] (Table 10.1). Laboratory tests of platelet function such as light transmission aggregation may show a wide range of abnormalities, and there is currently poor consensus about minimal diagnostic criteria for many disorders in this group [30]. Molecular genetic defects have been identified in only a small proportion of reported families [31].

By contrast to severe GT and BSS, the non-severe PFDs typically show a mild bleeding phenotype that often manifests in later childhood or adulthood with mucocutaneous bleeding and prolonged bleeding after trauma or surgery. Non-severe PFDs are prevalent in women with otherwise unexplained menorrhagia [32, 33]. It is likely that the prevalence of this group of disorders is high and that many non-severe PFDs are not recognized. Some non-severe PFDs such as Hermansky-Pudlak syndrome are associated with syndromic feature (oculocutaneous albanism and nystagmus in the case of Hermansky Pudlak syndrome) which may aid clinical diagnosis [24].

10.5 Platelet Function Disorders and Pregnancy Outcomes

Data on pregnancy outcome in women with PFDs are sparse in the literature and comprise single case reports or single-center case series with small numbers of patients. Therefore, the absolute risk of adverse maternal and fetal outcomes is difficult to quantify, and there may be significant reporting bias toward adverse outcomes. However, despite these limitations, it is clear that severe GT and BSS confer an increased maternal risk of postpartum hemorrhage (PPH) and increased fetal bleeding risk from fetal alloimmune thrombocytopenia. Reports of pregnancy outcomes for the non-severe PFDs are infrequent and contain anecdotal descriptions of adverse maternal outcomes because of bleeding.

10.5.1 Maternal Bleeding in Platelet Function Disorders

There are detailed descriptions of clinical course and outcomes in approximately 40 pregnancies in women with severe GT and approximately 15 further pregnancies which are reported in larger single-center cohort studies [21, 34]. Abnormal bleeding before the onset of labor was described in approximately 75 % of the reports that documented the antenatal course in GT pregnancies and was usually mild. Bleeding episodes occurring throughout pregnancy included epistaxis, urinary tract bleeding, skin bruising, and gingival bleeding which are similar to bleeding symptoms in nonpregnant women with severe GT. Antenatal vaginal bleeding has been reported after vaginal examination [35] and in association with placenta previa [36].

The majority of pregnant women with severe GT received prophylaxis against PPH, usually with platelet transfusion and antifibrinolytics (see Sect. 10.7.3.1) as well as obstetric active management of the third stage of labour. However, despite these measures, PPH was reported in approximately 50 % of reported pregnancies in severe GT of which half occurred between 24 h and 2 weeks after delivery (namely 'secondary' PPH) [37]. Severe PPH has been reported after vaginal laceration during a forceps delivery [38] and after perineotomy [39]. There is a single report of hysterectomy that was performed during pregnancy for severe obstetric sepsis [40].

A systematic review has been performed of similar data available for approximately 30 pregnancies in women with BSS, including both severe and non-severe BSS variants [41]. Mild antenatal bleeding was reported in less than 15 % of all BSS pregnancies. However, primary PPH occurred in approximately 33 % and secondary PPH up to 6 weeks after delivery in approximately 40 % despite the widespread use of platelet transfusion as prophylaxis against PPH [41]. Caesarean hysterectomy for bleeding was reported in two pregnancies [42, 43].

Reports of maternal outcomes in women with non-severe PFDs include descriptions of primary PPH or bleeding at caesarean section in Hermansky-Pudlak syndrome [44, 45] and nonsyndromic δ-storage pool disease [46]. In a case series that reported seven women with non-severe PFDs, there was no abnormal maternal bleeding although most women received intrapartum platelet transfusion and oral antifibrinolytics [47].

10.5.2 Fetal Bleeding in Platelet Function Disorders

Severe GT and BSS and many other non-severe PFDs are autosomal recessive traits. Therefore, affected women are unlikely to carry an affected fetus unless from a consanguineous partner. In this circumstance, major fetal bleeding such as intracranial hemorrhage is rare although a single-center case series identified petechiae and scalp hematomas in approximately 25 % of neonates with severe GT who were delivered vaginally [48]. Some non-severe PFDs, including some BSS variants and storage pool disorders, show autosomal dominant inheritance. For these disorders, it is predicted that 50 % of fetuses from an affected mother will also have a non-severe PFD. Delivery of fetuses with autosomal dominant non-severe PFDs carries low risk of intracranial or other major bleeds [24].

10.5.3 Fetal Alloimmune Thrombocytopenia

Women with PFDs who have previously received donor platelets for the treatment of bleeding are at increased risk of developing alloantibodies against the human platelet antigen (HPA) or human leucocyte antigen (HLA) systems. This may be more common in women with severe GT or BSS because women with these disorders usually have frequent exposures to donor platelets [21, 26]. Absent expression of GPIIb-IIIa or GPIb/IX/V in severe GT or BSS may also promote alloantibody formation against HPA epitopes within these glycoproteins [41, 49]. Both HPA and HLA alloantibodies may cause refractoriness to further platelet transfusion and may jeopardize future treatment of bleeding.

Alloantibodies against GPIIb-IIIa and GPIb-IX-V may also cross the placenta and cause severe fetal thrombocytopenia through immune-mediated consumption of platelets in the fetal circulation. This has been associated with intracranial hemorrhage or other severe fetal bleeds in both severe GT [35, 49, 50] and BSS [43, 51] sometimes resulting in intrauterine or early postnatal death [43, 49, 52]. In most of the reported pregnancies with fetal alloimmune thrombocytopenia, the affected women had previously received platelet transfusions and had detectable alloantibodies against GPIIb-IIIa or GPIb-IX-V before pregnancy.

An anamnestic rise in the titer of alloantibodies against GPIIb-IIIa has also been reported during pregnancy in GT [35, 53] suggesting that exposure to fetal platelet antigens may also be a significant cause of alloimmunization in women with severe GT and BSS. Therefore, the absence of platelet alloantibodies at the start of pregnancy does not preclude alloimmunization later in pregnancy.

10.6 Approaches to Treatment or Prevention of Bleeding in Platelet Function Disorders

The choice of agent to treat or prevent bleeding in the PFDs during pregnancy requires evaluation of the site and severity of bleeding or anticipated bleeding. It is also essential to consider previous clinical responses to different agents. For platelet transfusion, the recoveries or corrected count increments following previous platelet transfusions should be calculated, and it should be determined whether platelet alloantibodies are present. The relative safety of different therapies should also be considered, particularly platelet transfusion which may carry particular hazards for pregnant women with PFDs.

In this section, the mode of action, indications, and safety of different pro-hemostatic agents are discussed. Management approaches are also suggested for the treatment or prevention of bleeding in nonpregnant and pregnant women. Specific measures to prevent or treat PPH are described in Sect. 10.7.3.

10.6.1 Local Measures and Antifibrinolytics

For minor mucocutaneous bleeds that occur commonly throughout pregnancy in severe GT and BSS, local measures and oral antifibrinolytics such as tranexamic acid, 1–1.5 g (or 15–25 mg/kg) tds for 5–7 days, may be sufficient [24, 54]. Local therapies such as topical thrombin or antifibrinolytics may also improve local hemostasis [55]. Intravenous preparations of tranexamic acid or the alternative antifibrinolytic ε-aminocaproic acid are available, but it should be emphasized that all antifibrinolytics are unsuitable for urinary tract bleeding because of the risk of ureteric obstruction with clot.

10.6.2 Desmopressin

Desmopressin (DDAVP; 1-deamino-8-D-arginine vasopressin) is a selective agonist of the endothelial V2 vasopressin receptor that stimulates release of VWF and tissue plasminogen activator (t-PA) and also causes plasma factor VIII activity to increase [56]. This agent promotes primary hemostasis in a variety of platelet function disorders [57] probably through an indirect VWF-mediated effect through activation of platelet GPIb-IX-V [56].

In women with non-severe PFDs outside of pregnancy, desmopressin 0.3 µg/kg in combination with antifibrinolytics may be sufficient for mild or moderate bleeding. This agent is usually administered by intravenous infusion or subcutaneous injection although a concentrated nasal spray preparation also enables home treatment by women with frequent minor bleeds or menorrhagia [24]. Since desmopressin has very little activity against the V1 vasopressin receptor, there is negligible vasoconstrictor or pro-oxytocic effect on uterine contraction [57]. Therefore, concerns that this agent might cause placental arterial insufficiency or preterm labor appear to be unfounded [58]. Instead, the clinical experience of desmopressin in women with diabetes insipidus [59] or von Willebrand disease [60] in pregnancy is favorable.

Desmopressin may therefore be considered as a pro-hemostatic agent throughout pregnancy for mild PFDs. In common with the use of this agent outside pregnancy, desmopressin may exert a potent antidiuretic effect [61]. Therefore, all pregnant women who receive desmopressin should be advised to avoid excessive fluid intake for 24 h after therapy. A significant clinical response to desmopressin is unlikely in severe GT or BSS, and even in mild PFDs, the clinical response is often unpredictable.

Laboratory testing of platelets after trial doses of desmopressin is uninformative, but a previous satisfactory clinical response to treatment may be helpful in predicting a good response in pregnancy. If a desmopressin infusion fails to control bleeding, then repeated treatment is unlikely to be successful because there is significant tachyphylaxis in the pro-hemostatic response [56].

10.6.3 Recombinant FVIIa

Recombinant FVIIa promotes hemostasis in severe GT and BSS by enhancing thrombin generation on the platelet surface which leads to increased platelet activation [62].

An international registry has reported the safe and effective use of rFVIIa as a pro-hemostatic therapy in GT outside of pregnancy [63].

Accordingly, rFVIIa is licensed by the European Medicines Agency for GT with antibodies to GPIIb-IIIa or HLA and with past or present refractoriness to platelet transfusion. There is also some favorable experience of rFVIIa in severe BSS [64], and it is now recommended that rFVIIa is considered either alone or in combination with platelet transfusion in both severe GT and BSS even if there are no alloantibodies or platelet refractoriness [24]. rFVIIa may have greater efficacy in severe GT and BSS if doses of at least 90 μg/kg bodyweight are given early after the start of bleeding or immediately before an invasive procedure such as chorionic villus sampling (CVS) or amniocentesis. It is also recommended that rFVIIa doses are repeated at 90–120-min intervals until hemostasis is achieved [24, 65]. rFVIIa has a good safety record in pregnancy and is an attractive treatment option in women with severe GT and BSS since it may avoid exposure to donor platelets. However, rFVIIa has been associated with venous thromboembolism and arterial thrombosis during "off-label" use for severe PPH in women without PFDs [66, 67]. Therefore, in women with other thrombosis risk factors, this agent should be used with caution, particularly in women with other thrombotic risk factors.

10.6.4 Platelet Transfusion

Platelet transfusion is an alternative or adjunct to rFVIIa and antifibrinolytics for the management of bleeding in severe GT and BSS and refractory bleeding in any PFD. Standard platelet components are now supplied in the UK either as a pooled product from the buffy coats of four whole blood donations or from a single donor prepared by apheresis [68]. For most bleeding episodes in the PFDs, one or two standard adult therapeutic doses, each of which contains $>240 \times 10^9$ platelets, will achieve initial hemostasis although further treatments may be necessary according to clinical response [24].

Platelet transfusion also confers risk of alloimmunization, allergy, and transfusion-transmitted infection which in the UK includes the prion associated with variant Creutzfeldt-Jakob disease which is transmissible through cellular blood products [69]. These risks increase with multiple donor exposures, and so platelet transfusion in severe GT and BSS is now usually reserved for refractory bleeding or prevention of bleeding in high-risk surgical procedures. If platelets are unavoidable, then the incidence of alloimmunization in women with PFDs may be reduced by prestorage leucodepletion of blood products, which is now performed on all the UK platelet components [70]. This risk may be reduced further by using HLA-selected platelets which is now the preferred component for all women with severe GT or BSS who require platelets [24, 54]. It should be emphasized that HLA-selected platelets will not prevent alloimmunization against HPA epitopes in severe GT or BSS. Random donor pool platelets may be the only available option for the emergency treatment of bleeding that is unanticipated.

In women who already have platelet alloantibodies detected by platelet immunofluorescence testing (PIFT), it is essential to define the specificity of the antibodies using a monoclonal antibody immobilization of platelet antigen (MAIPA) assay. If platelet transfusion is required, then HLA- or HPA-selected platelets should be supplied, and the platelet recovery or corrected count increment in response to each treatment episode should be documented [68]. Close liaison with a specialist transfusion laboratory is required.

10.7   Management of Pregnancy and Delivery

10.7.1 Preconception Counseling

Most women with severe GT or BSS will have received a diagnosis well before pregnancy and ideally, should undergo preconception counseling during which the risks of maternal PPH and alloimmunization are discussed. When a woman with severe GT or BSS is in a consanguineous partnership, the risk that the fetus may also have severe GT or BSS is significant. Counseling should therefore include specific discussion of the lifelong impact of these disorders. It is preferable for preconception counseling to be performed after genetic diagnosis of severe GT or BSS in the maternal proband and after genetic testing of partners in consanguineous families. Antenatal diagnosis of severe GT or BSS should be considered although chorionic villus sampling or amniocentesis requires pro-hemostatic therapy to prevent maternal bleeding, usually with platelet transfusion. The benefits and relative hazards of this approach should be considered carefully with the individual woman.

Diagnosis of the non-severe PFDs is also made in most affected women before pregnancy. Preconception counseling in these highly heterogeneous disorders should explore the fact that the prediction of maternal bleeding risk may be difficult and that the fetal risk of also having a PFD may be difficult to estimate if the inheritance pattern in the affected family is unclear. For women who present during pregnancy with a family history of a non-severe PFD, attempts should be made to offer definitive diagnosis well before delivery. This will usually require a detailed symptomatic inquiry and laboratory testing of platelets. However, it should be recognized that changes in platelet responsiveness to laboratory agonists during pregnancy may hamper diagnosis, particularly if pregnancy is complicated by disorders such as preeclampsia. Molecular diagnosis in the non-severe PFDs is seldom possible since the genetic basis of these disorders is usually unknown.

10.7.2 General Measures

When pregnancy is confirmed, it is preferable that antenatal management occurs in a center with specific expertise in hemostatic disorders and with readily available access to platelets and other pro-hemostatic therapies. Close collaboration is required between hemostasis clinicians, obstetricians, anesthetists and neonatologists, and a written delivery plan should be generated and discussed with the family.

Previous reports of pregnancy in women with severe GT or BSS indicate that PPH may complicate both caesarean and vaginal delivery, and it is therefore not currently possible to recommend the optimum mode of delivery. Since fetal intracranial hemorrhage in pregnancies complicated

by maternal alloimmunization frequently antecedes delivery [49, 52], caesarean section will not guarantee against adverse fetal outcomes. However, many obstetricians prefer this route of delivery in women with alloantibodies in order to minimize the potential further risk of fetal bleeding during vaginal birth. Caesarean section can be performed for standard obstetric indications in all women with PFDs, and in situations where difficult instrumental delivery is anticipated, consideration should be given to performing caesarean section in preference [24, 41].

Regional analgesia is contraindicated in women with severe GT or BSS because of the difficulty in guaranteeing hemostasis with current therapies [24, 41]. Caesarean section in women with these severe disorders therefore requires general anesthesia. In women with non-severe PFDs, the contraindication to regional anesthesia is less absolute, and the risk of spinal hematoma must be weighed against the individual's risk of general anesthesia for caesarean section [47].

Delivery plans should include specific measures to ensure uterine contraction which is essential for peripartum hemostasis, especially in women with hemostatic disorders. The most widely used uterotonic syntometrin requires intramuscular injection and is therefore not ideal for most women with PFDs. However, intravenous oxytocin (10IU) is equally effective and is a reasonable alternative in this circumstance. Misoprostol is another uterotonic that can be administered rectally, vaginally, orally (sublingual) or, at caesarean section, directly into the uterine cavity. During caesarean section or surgical repair of episiotomy or perineal trauma, there should be meticulous attention to surgical hemostasis.

10.7.3 Prevention and Treatment of Postpartum Hemorrhage

10.7.3.1 Severe Platelet Function Disorders

Postpartum hemorrhage is a major hazard for women with severe GT or BSS, and pro-hemostatic therapy is required to minimize maternal risk. Platelet transfusion has been used widely in women with these disorders, usually in combination with antifibrinolytics [36, 41, 71]. rFVIIa has been also used in combination with platelet transfusion in GT [72, 73], but there is less published experience in severe BSS.

For vaginal delivery, it is currently recommended that rFVIIa with an oral antifibrinolytic is considered as a first-line agent for both severe GT and BSS. rFVIIa 90 μg/kg (early pregnancy weight) should be administered as soon as possible and repeated every 2 hours for at least 3 doses or until hemostasis is secure. An alternative approach is to combine an oral antifibrinolytic with one or two adult therapeutic doses of HLA-selected platelets immediately before delivery and repeated if necessary according to clinical hemostasis. For refractory PPH, or if there are platelet alloantibodies, then rFVIIa in conjunction with HLA-selected platelets and an oral antifibrinolytic may be effective [49, 72, 74]. This combination of therapies should be considered in women with platelet alloantibodies even if platelet refractoriness has not been documented. Severe secondary PPH several weeks after delivery has been recognized in severe GT and BSS, even following apparently uncomplicated deliveries [21, 41]. Therefore, it is recommended that oral antifibrinolytics are continued weeks postpartum and that women are observed closely throughout weeks after the birth [24].

Caesarean section caries major bleeding risk in this group, and HLA-selected platelets are justified before and after delivery. All women require prolonged treatment with oral antifibrinolytics and careful inpatient observation for bleeding. rFVIIa should be considered as additional treatment if there is any clinical concern about the efficacy of platelet transfusion alone [24, 36]. Approaches such as uterine artery embolisation or hysterectomy may be necessary for uncontrolled PPH that is refractory to therapy or other conservative surgical measures [42, 43].

10.7.3.2 Non-severe Platelet Function Disorders

For the non-severe PFDs, the individual risk of PPH and the efficacy of different therapies are difficult to estimate before delivery. However, women who have a history before pregnancy of frequent or severe bleeding are anticipated to be a greater risk of PPH and to require pro-hemostatic therapy. In previous reports, oral antifibrinolytics, desmopressin, and platelet transfusion have been administered with variable success in preventing PPH [44, 46, 47].

For vaginal delivery in women with mild PFDs, careful observation may be adequate or oral antifibrinolytics alone may prevent PPH. However, in women with a more significant bleeding history, and particularly a previous history of PPH, desmopressin should be considered during the second stage of labor. Platelet transfusion may also be necessary if PPH occurs despite desmopressin. For caesarean section, most women require preoperative platelet transfusion with an oral antifibrinolytic repeated as necessary after delivery. There is limited experience of rFVIIa in mild platelet function disorders, and this agent should be considered only if there is refractory bleeding despite platelet transfusion [24].

10.7.4 Surveillance and Management of Alloantibody Formation

Maternal alloimmunization against HPA and HLA antigens is highly significant because of the associations with maternal refractoriness to platelet transfusion and with fetal thrombocytopenia and intracranial hemorrhage. Therefore, all women with severe GT or BSS, in which the risk of alloimmunization against clinically significant alloantigens is greatest, should be tested for anti-HPA and anti-HLA alloantibodies at the start of pregnancy and after any exposure to donor platelets during pregnancy (the reader should also refer to Chapter 12). Initial testing should be by PIFT, and the specificities of antibodies should be determined using a MAIPA assay. Testing should be repeated periodically through pregnancy even if there is no further exposure to donor platelets [24] because of the possibility of alloimmunization from fetal platelets crossing the placenta into the maternal circulation.

It should be recognized that there is little relationship between antibody specificity or titer, and the risk of fetal bleeding and that adverse fetal outcomes have been reported in pregnancies without demonstrable maternal alloantibodies [51]. However, a rising maternal alloantibody titer, platelet refractoriness, or a previous pregnancy complicated by fetal thrombocytopenia or intracranial hemorrhage should be considered as indications for intervention. Maternal intravenous immunoglobulin [51, 75], oral corticosteroids [43, 50], and plasma exchange or immunoabsorption [35, 75, 76] have been reported as successful interventions in this setting. Fetal cordocentesis to detect thrombocytopenia or to administer platelets or immunoglobulin may have benefit in neonatal alloimmune thrombocytopenia in women without PFDs [77]. However, in women with PFDs, cordocentesis confers additional bleeding risk in both the fetus (umbilical cord haematoma or haemorrhage can be fatal) and in the woman herself the needle passes through both the abdominal wall and the uterine wall. Therefore, the benefits of these fetal interventions remain undertain, even in severe alloimmunization.

10.7.5 Measures to Minimize the Risk of Fetal Bleeding

For pregnancies in which the fetus is also at risk of a PFD or of neonatal thrombocytopenia, interventions during labor such as application of a fetal scalp electrode (FSE), fetal scalp, blood sampling (FBS), and instrumentation by vacuum (for example ventouse) or rotational forceps should be avoided. Ideally, a prolonged second stage of labor should also be avoided, but each case should be judged individually. If, for example, there is steady, albeit slow, progress in the second stage, waiting a little longer for normal delivery will be preferable to instrumental or caesarean delivery. After delivery, oral or intravenous rather than intramuscular vitamin K for the baby is preferred. The cord blood platelet count should be measured and a cranial ultrasound considered in all neonates at risk of thrombocytopenia. Cord blood may also be used to identify neonates who have inherited severe GT or BSS although platelet function and flow cytometry results should be interpreted with care because normal laboratory reference ranges differ markedly between neonates and older children or adults.

Case Study 1

A 24-year-old Pakistani woman presented at 8-week gestation in her first pregnancy. She had been diagnosed to have Bernard-Soulier syndrome at another center and gave a history of lifelong easy bruising, occasional prolonged epistaxis, and menorrhagia. She had previously received platelet transfusions before a dental extraction, after a traumatic skin bleed, and for prolonged bleeding after a previous miscarriage. Consistent with her previous diagnosis, repeat investigations showed that her platelets failed to agglutinate with ristocetin and failed to express GPIb-IX-V. A causative mutation was identified in the *GPIBA* gene, and this was also present in the woman's current partner. Antenatal diagnosis was declined. The platelet count was 105×10^9/l, and platelet alloantibodies against class II HLA epitopes were identified by MAIPA assay. Surveillance blood tests at 6 weekly intervals throughout pregnancy showed no change in the platelet count or maternal alloantibody titer. There was no abnormal antenatal bleeding.

The woman presented at 39^{+1} weeks in spontaneous labor. In accordance with the delivery plan, she received tranexamic acid 1 g every 6 hours. Two adult doses of random donor pool platelets were moved from the blood transfusion laboratory to a platelet agitator within the delivery suite for use only in the event of uncontrolled bleeding. When cervical dilation has progressed to 5 cm, the woman received an intravenous infusion of rFVIIa 90 μg/kg and vaginal delivery proceeded without regional anesthesia. The delivery was not instrumented although an episiotomy was required that was repaired using local anesthetic. A second infusion of rFVIIa 90 μg/kg was given 30 min after delivery, and the woman received an intravenous syntocinon infusion. Postpartum blood loss was 500 mL. The neonate was well with no evidence of abnormal bleeding on clinical examination or by cranial ultrasound. Cord blood was obtained for flow cytometry and genetic testing and later confirmed that the neonate was unaffected with severe BSS.

Tranexamic acid 1 g every 6 h was continued after delivery, and mother and baby were observed in hospital for a further 7 days before discharge home with instructions to continue tranexamic acid for a further 3 weeks. At 22 days after delivery, the patient was readmitted with a 400-mL-secondary PPH that was managed by infusion of two adult doses of random donor pool platelets and rFVIIa 90 μg/kg. There was a satisfactory platelet recovery of 50 % at 1 h and 35 % at 24 h after transfusion. The rFVIIa infusion was repeated at 2, 4, and 6 h. There was no further bleeding, and mother and baby were discharged home after a further 7-day observation period in hospital.

Case Study 2

A 36-year-old Caucasian woman with a lifelong history of mild mucocutaneous bleeding and menorrhagia presented at 8-week gestation in her second pregnancy. There was a history of similar symptoms in her mother and older sister. During a previous evaluation as a teenager, she showed reduced platelet aggregation and absent ATP secretion in response to multiple platelet agonists and reduced platelet ADP consistent with a δ-storage pool disorder. Wisdom teeth extraction at 18 years was managed successfully with desmopressin. Her previous pregnancy at 32 years was managed at her local maternity unit and was uncomplicated. However, before delivery, she received a single adult dose of random donor pool platelets. Investigation by PIFT in her current pregnancy showed no platelet alloimmunization. Since her non-severe PFD was tracking in her family as

an autosomal dominant trait, she was counseled that the fetus in her current pregnancy had a 50 % probability of a similar disorder and that delivery would be performed using standard hemostatic precautions.

At 32-week gestation, the woman developed persistent nose bleeds that initially responded to local compression and ice. However, at 33 + 2 weeks, she attended the maternity unit with persistent bleeding of 4 h duration. She was not hemodynamically compromised, and she was managed with oral tranexamic acid 1 g every 6 hours and 0.3 μg/kg (pre-pregnancy weight) desmopressin by subcutaneous injection. There was a rapid resolution of bleeding, and the woman was observed in hospital overnight during which time she was instructed to avoid excessive fluid intake. The woman continued oral tranexamic acid at home.

She re-presented at 40 + 2 weeks in established second stage of labor. Oral tranexamic acid was continued, and she received a further dose of 0.3 μg/kg desmopressin. Uncomplicated vaginal delivery proceeded without regional anesthesia. After delivery, the woman received intravenous syntocinon. Blood loss after delivery was 150 mL, and the fetus was well with no clinical evidence of bleeding. The woman was discharged from hospital at 48 h after with instructions to continue oral tranexamic acid for 2 weeks.

Learning Points

1. The obstetric management of all women with PFDs requires a multidisciplinary approach between hemostasis clinicians, obstetricians, anesthetists and neonatologists.
2. Women with severe GT or BSS are at high risk of postpartum hemorrhage and require meticulous pro-haemostatic support with oral antifibrinolytics, rFVIIa, and/or HLA-selected platelet transfusions that should continue after delivery.

3. Maternal alloimmunization against platelet antigens is common in severe GT and BSS and may cause maternal platelet refractoriness and fetal bleeding through alloimmune thrombocytopenia. All women with severe GT or BSS should be screened for platelet alloantibodies throughout pregnancy.

4. The maternal and fetal risks of bleeding in non-severe PFDs vary markedly between affected women. Each pregnancy requires an individualized management plan based on the previous clinical severity of maternal bleeding and response to pro-hemostatic therapies.

5. Delivery in all women with PFDs should be performed using careful hemostatic precautions and active management of the third stage of labor. Regional anesthesia is contraindicated in severe GT or BSS and should be considered cautiously in women with non-severe PFDs.

References

1. Morrison R, Crawford J, MacPherson M, Heptinstall S. Platelet behaviour in normal pregnancy, pregnancy complicated by essential hypertension and pregnancy-induced hypertension. Thromb Haemost. 1985;54: 607–11.

2. Louden KA, Broughton Pipkin F, Heptinstall S, Fox SC, Mitchell JR, Symonds EM. A longitudinal study of platelet behaviour and thromboxane production in whole blood in normal pregnancy and the puerperium. Br J Obstet Gynaecol. 1990;97:1108–14.

3. Sheu JR, Hsiao G, Shen MY, Lin WY, Tzeng CR. The hyperaggregability of platelets from normal pregnancy is mediated through thromboxane A2 and cyclic AMP pathways. Clin Lab Haematol. 2002;24:121–9.

4. Bagamery K, Landau R, Kvell K, Graham J. Different platelet activation levels in non-pregnant, normotensive pregnant, pregnancy-induced hypertensive and pre-eclamptic women. A pilot study of flow cytometric analysis. Eur J Obstet Gynecol Reprod Biol. 2005; 121:117–8.

5. Janes SL, Goodall AH. Flow cytometric detection of circulating activated platelets and platelet hyper-responsiveness in pre-eclampsia and pregnancy. Clin Sci (Lond). 1994;86:731–9.

6. Douglas JT, Shah M, Lowe GD, Belch JJ, Forbes CD, Prentice CR. Plasma fibrinopeptide A and beta-thromboglobulin in pre-eclampsia and pregnancy hypertension. Thromb Haemost. 1982;47:54–5.

7. Star J, Rosene K, Ferland J, DiLeone G, Hogan J, Kestin A. Flow cytometric analysis of platelet activation throughout normal gestation. Obstet Gynecol. 1997;90:562–8.

8. Harlow FH, Brown MA, Brighton TA, Smith SL, Trickett AE, Kwan YL, Davis GK. Platelet activation in the hypertensive disorders of pregnancy. Am J Obstet Gynecol. 2002;187:688–95.

9. Nicolini U, Guarneri D, Gianotti GA, Campagnoli C, Crosignani PG, Gatti L. Maternal and fetal platelet activation in normal pregnancy. Obstet Gynecol. 1994;83:65–9.

10. Oron G, Ben-Haroush A, Hod M, Orvieto R, Bar J. Serum-soluble CD40 ligand in normal pregnancy and in preeclampsia. Obstet Gynecol. 2006;107:896–900.

11. Horn EH, Cooper JA, Hardy E, Heptinstall S, Rubin PC. Longitudinal studies of platelet cyclic AMP during healthy pregnancy and pregnancies at risk of pre-eclampsia. Clin Sci (Lond). 1995;89:91–9.

12. Konijnenberg A, Stokkers EW, van der Post JA, Schaap MC, Boer K, Bleker OP, Sturk A. Extensive platelet activation in preeclampsia compared with normal pregnancy: enhanced expression of cell adhesion molecules. Am J Obstet Gynecol. 1997;176: 461–9.

13. Halim A, Kanayama N, el Maradny E, Nakashima A, Bhuiyan AB, Khatun S, Terao T. Plasma P selectin (GMP-140) and glycocalicin are elevated in preeclampsia and eclampsia: their significances. Am J Obstet Gynecol. 1996;174:272–7.

14. Mellembakken JR, Solum NO, Ueland T, Videm V, Aukrust P. Increased concentrations of soluble CD40 ligand, RANTES and GRO-alpha in preeclampsia – possible role of platelet activation. Thromb Haemost. 2001;86:1272–6.

15. Norris LA, Gleeson N, Sheppard BL, Bonnar J. Whole blood platelet aggregation in moderate and severe pre-eclampsia. Br J Obstet Gynaecol. 1993;100:684–8.

16. Takeuchi T, Yoneyama Y, Suzuki S, Sawa R, Otsubo Y, Araki T. Regulation of platelet aggregation in vitro by plasma adenosine in preeclampsia. Gynecol Obstet Invest. 2001;51:36–9.

17. Ahmed Y, Sullivan MH, Elder MG. Detection of platelet desensitization in pregnancy-induced hypertension is dependent on the agonist used. Thromb Haemost. 1991;65:474–7.

18. Plow EF, Pesho MM, Ma Y-Q. Integrin alphaIIbBeta3. 2nd ed. Boston: Elsevier; 2007.

19. Kottke-Marchant K, Corcoran G. The laboratory diagnosis of platelet disorders. Arch Pathol Lab Med. 2002;126:133–46.

20. French DL. The molecular genetics of Glanzmann's thrombasthenia. Platelets. 1998;9:5–20.

21. George JN, Caen JP, Nurden AT. Glanzmann's thrombasthenia: the spectrum of clinical disease. Blood. 1990;75:1383–95.

22. Markovitch O, Ellis M, Holzinger M, Goldberger S, Beyth Y. Severe juvenile vaginal bleeding due to Glanzmann's thrombasthenia: case report and review of the literature. Am J Hematol. 1998;57:225–7.

23. Andrews RK, Berndt MC, Lopez JA. Platelets. London: Elsevier; 2007.

24. Bolton-Maggs PH, Chalmers EA, Collins PW, Harrison P, Kitchen S, Liesner RJ, Minford A, Mumford AD, Parapia LA, Perry DJ, Watson SP,

Wilde JT, Williams MD. A review of inherited platelet disorders with guidelines for their management on behalf of the UKHCDO. Br J Haematol. 2006;135: 603–33.

25. Kunishima S, Kamiya T, Saito H. Genetic abnormalities of Bernard-Soulier syndrome. Int J Hematol. 2002;76:319–27.

26. Lopez JA, Andrews RK, Afshar-Kharghan V, Berndt MC. Bernard-Soulier syndrome. Blood. 1998;91:4397–418.

27. Savoia A, Balduini CL, Savino M, Noris P, Del Vecchio M, Perrotta S, Belletti S. Poggi, iolascon A: autosomal dominant macrothrombocytopenia in Italy is most frequently a type of heterozygous Bernard-Soulier syndrome. Blood. 2001;97:1330–5.

28. Rao AK, Jalagadugula G, Sun L. Inherited defects in platelet signaling mechanisms. Semin Thromb Hemost. 2004;30:525–35.

29. Nurden P, Nurden AT. Congenital disorders associated with platelet dysfunctions. Thromb Haemost. 2008;99:253–63.

30. Hayward CP, Pai M, Liu Y, Moffat KA, Seecharan J, Webert KE, Cook RJ, Heddle NM. Diagnostic utility of light transmission platelet aggregometry: results from a prospective study of individuals referred for bleeding disorder assessments. J Thromb Haemost. 2009;7:676–84.

31. Watson S, Daly M, Dawood B, Gissen P, Makris M, Mundell S, Wilde J, Mumford A. Phenotypic approaches to gene mapping in platelet function disorders – identification of new variant of P2Y12, TxA2 and GPVI receptors. Hamostaseologie. 2010;30:29–38.

32. Kouides PA, Kadir RA. Menorrhagia associated with laboratory abnormalities of hemostasis: epidemiological, diagnostic and therapeutic aspects. J Thromb Haemost. 2007;5 Suppl 1:175–82.

33. Philipp CS, Dilley A, Miller CH, Evatt B, Baranwal A, Schwartz R, Bachmann G, Saidi P. Platelet functional defects in women with unexplained menorrhagia. J Thromb Haemost. 2003;1:477–84.

34. Toogeh G, Sharifian R, Lak M, Safaee R, Artoni A, Peyvandi F. Presentation and pattern of symptoms in 382 patients with Glanzmann thrombasthenia in Iran. Am J Hematol. 2004;77:198–9.

35. Vivier M, Treisser A, Naett M, Diemunsch P, Schmitt JP, Waller C, Tongio MM, Hemmendinger S, Lutz P. Glanzmann's thrombasthenia and pregnancy. Contribution of plasma exchange before scheduled cesarean section. J Gynecol Obstet Biol Reprod (Paris). 1989;18:507–13.

36. Bell JA, Savidge GF. Glanzmann's thrombasthenia proposed optimal management during surgery and delivery. Clin Appl Thromb Hemost. 2003;9:167–70.

37. Malhotra N, Chanana C, Deka D. Pregnancy in a patient of Glanzmann's thrombasthenia. Indian J Med Sci. 2006;60:111–3.

38. Caen JP, Castaldi PA, Leclerc JC, Inceman S, Larrieu MJ, Probst M, Bernard J. Congenital bleeding disorders with long bleeding time and normal platelet count I. Am J Med. 1966;41:4–26.

39. Cézar Alencar de Lima R, Ana Lúcia de Castro F M, Regina Amélia Lopes P A, Vitor Hugo de M, Madalena Maria Ferreira M, Eduardo Barçante R, Lúcia Jamille A, Darci Ribeiro da S. Glanzmann's thrombasthenia and pregnancy: a case report. J Bras Ginecol. 1998; 108:375–8.

40. Heyes H, Scheck R, Rasche H. Obstetrical problems in patients with Glanzmann's thrombasthenia. A casuistic presentation (author's transl). Geburtshilfe Frauenheilkd. 1979;39:68–74.

41. Peitsidis P, Datta T, Pafilis I, Otomewo O, Tuddenham EG, Kadir RA. Bernard Soulier syndrome in pregnancy: a systematic review. Haemophilia. 2010;16:584–91.

42. Michalas S, Malamitsi-Puchner A, Tsevrenis H. Pregnancy and delivery in Bernard-Soulier syndrome. Acta Obstet Gynecol Scand. 1984;63:185–6.

43. Fujimori K, Ohto H, Honda S, Sato A. Antepartum diagnosis of fetal intracranial hemorrhage due to maternal Bernard-Soulier syndrome. Obstet Gynecol. 1999;94:817–9.

44. Zatik J, Poka R, Borsos A, Pfliegler G. Variable response of Hermansky-Pudlak syndrome to prophylactic administration of 1-desamino 8D-arginine in subsequent pregnancies. Eur J Obstet Gynecol Reprod Biol. 2002;104:165–6.

45. Beesley RD, Robinson RD, Stewart TL. Two successful vaginal births after cesarean section in a patient with Hermansky-Pudlak syndrome who was treated with 1-deamino-8-arginine-vasopression during labor. Mil Med. 2008;173:1048–9.

46. Rahman SS, Myers JE, Gillham JC, Fitzmaurice R, Johnston TA. Post partum haemorrhage secondary to uterine atony, complicated by platelet storage pool disease and partial placenta diffusa: a case report. Cases J. 2008;1:393.

47. Chi C, Lee CA, England A, Hingorani J, Paintsil J, Kadir RA. Obstetric analgesia and anaesthesia in women with inherited bleeding disorders. Thromb Haemost. 2009;101:1104–11.

48. Awidi AS. Delivery of infants with Glanzmann thrombasthenia and subsequent blood transfusion requirements: a follow-up of 39 patients. Am J Hematol. 1992;40:1–4.

49. Leticee N, Kaplan C, Lemery D. Pregnancy in mother with Glanzmann's thrombasthenia and isoantibody against GPIIb-IIIa: is there a foetal risk? Eur J Obstet Gynecol Reprod Biol. 2005;121:139–42.

50. Kashyap R, Kriplani A, Saxena R, Takkar D, Choudhry VP. Pregnancy in a patient of Glanzmann's thrombasthenia with antiplatelet antibodies. J Obstet Gynaecol Res. 1997;23:247–50.

51. Uotila J, Tammela O, Makipernaa A. Fetomaternal platelet immunization associated with maternal Bernard-Soulier syndrome. Am J Perinatol. 2008; 25:219–23.

52. Peng TC, Kickler TS, Bell WR, Haller E. Obstetric complications in a patient with Bernard-Soulier syndrome. Am J Obstet Gynecol. 1991;165: 425–6.

53. Monrigal C, Beurrier P, Mercier FJ, Boyer-Neumann C, Gillard P. Glanzmann's thrombasthenia and pregnancy: a case and review of the literature. Ann Fr Anesth Reanim. 2003;22:826–30.

54. Alamelu J, Liesner R. Modern management of severe platelet function disorders. Br J Haematol. 2010;149: 813–23.

55. Bellucci S, Caen J. Molecular basis of Glanzmann's Thrombasthenia and current strategies in treatment. Blood Rev. 2002;16:193–202.

56. Kaufmann JE, Vischer UM. Cellular mechanisms of the hemostatic effects of desmopressin (DDAVP). J Thromb Haemost. 2003;1:682–9.

57. Mannucci PM. Desmopressin (DDAVP) in the treatment of bleeding disorders: the first 20 years. Blood. w1997;90:2515–21.

58. Cohen AJ, Kessler CM, Ewenstein BM. Management of von Willebrand disease: a survey on current clinical practice from the haemophilia centres of North America. Haemophilia. 2001;7:235–41.

59. Ray JG. DDAVP use during pregnancy: an analysis of its safety for mother and child. Obstet Gynecol Surv. 1998;53:450–5.

60. Mannucci PM. Use of desmopressin (DDAVP) during early pregnancy in factor VIII-deficient women. Blood. 2005;105:3382.

61. Nolan B, White B, Smith J, O'Reily C, Fitzpatrick B, Smith OP. Desmopressin: therapeutic limitations in children and adults with inherited coagulation disorders. Br J Haematol. 2000;109:865–9.

62. Hers I, Mumford A. Understanding the therapeutic action of recombinant factor VIIa in platelet disorders. Platelets. 2008;19:571–81.

63. Poon MC, D'Oiron R, Von Depka M, Khair K, Negrier C, Karafoulidou A, Huth-Kuehne A, Morfini M. Prophylactic and therapeutic recombinant factor VIIa administration to patients with Glanzmann's thrombasthenia: results of an international survey. J Thromb Haemost. 2004;2:1096–103.

64. Almeida AM, Khair K, Hann I, Liesner R. The use of recombinant factor VIIa in children with inherited platelet function disorders. Br J Haematol. 2003;121: 477–81.

65. Poon MC. The evidence for the use of recombinant human activated factor VII in the treatment of bleeding patients with quantitative and qualitative platelet disorders. Transfus Med Rev. 2007; 21:223–36.

66. Alfirevic Z, Elbourne D, Pavord S, Bolte A, Van Geijn H, Mercier F, Ahonen J, Bremme K, Bodker B, Magnusdottir EM, Salvesen K, Prendiville W, Truesdale A, Clemens F, Piercy D, Gyte G. Use of recombinant activated factor VII in primary postpartum hemorrhage: the Northern European registry 2000-2004. Obstet Gynecol. 2007;110:1270–8.

67. Franchini M, Franchi M, Bergamini V, Montagnana M, Salvagno GL, Targher G, Lippi G. The use of recombinant activated FVII in postpartum hemorrhage. Clin Obstet Gynecol. 2010;53:219–27.

68. British Committee for Standards in Haematology, Blood Transfusion Task Force. Guidelines for the use of platelet transfusions. Br J Haematol. 2003;122: 10–23.

69. Ponte ML. Insights into the management of emerging infections: regulating variant Creutzfeldt-Jakob disease transfusion risk in the UK and the US. PLoS Med. 2006;3:e342.

70. Novotny VM. Prevention and management of platelet transfusion refractoriness. Vox Sang. 1999;76:1–13.

71. Dede M, Ural AU, Yenen M, Mesten Z, Baser I. Glanzmann's thrombasthenia in two pregnant females. Am J Hematol. 2007;82:330–1.

72. Kale A, Bayhan G, Yalinkaya A, Yayla M. The use of recombinant factor VIIa in a primigravida with Glanzmann's thrombasthenia during delivery. J Perinat Med. 2004;32:456–8.

73. Monte S, Lyons G. Peripartum management of a patient with Glanzmann's thrombasthenia using Thrombelastograph. Br J Anaesth. 2002;88: 734–8.

74. Sugihara S, Katsutani S, Hyodo H, Hyodo M, Kudo Y, Fujii T, Kimura A. Postpartum hemorrhage successfully treated with recombinant factor VIIa in Glanzmann thromboasthenia. Rinsho Ketsueki. 2008;49:46–50.

75. Peaceman AM, Katz AR, Laville M. Bernard-Soulier syndrome complicating pregnancy: a case report. Obstet Gynecol. 1989;73:457–9.

76. Ito K, Yoshida H, Hatoyama H, Matsumoto H, Ban C, Mori T, Sugiyama T, Ishibashi T, Okuma M, Uchino H, et al. Antibody removal therapy used successfully at delivery of a pregnant patient with Glanzmann's thrombasthenia and multiple anti-platelet antibodies. Vox Sang. 1991;61:40–6.

77. Birchall JE, Murphy MF, Kaplan C, Kroll H. European collaborative study of the antenatal management of feto-maternal alloimmune thrombocytopenia. Br J Haematol. 2003;122:275–88.

Thrombocytopenia in Pregnancy: Gestational Thrombocytopenia and Idiopathic Thrombocytopenic Purpura

11

Stavroula Tsiara, Catherine Nelson-Piercy, and Nichola Cooper

Abstract

The management of idiopathic thrombocytopenic purpura (ITP) during pregnancy can be challenging. The diagnosis and distinction between gestational thrombocytopenia and ITP is important and requires assessment of the timing and degree of thrombocytopenia. Exclusion of thrombocytopenia of another origin and of secondary causes of ITP is also vital before embarking on treatment, and current therapeutic options are discussed in this chapter. The mode of delivery should be dictated by obstetric indications and not related to the platelet count. Fetal blood sampling is not recommended as the incidence of neonatal bleeding remains low, but a cord-derived blood count should be taken at birth. In babies who are thrombocytopenic, intravenous immunoglobulin treatment is recommended and counts should be repeated daily until normalization of the platelet count.

The most common isolated disorder of platelets observed during pregnancy is thrombocytopenia. This abnormality is of particular interest because it can affect both mother and fetus causing maternal and neonatal hemorrhagic complications. Although

S. Tsiara, PhD, FRCP
Department of Internal Medicine,
University of Ioannina, School of Medicine Ioannina,
Ioannina, Greece

C. Nelson-Piercy, MA, FRCP, FRCOG
Department of Obstetrics and Gynaecology,
Maternity Services, Guy's and St Thomas' NHS
Foundation Trust and Imperial Health Care Trust,
London, UK

N. Cooper, MD, MRCP, FRCPath (✉)
Department of Haematology,
Imperial Health Care Trust, London, UK
e-mail: nicholacooper@yahoo.com

the majority of women have normal platelet counts during pregnancy, there is frequently a slight platelet fall, particularly during the third trimester of the pregnancy, with platelet counts fluctuating from 109 to 341×10^9/L [4, 8–10]. This mild thrombocytopenia reflects a benign condition called incidental or gestational thrombocytopenia (GT) [9, 10]. Other causes of isolated thrombocytopenia during pregnancy are immune thrombocytopenia (ITP); preeclampsia; hemolysis, elevated liver enzymes, low platelet (HELLP) syndrome; HIV or malaria infection; thrombocytopenia induced by drugs, such as heparin (HIT); microangiopathic hemolytic anemias (MAHA), including hemolytic uremic syndrome (HUS) and thrombotic thrombocytopenic purpura (TTP); antiphospholipid syndrome (APS); sepsis; type IIb von Willebrand disease; and the congenital thrombocytopenias [9–12].

H. Cohen, P. O'Brien (eds.), *Disorders of Thrombosis and Hemostasis in Pregnancy*,
DOI 10.1007/978-1-4471-4411-3_11, © Springer-Verlag London 2012

Following the widespread use of automatic hematologic counters, another cause of thrombocytopenia has emerged: spurious thrombocytopenia or "pseudothrombocytopenia." This in vitro phenomenon, which is not of clinical significance, condition occurs when EDTA (ethylenediamine-tetraacetic acid) is used as the anticoagulant for blood collection. Platelets agglutinate or form clumps and the real platelet number cannot be recognized by the automatic analyzer. This phenomenon is related to the activation of certain platelet membrane glycoprotein receptors and occurs only "ex vivo," when platelets are exposed to the EDTA. For the exclusion of this spurious thrombocytopenia related to EDTA, the blood must be collected in tubes containing sodium citrate or heparin as anticoagulant, although these anticoagulants may also induce platelet clumping.

Another type of spurious thrombocytopenia is satellitism, when platelets form rosettes around white blood cells and cannot be accurately counted. Also, when there are large platelets in the circulation, these may be misdiagnosed as red cells by the automatic analyzer. In all thrombocytopenic patients, a careful examination of a blood smear is the best method to exclude misleading conditions in order to avoid unnecessary investigations and treatment [9–12, 66].

11.1 Gestational Thrombocytopenia

Gestational thrombocytopenia (GT) was first described by Burrows and Kelton in 1988 and reflects a condition that occurs during the second and third trimesters of pregnancy [9–12, 45, 63]. In patients with GT, the antenetal booking platelet count is normal, and, in the majority, the platelet count is mildly decreased to between 100 and 150×10^9/L. In rare cases, platelets might fall below 80×10^9/L [8–12]. The lower platelet count usually returns to normal within 12 weeks of delivery [45, 63]. Differences in the timing of the platelet fall and the degree of thrombocytopenia, shown in Table 11.1, help to differentiate between GT and ITP [33]. Overall, when isolated mild thrombocytopenia appears during the last trimester of pregnancy, it is most commonly due to GT or preeclampsia, rather

Table 11.1 Variables significantly differentiating gestational thrombocytopenia and ITP

Variable	GT	ITP
Gestational age at diagnosis (weeks)	32.8 ± 7.6	20.1 ± 11.1
Gestational age when platelet counts at nadir (weeks)	35.7 ± 5.5	27.0 ± 11.2
Platelet counts at diagnosis ($\times 10^9$/L)	71.3 ± 19.2	40.0 ± 25.5
Platelet count at nadir ($\times 10^9$/L)	58.6 ± 24.1	24.3 ± 15.5
Platelet count on day of delivery ($\times 10^9$/L)	70.1 ± 28.2	37.3 ± 24.0
Platelet count at postpartum day 3 ($\times 10^9$/L)	100.9 ± 1.6	81.9 ± 26.3

than to ITP or other causes of thrombocytopenia [9–12, 33]. Similarly, the platelet count on the day of delivery is significantly higher in patients with GT, relative to that of patients with ITP [33].

The incidence of GT has been investigated by several authors. In two population studies including almost 7,000 and over 4,000 women, the rate of GT was found to be 10.9 and 5.9 %, respectively, while in another study it was estimated at 5.4 % [8–12, 45]. Although the pathogenesis of this phenomenon is unknown, it has been proposed that thrombocytopenia results from relative hemodilution that occurs in pregnancy in combination with the capture and destruction of platelets in the placental bed [40]. Women with GT are usually asymptomatic, and do not have a previous history of thrombocytopenia, although if they have previously been pregnant, are likely to have also had GT in the previous pregnancy. Usually the diagnosis is made when a low platelet count is discovered incidentally on routine laboratory testing, during the second or the third trimester of pregnancy, or when delivery is imminent [8–12]. Other hematological and biochemical parameters are usually normal [8–12].

In the majority of women with GT, pregnancy and the peripartum period are uneventful, and there are no complications either for the mother or baby related to the low platelet count [8–12, 63]. The risk of developing a low platelet count in neonates of mothers with GT has been determined from cord blood samples and was found to be 4 %, similar to that observed in infants born to women with normal platelet counts [8–12]. Although GT is a benign condition, platelet counts should be monitored during pregnancy, in order to detect a sudden decline with the potential for subsequent hemorrhagic manifestations [8–12].

11.2 Immune Thrombocytopenic Purpura

Immune thrombocytopenic purpura (ITP) is an acquired disorder of platelet number that is characterized by immune-mediated platelet destruction [8–12, 60].

The disease is mostly benign with the majority of patients being asymptomatic [9–12]. It is not infrequent in women of childbearing age, although the prevalence increases with age [1, 24, 47]. The main clinical feature of the disease is hemorrhagic manifestations ranging from mild cutaneous bleeding lesions such as petechiae and ecchymoses to, rarely, severe intracranial hemorrhage [8, 41, 43, 60]. Although in children the disease is usually self-limited, in adults, it usually runs a relapsing-remitting course [8, 41, 43].

11.2.1 Terminology and Classification

An international working group on ITP defined that the term ITP requires a platelet count lower than $100 \times 10^9/L$ [43] and that the thrombocytopenia should be isolated, with an otherwise normal full blood count, peripheral blood smear, and biochemical indices [43]. Additionally, on clinical examination there should be no pathological features indicative of an underlying disease, which may precipitate thrombocytopenia [43]. In borderline conditions, when the platelet count ranges between 100 and $150 \times 10^9/L$, patients have a low probability, 6.9 %, of developing more profound thrombocytopenia and hemorrhagic complications [43]. These patients should be regularly monitored and usually they do not need treatment [43, 54, 55]. ITP is termed 'persistent' when it lasts between 3 and 12 months and 'chronic' when low platelet counts are observed for more than 12 months [43]. It is very important to distinguish between primary or secondary ITP [43]. Secondary ITP has a different natural history and usually resolves when the underlying condition is treated [43].

The same definitions should be applied to pregnant women with ITP [32].

11.2.2 Epidemiology

The incidence of ITP is not well defined. In a study based on the UK General Practice Research Database, the incidence of ITP in the general population has been determined as 3.9 cases/100,000 person-years. The incidence of ITP in women ranges from 4.9 cases/100,000 person-years in the second decade of life to 3.5 and 3.0 in the fourth and fifth decades, respectively [1, 24, 47].

During pregnancy, determination of the incidence of ITP is even more challenging because of the difficulty in distinguishing ITP from other causes of thrombocytopenia including GT [8–12]. Some authors estimate the prevalence of ITP as approximately 1–5 cases/10,000 pregnancies, whereas the prevalence of GT in the same population is 100 times greater [8–12, 27, 35, 62]. Other investigators estimated that ITP occurs in 1/1,000–1/10,000 pregnant women [1, 8–12, 27, 35, 62]. In a Korean study, among 31,309 women who were reviewed, 25 (0.07 %) were diagnosed with ITP, and 33 (0.1 %) were diagnosed with GT [33].

Similar results were obtained from a study enrolling 62,441 pregnant women: The diagnosis of ITP was established in 55 women (0.08 %), 24 of whom had a previous history of ITP [44].

11.2.3 Pathophysiology

Although the underlying pathophysiologic disorder in ITP remains unknown, there are several studies that convincingly demonstrate an altered immune response, as reviewed by Cines and Mc Millan [15]. The major feature of ITP has been considered to be the production of antiplatelet antibodies (IgG or IgM) by activated B lymphocytes. The target of these antibodies is most frequently platelet membrane glycoproteins GPIIb/IIa and Ib/IX [7, 15], although other platelet membrane glycoprotein antibodies have also been described [7, 15]. Immune complexes containing platelets coated by antiplatelet antibodies are cleared by the Fcγ receptors of the mononuclear cells in the reticuloendothelial system [42]. These cells are located primarily in the spleen but also in other organs such as the liver and the bone marrow [19, 42]. Specific genetic polymorphisms of the Fcγ receptors have been observed in patients with ITP, which may result in enhanced clearance of the antibody-coated platelet [6, 7, 19, 20, 42]. Although antiplatelet antibodies had been considered the hallmark of ITP, they have characteristically been difficult to measure and it is clear that T lymphocytes contribute to, if not initiate, ITP pathogenesis [15, 19, 39, 48, 49]. A number of studies have described polarization of T helper cells toward the Th1 immune response with an increase in the production of IL-2, IFN-γ, and TNF-α [15, 19, 39, 48, 49]. This response activates cytotoxic, inflammatory, and delayed hypersensitivity reactions [15, 19, 39, 48, 49]. In contrast, there is a reduction in Th2 response cells that produce IL-4, IL-5, IL-6, IL-9, IL-10, and IL-13 cytokines [15, 19, 20, 39, 42, 48, 49]. Activated T cells not only increase the biogenesis of B cells producing antiplatelet antibodies but also show direct CD8-mediated cytotoxicity against platelets and megakaryocytes in some patients with ITP [14, 39]. More recently, regulatory T cells have been found to be decreased in both number and functional activity when compared to healthy individuals, indicating loss of the immune tolerance [57, 65]. Ongoing interaction between B cells and T cells is also suggested by elevated CD40 and CD40L (CD154) on the surface of B and T cells. CD154 was also found in increased levels on the platelet surface in patients with ITP, suggesting that the in vivo activation of autoreactive B lymphocytes may be driven by the platelets [52].

There are also signals that impaired thrombopoiesis contributes to the thrombocytopenia in ITP [15, 19, 28, 32]. Platelet survival studies have revealed a low or inappropriately normal production of platelets in patients with ITP

[15, 19, 28, 32, 36]. Electron microscope images and in vitro studies suggest increased apoptotic indexes and poor differentiation, presumably driven by antiplatelet antibodies directed at the megakaryocytes [29]. In addition, it has been reported that in bone marrow biopsy specimens from ITP patients, there is an increased proportion of megakaryocytes with activated caspase-3, reflecting a direct effect of B and T cells on megakaryocytes [30].

Moreover, thrombopoietin, the growth factor for megakaryocytes and platelets, is inappropriately low for the platelet count when compared to the thrombopoietin levels in patients with other thrombocytopenia due to other causes such as aplastic anemia [32].

Although in the majority of patients with ITP the precipitating cause remains obscure, it has been observed that viral and bacterial infections may initiate the condition [15, 19, 58]. Viruses may cause secondary ITP, inducing loss of immune tolerance, a decrease in T helper cells, direct proliferation of B cells leading to increased antibody production, and macrophage activation which contributes to the disease severity [15, 19]. Bacterial infections, such as H. pylori infection, are also implicated in the pathogenesis of ITP, and eradication therapy can result in prolonged remissions [58]. In this situation ITP may be caused by molecular mimicry, where instead of additional production of antibodies against H. pylori, there is antibody production to self. Moreover, alterations in the cytokine milieu stimulate B cell activation and loss of immune tolerance [15, 19, 58].

Overall, it is clear that ITP is characterized by a pathogenetic diversity. Several factors can provoke the initiation of the disease and contribute to thrombocytopenia. This pathogenetic diversity observed in ITP leads to a similar variability in the clinical expression of the disease. The variation observed in the clinical picture is irrespective of the severity of thrombocytopenia and the existence of antiplatelet antibodies [41].

Better understanding of the pathogenesis of the disease will hopefully lead to treatment targeted at many of these pathophysiological alterations and amelioration of the hemorrhagic tendency [15, 19].

11.2.4 Clinical Features and Differential Diagnosis

As also occurs in the general population, pregnant women with ITP may present with hemorrhagic manifestations of variable severity, or thrombocytopenia might be an incidental finding on routine laboratory testing. Occasionally, there is a preceding history of ITP with or without treatment [2, 8–12, 60].

Women with a previous history of ITP may present with an exacerbation during any of the trimesters, or the disease may remain quiescent [9–12]. As in the nonpregnant population, the diagnosis of ITP is one of exclusion [26, 27, 41]. In accordance with the International consensus report guidance on the diagnosis and treatment of ITP, other causes of maternal thrombocytopenia during pregnancy should be excluded [41, 60]. In Table 11.2, the causes of thrombocytopenia associated only with pregnancy are shown. Thrombocytopenic conditions not necessarily associated with pregnancy are listed in Table 11.3 and laboratory investigations that should be performed in pregnant women with suspected ITP for the exclusion of underlying diseases are shown in Table 11.4. Serum antiplatelet antibodies cannot clearly establish the diagnosis of ITP because they lack specificity. During pregnancy, they are equally uninformative and they do not predict the risk of maternal or fetal hemorrhage [2, 41]. In a study including 6,770 pregnant women, 566 of whom had thrombocytopenia, antiplatelet antibodies detected using the monoclonal antibody-specific immobilization of platelet antigens assay (MAIPA), were identified in 6.7 % of thrombocytopenic women; this was no different to the incidence of detection of antibodies in nonthrombocytopenic women [5]. Other investigators found that antiplatelet antibodies were evident at a similar rate of 20.8 % of pregnant patients with ITP and 16.7 % of those with GT [33]. Similar inconclusive results have been reported in other studies [44, 45]. In this context, the International consensus report does not recommend serum antiplatelet antibody testing as a valuable method to establish the diagnosis of ITP in pregnancy [41, 60]. Similarly, bone marrow examination is not necessary for the confirmation of ITP in pregnancy,

Table 11.2 Causes of thrombocytopenia exclusively associated with pregnancy

Preeclampsia
HELLP syndrome
Acute fatty liver of pregnancy
Obstetric hemorrhage
Gestational thrombocytopenia

Table 11.3 Causes of thrombocytopenia not necessarily associated with pregnancy

Spurious – EDTA-dependent platelet agglutination
Drug-related thrombocytopenia (e.g., unfractionated heparin)
Thrombotic microangiopathies (HUS, TTP, DIC)
SLE and antiphospholipid syndrome
Autoimmune diseases (autoimmune hepatitis, Crohn's disease, thyroiditis)
Lymphoproliferative diseases (CLL and lymphomas)
Infections (HIV, HCV, H. Pylori)
Immunodeficiencies (common variable immunodeficiency, IgA deficiency)
Nutritional deficiencies (folate and B12 deficiency)
Concurrent bone marrow disorders
Congenital platelet disorders
Type II vWD
Hypersplenism

Table 11.4 Investigation of suspected ITP

Peripheral blood film
Normal blood coagulation screening (PT, aPTT, fibrinogen, D-dimers)
Liver function tests
Antinuclear antibodies (ANA)
Antiphospholipid antibodies (lupus anticoagulant, anticardiolipin and anti-beta 2 glycoprotein 1 antibodies)

unless there are clinical or laboratory indications of another underlying hematologic disease [41, 60]. In patients who fail to respond to conventional therapeutic strategies, or when splenectomy is planned for curative purposes, bone marrow aspiration and biopsy should be considered [41, 60].

11.2.5 Risks of ITP During Pregnancy

Although sometimes difficult, it is critical to determine the cause of thrombocytopenia, because women with GT usually have an uneventful pregnancy and peripartum period. In contrast, women with ITP sometimes develop severe thrombocytopenia and experience hemorrhagic complications during delivery and postpartum and require more careful monitoring [8, 41, 60].

The platelet count is an important predictor of hemorrhage in these patients [8, 41, 60].

The risk of significant hemorrhage is related to the severity of the thrombocytopenia and the gestational age at the time of diagnosis of ITP [8, 41, 60]. Women with thrombocytopenia also have a higher rate of nonhemorrhagic maternal and fetal complications. In one study which compared 199 pregnant women with thrombocytopenia due to a variety of causes (mainly GT and to a lesser extent ITP, preeclampsia, disseminated intravascular coagulation, HELLP syndrome, and antiphospholipid syndrome), to 201 women with normal platelet counts, the following complications were significantly more common (p<0.001) in the thrombocytopenia group: preterm delivery (<37 weeks), placental abruption, intrauterine growth restriction (P<0.003), stillbirth, need for induction of labor, low neonatal Apgar scores (<7) at 1 and 5 minutes, and need for blood or blood component transfusion in the mother [40].

11.2.6 Treatment of ITP During Pregnancy

The management of ITP in pregnancy is based on the estimated risk of significant maternal hemorrhage [8, 41, 46, 60]. As the platelet count usually declines during the third trimester, careful monitoring of the platelet count is required to ensure that the platelet count is adequate around the time of delivery [8, 41, 60]. The frequency of platelet count determination is based on the absolute number of platelets and the gestation [41, 60].

11.2.6.1 Indications for Treatment
Throughout the first and the second trimesters, treatment for ITP is not indicated unless:
• Hemorrhagic manifestations are evident.
• The platelet count is lower than 20–30×10^9/L.
• There is a need to increase the platelet count to a level safe for an invasive procedure (such as amniocentesis).

During the second and the third trimesters or when delivery is imminent, the platelet count should exceed 20×10^9/L [3, 8, 38, 41]. There are some variations in guidance on platelet count thresholds around delivery (detailed below). The 2010 international consensus report states that haematologists believe that the platelet count considered safe for Caesarean section is at least 50 × 10^9/L (which is therefore also required for normal vaginal delivery as emergency Caesarean section may be required); and that obstetric anaesthetists generally recommend a platelet count of at least 75 × 10^9/L for spinal or epidural anaesthesia. The authors of the 2011 ASH guidelines state that they found no evidence to support specific platelet count thresholds that are 'safe' in the antenatal or peripartum periods [3, 4, 41].

11.2.6.2 Recommended Medical Treatment
Therapeutic options used for the treatment of ITP in pregnancy are similar to those used outside of pregnancy [8, 41, 60]. Drugs of choice for first-line treatment are corticosteroids and intravenous immunoglobulin (IVIg). There is also limited evidence for the use of intravenous (IV) anti-D immunoglobulin (anti-D) [8, 18, 60]. Splenectomy, azathioprine, or combinations of the above mentioned first-line treatment options can be used in unresponsive or relapsing patients [8, 41, 60].

Other therapeutic modalities such as rituximab, vinca alkaloids, danazol, recombinant thrombopoietin receptor agonists, and immunosuppressive drugs should generally be avoided during pregnancy because of lack of evidence of benefit and the risks of possible harmful effects for the fetus [41].

11.2.6.3 Corticosteroids
Prednisolone is the most commonly used therapy in both pregnant and nonpregnant patients [8, 41, 60]. Although the standard therapy for ITP is oral administration of prednisolone in a dose of 0.5–1 mg/kg/day [8, 41, 60], during pregnancy, a lower dose such as 10–20 mg is frequently used [41]. Prednisolone is extensively metabolized in the placenta with only 10 % reaching the fetus, so is considered safe for both the mother and the fetus [10, 41, 60].

Concerns about the use of steroids include hypertension, hyperglycemia, osteoporosis, excessive weight gain, and psychosis in the mother. If higher doses are used for initial therapy, the dose should be carefully tapered to the minimum required for maintaining a safe count for delivery [8, 27, 34].

Corticosteroid administration has been described in an observational study including 110 women, 37 of whom required therapy [62]. Prednisone alone was administered in eight patients, and in seven, the drug was administered in combination with IVIg [62]. Treatment was effective in increasing the platelet count, but the increase was transient. No severe side effects were observed [62]. In another study in 284 pregnant women, 94 patients required therapy. Eighty-five patients received corticosteroids in various dose regimens [25]. Women treated with doses exceeding 15 mg/day delivered infants with abnormal body weight, either small or large for dates ($p = 0.017$) [25]. Although corticosteroids are considered safe therapy for the fetus, a slightly increased incidence of fetal death and congenital abnormalities ($p = 0.043$) was observed in one group of patients treated with larger doses (exceeding 15 mg/day) compared with the non-treated patients [25]. It seems sensible therefore, that the lowest dose of steroids required to maintain a "safe" platelet count should be used [2, 25, 62].

Platelet counts should be carefully monitored, during pregnancy and after delivery, particularly during the phase of dose tapering, to avoid a rapid fall in levels [41].

11.2.6.4 Intravenous Immunoglobulin (IVIg)

When corticosteroid therapy is ineffective, or has unacceptable side effects, or high dose and prolonged duration of therapy is required to achieve an adequate platelet count, IVIg should be considered as an alternative [16–18]. Similarly, IVIg should be administered whenever a rapid rise in platelet count is needed. [41]. Studies comparing the safety and efficacy of prednisone and IVIg are not available [16, 17]. However, data from observational studies on the administration of IVIg during pregnancy show that response rates are similar to those in the nonpregnant population with an excellent safety profile for both fetus and mother [16, 18]. Although the response rate in pregnancy exceeds that of corticosteroids, with an increase in the platelet count of up to 80 %, the effect is usually transient [16]. The mode of activity of IVIg in ITP is complicated and relates to increased expression of the inhibitory receptor FcRIIb, possibly just from the activity of a small fraction of the IVIg used [18, 51]. The recommended dose is 1 g/kg infused over the course of 1 day [41]. A small number of patients who do not respond to this dose may respond to a second infusion [18, 41]. If patients do not tolerate this large volume of infusion, smaller doses, given over a number of days, may be administered [18]. The infusion may be repeated, if needed, to prevent hemorrhage and maintain platelet counts levels safe for delivery [18].

The International consensus recommendations suggest that IVIg should be administered as initial treatment in pregnant women when the platelet count is less than 10×10^9/L and there is active bleeding or during the third trimester of pregnancy or when delivery is imminent [3, 41].

As second-line treatment after steroid failure, IVIg should be administered when the platelet count falls below 10×10^9/L, or the platelet count is $10–30 \times 10^9$/L and there is active bleeding, or in asymptomatic women with a platelet count $10–30 \times 10^9$/L when delivery is imminent [3, 27, 41].

Although generally well tolerated, IVIg causes adverse effects in approximately 5 % of patients; these include headaches, chills, myalgia, arthralgia, and back pain [41]. Headaches can be severe with acute aseptic meningitis occurring within 72 h of administration in a minority of individuals. Nonsteroidal anti-inflammatory agents which are usually used to ameliorate symptoms are contraindicated in pregnancy particularly after 32 weeks' gestation [41]. More serious adverse events such as intravascular hemolysis, renal failure, strokes, and myocardial infarctions are very rare [41]. IVIg undergoes a very rigorous production process, and transmission of viruses through IVIg has not been reported since the hepatitis C transmission reported in the 1990s [41].

11.2.6.5 Intravenous anti-D Immunoglobulin (IV anti-D)

Although IV anti-D is widely used in patients with ITP, there are few published series describing its use during pregnancy [18, 20, 22, 37]. It has been administered for ITP in pregnancy, either alone or in combination with other therapies, when an immediate rise in platelet count is required [18, 22, 37, 59]. In a small study including ten pregnant women with ITP, IV anti-D was administered during the second and the third trimesters [22]. Many of the women were taking concomitant therapy and received the drug in an attempt to increase the platelet count. In all patients, the platelet count increased above 30×10^9/L without severe side effects [22, 37]. There were no adverse events in the neonates. In particular, none of the neonates became anemic or jaundiced even though the direct test (DAT) was positive in three of the seven RhD (Rhesus) positive newborns [37].

Intravenous anti-D was also administered in a woman resistant to treatment with steroids and IVIg. She achieved a platelet count of $>40 \times 10^9$/L and had an uneventful vaginal delivery [50]. The platelet count remained high 1-week postpartum [50]. The International consensus recommendations suggest that anti-D may be administered during the second and the third trimesters in doses of 50–75 μg/kg, as a second-line therapy (evidence level IIb) [41]. However, monitoring of the neonate for neonatal jaundice, anemia, and a positive DAT is required in the postdelivery period [41, 50, 59].

The mode of action of IV anti-D immunoglobulin is different to that of IVIg [18, 20, 53]. Anti-D immunoglobulin is generally ineffective in splenectomized patients and responses can vary; patients with HIV have a better and longer-lasting response to anti-D immunoglobulin than to IVIg [18, 20, 41, 53]. Anti-D does not work through the inhibitory FcRIIb receptor but through the activating receptors [20, 23, 53].

Like IVIg, IV anti-D is usually well tolerated. As the mode of activity relates to the destruction of antibody-coated red blood cells, a fall in hemoglobin is usually seen, with a median fall of 1.5 g/dL [18, 41]. However, most individuals recover their hemoglobin levels well and only infrequently do patients develop significant anemia [18, 41, 53]. Shivers and shakes, which can accompany the infusion, are ameliorated by the use of antihistamines, paracetamol, and prednisolone premedication [18, 41]. Much more rarely, intravascular hemolysis has been reported, although not during pregnancy [18, 41]. The cases described were almost exclusively associated with other comorbidity, and it is recommended that IV anti-D is avoided during episodes of sepsis or if there is overt evidence of hemolysis or a positive DAT [41].

11.2.7 Second-Line Treatment Options

As in the nonpregnant individuals, combinations of first-line therapeutic options or splenectomy are appropriate in severely antiglobulin thrombocytopenic patients, in patients with hemorrhage, or prior to delivery (evidence level IV) [41].

11.2.7.1 Splenectomy

Splenectomy is a technically difficult procedure in pregnancy, particularly beyond the 20th week, and carries an increased risk of pregnancy loss [8, 41]. Hence, it is reserved for patients with disease resistant to other therapeutic options [41]. It may be performed during the second and the third trimesters preferably using a laparoscopic technique (evidence level III, International consensus recommendations) [41].

11.2.7.2 Use of Rituximab in Pregnancy

Rituximab has been given during pregnancy for a variety of indications including ITP, autoimmune haemolytic anaemia, and thrombotic thrombocytopenic purpura, and to treat lymphoma [41, 56]. A summary of eight case reports of rituximab given during pregnancy described no adverse events for the fetus or the neonate, despite passage of rituximab across the placenta [31]. Rituximab was given at all stages of gestation (from week 1 to week 34), and in this series, three babies were delivered prematurely (at 30, 33 and 35) with no adverse events reported [31]. B cells were depleted in four of five babies who were tested and normalized in at least one of these cases (the tests in the remaining patients were not reported) [31].

One additional child had normal levels of B cells 1 month after birth, when the mother had been treated at 21 weeks [31]. Vaccination titers were adequate in the four babies who were assessed, and immunoglobulin levels were appropriate in three children. One child, whose mother had received rituximab between 30 and 34 weeks' gestation, had low immunoglobulin levels at 1–2 months, but with partial recovery by 6 months [31]. No infectious complications were reported [31]. Although not recommended during pregnancy and not licensed for use in ITP, rituximab can be considered in refractory cases and may be safer than splenectomy and other immunosuppressive agents [41]. Although there have been reports of increased infections and rare cases of progressive multifocal leucoencephalopathy (PML) following rituximab, this appears to be more frequent in patients receiving treatment for lymphoproliferative disorders or SLE and has only very rarely been reported in adults with ITP treated with rituximab [21].

11.2.7.3 Other Immunosuppressive Drugs

As a general rule, immunosuppressive or cytotoxic agents should be avoided during pregnancy [41]. However, there are reports that come mainly from the use of azathioprine in patients with inflammatory bowel disease, lupus, and transplant recipients [41]. In these cases, the drug has been proved safe for the fetus and the mother and may safely be administered during pregnancy in all three trimesters (evidence level III) [41].

Although cyclosporine A appears safe for the fetus, it is not recommended for the treatment of ITP in pregnancy [41].

Vincristine and cyclophosphamide have been used to treat pregnant women with lymphomas and cancer, however their use should generally be avoided especially during the first trimester of pregnancy [41, 59].

11.2.7.4 Platelet Transfusions

Prophylactic platelet transfusions are not indicated in the management of ITP [41]. Transfused platelets are cleared by the macrophages soon after infusion. Platelets should be infused only in cases of severe hemorrhage or immediately before the delivery, regional anesthesia, or other invasive procedures in thrombocytopenic women, in whom other treatment options have failed [41].

11.2.7.5 Mode of Delivery

Although moderate thrombocytopenia ($<50 \times 10^9$/L) may occur in up to 10 % of neonates [60, 62], intracranial hemorrhage occurs in only 0–1.5 % of newborns with thrombocytopenia [10, 13, 25, 35, 41, 61–64]. Data from retrospective reports and small studies including 608 pregnant women with thrombocytopenia (most of whom had ITP) showed that 417 (68.5 %) of them had vaginal delivery and 191 (31.5 %) had Cesarean section [2, 17, 25, 33, 45, 62]. Patients who underwent Cesarean section had more perioperative complications mainly at the site of surgical incisions [2, 17, 25, 33, 44, 45]. Although there was evidence that uncomplicated vaginal delivery was safer for the woman, mild hemorrhagic complications such as soft tissue hematomas were observed [2, 9–13, 17, 25, 33, 44, 45].

Given the low incidence of hemorrhagic complications in the newborn, the International consensus report and 2011 ASH guidelines recommend that the mode of delivery should be primarily decided on the basis of obstetric indications [38, 41]. Platelet counts of at least 50×10^9/L are considered safe for vaginal delivery to [60] and the International consensus recommendations suggest that a platelet count of at least 50×10^9/L is also considered safe for Cesarean section [41].

The International consensus recommendations also state that vaginal delivery is previous safer for both mother and fetus [41].

11.2.7.6 Anesthetic Options

BCSH guidelines (2003, now archived) suggested that the safe platelet count for regional/neuraxial anesthesia is 80×10^9/L [8]. However, the current trend is to accept a lower threshold [3]. In a study including 80 women with platelet counts lower than 100×10^9/L during the peripartum period, 52 received epidural anaesthesia and 28 did not [3]. In this series, although platelet count was lower than 100×10^9/L, hemorrhagic complications or neurological sequelae were not recorded [3]. Although, there are insufficient data to indicate a safe platelet count required for these procedures, the International consensus report from 2010 states that a small consensus of obstetric anaesthetists agree that the minimum required platelet count is 50×10^9/L, in the absence of bruising, bleeding history, and recent anticoagulation. The international normalized ratio (INR) and the activated partial thromboplastin time test should be within normal values (evidence grade IV) [41].

11.2.8 Venous thromboembolism

Some patients with ITP in pregnancy may be at increased risk of venous thromboembolism (VTE) because of associated antiphospholipid syndrome, or as a result of other patient- or pregnancy-related factors. All patients should be assessed for their risk of VTE and managed accordingly (see chapter 3), taking into account the level of thrombocytopenia.

11.2.9 Risk of Fetal and Neonatal Thrombocytopenia

One major concern in managing ITP during pregnancy is the risk of severe thrombocytopenia and intracranial hemorrhage in the newborn. The incidence of severe thrombocytopenia in the newborn of mothers with ITP is very low. Several studies show that the incidence of severe neonatal thrombocytopenia (platelet count lower than 50×10^9/L) ranges from 9 to 15 % [10, 13, 25, 35, 41, 61, 64]. Retrospective studies, including 1,109 newborns in total, show that 119 (10 %) neonates had a platelet count lower than 50×10^9/L [2, 5, 17, 25, 40, 44, 45, 61, 62, 64]. Hemorrhagic complications have been observed in 0–1.5 % of the neonates [2, 5, 17, 25, 40, 43, 44, 59, 61, 63, 64]. The risk of severe intracranial hemorrhage in these studies is quoted as less than 1 % [61].

Moreover, it is clear that the majority of hemorrhagic complications in the newborn where the mother has ITP occur postpartum, when the neonatal platelet count is at its nadir, between the second and the fifth day of life. The risk remains high until platelet counts begins to rise; this usually occurs by the seventh day of life [41, 59, 61].

11.2.10 Assessment of the Neonatal Platelet Count

Although neonatal thrombocytopenia and related hemorrhagic complications are rare, it is well documented that infants born to mothers with ITP are at greater risk of severe bleeding compared to other babies [17, 27, 59, 61–64]. Following delivery, umbilical cord blood (which is fetal blood) should be taken for a platelet count. If the baby is thrombocytopenic (platelet count lower than 50×10^9/L), daily monitoring is recommended (ASH guidelines, level III, grade C recommendation) [41]. The International consensus report guidance recommends that offspring with platelet count below 50×10^9/L should be evaluated with transcranial ultrasound for evidence of intraventricular hemorrhage (evidence level IV) [27, 41, 60].

Several attempts have been made to predict which neonates will be born with low platelet count. Circulating maternal antiplatelet antibodies and maternal platelet count do not predict the risk of neonatal thrombocytopenia [5]. One report indicates that women with a pre-gestational history of ITP and a previous thrombocytopenic infant are more likely to deliver neonates with low platelet count [59]. Additionally, a history of severe maternal disease requiring splenectomy during pregnancy is another risk factor for neonatal thrombocytopenia [59].

11.2.11 Fetal Blood Sampling

Since maternal characteristics have been proven to be unreliable in predicting the platelet count in the newborn, direct platelet count determination, before delivery, by fetal blood sampling, was previously employed. The methods used were fetal scalp sampling and umbilical cord blood sampling. However, fetal scalp blood sampling as a method can be technically difficult, is not accurate, and usually underestimates the platelet count because platelets may form in vitro microaggregates [59, 61–64]. Although umbilical cord blood sampling is a reliable method for the assessment of the fetal platelet count, it carries an increased risk of fetal morbidity and a 1–2 % risk of fetal death. It may cause cord hematoma or hemorrhage or scalp hemorrhage, such that immediate Cesarean section is necessary or indeed the pregnancy is lost. These risks are unacceptably higher than the risk of neonatal mortality observed in ITP and outweigh the benefits of determining the fetal platelet count [59, 61–64].

In this context, the International consensus report states that attempts to determine platelet counts before delivery are not recommended (level III evidence) [41]. Furthermore, procedures associated with an increased risk of intracranial hemorrhage or scalp hemorrhage or haematoma or scalp hemorrhage or haematoma in the neonate (application of a fetal scalp electrode, fetal scalp blood samping, ventouse delivery, rotational forceps) should be avoided (level IV evidence) [41].

11.2.12 Platelet Monitoring in the Neonate

The majority of infants born to mothers with ITP have satisfactory platelet counts at birth. However, during the first week of life, the platelet count may fall [9–12], usually reaching a nadir on the second- and the third-day postpartum [9–12]. Hemorrhagic complications are rare, but when they occur, it is most commonly during these days [9–12]. It is therefore recommended that all thrombocytopenic neonates, born to mothers with ITP, should have daily monitoring of their platelet count, until the thrombocytopenia resolves [8, 41, 60].

11.2.13 Treatment of the Thrombocytopenic Neonate

Although treatment of infants with low platelet counts is rarely required, the newborn with clinical evidence of hemorrhage and/or a platelet count less than 20×10^9/L should be treated [8, 41, 60]. The treatment of choice is IVIg 1 g/kg in repeated doses if it is necessary [30]. The administration of IVIg usually produces a rapid response [41].

The ASH guidelines from 1996 recommended corticosteroid administration additionally to IVIg [26, 60]. However, when life-threatening neonatal hemorrhage occurs and/or the CNS is involved, the infant should receive combined treatment with platelet transfusions and IVIg according to the International consensus report guidance [41].

11.3 Summary

In summary, the management of ITP during pregnancy can be challenging. The diagnosis of and distinction between GT and ITP is important particularly because of the different implications for the fetal/neonatal platelet count, and requires assessment of the timing and degree of thrombocytopenia. Exclusion of thrombocytopenia of another aetiology and of secondary causes of ITP is also vital before embarking on treatment.

In those patients who require treatment to bring the platelet count up to a level considered safe for pregnancy or delivery, options are limited. If possible, treatment should be restricted to low doses of steroids. Doses of 20 mg/day may be sufficient to maintain an adequate platelet count without causing excessive side effects to mother or fetus. IVIg is generally well tolerated and can be used when low doses of steroids are ineffective, not sufficient, or poorly tolerated. The use of intravenous anti-D, whilst, not supported by robust evidence, appears safe during pregnancy with little ill effect on the fetus, although further studies are warranted. Rituximab, although not recommended during pregnancy and not licensed for use in ITP, has been used during pregnancy with no ill effect on the fetus described so far. The data are limited, nevertheless, this may prove safer than other second-line therapies, although careful follow-up and safety data are required.

Finally, the mode of delivery should be dictated by obstetric indications and not in relation to the platelet count. A platelet count of at least 50×10^9/L is required for delivery; and a platelet count of at least 75×10^9/L in generally considered safe for spinal or epidural anaesthesia, (although a lower threshold may be adequate). Fetal cord blood sampling is not recommended as the incidence of neonatal bleeding remains low, but a cord-derived blood count should be taken at birth. In babies who are thrombocytopenic, IVIg treatment is recommended and counts should be repeated daily until normalization of the platelet count.

References

1. Abrahamson PE, Hall SA, Feudjo-Tepie M, Mitrani-Gold FS, Logie J. The incidence of idiopathic thrombocytopenic purpura (ITP) among adults: a population based study and literature review. Eur J Haematol. 2009;83(2):83–9.
2. Ali R, Ozkalemkac F, Ozcelik T, Ozkocaman V, Ozan U, Kimya T, Koksal N, Bulbul-Baskan E, Develioglu O, Tufekci M, Tunali A. Idiopathic thrombocytopenic purpura in pregnancy: a single institutional experience with maternal and neonatal outcomes. Ann Hematol. 2003;82:348–52.
3. Beilin Y, Zahn J, Comerford M. Safe epidural analgesia in thirty parturients with platelet counts between 69,000 and 98,000 mm^{-3}. Anesth Analg. 1997;85:385–8.
4. Boehlen F, Hohlfeld P, Extermann P. Platelet count at term pregnancy: a reappraisal of the threshold. Obstet Gynecol. 2000;95:29–33.
5. Boehlen F, Hohlfeld P, Extermann P, De Moerloose P. Maternal antiplatelet antibodies in predicting risk of neonatal thrombocytopenia. Obstet Gynecol. 1999;93:169–73.
6. Breunis WB, van Mirre E, Bruin M, Geissler J, de Boer M, Peters M, Roos D, de Haas M, Koene HR, Kuijpers TW. Copy number variation of the activating FcGR2C gene predisposes to idiopathic thrombocytopenic purpura. Blood. 2008;111:1029–38.
7. Brighton TA, Evans PA, Castaldi CN, Chesterman CN, Chong BH. Prospective evaluation of the clinical usefulness of an antigen-specific Assay (MAIPA) in idiopathic thrombocytopenic purpura and other immune cytopenias. Blood. 1996;88:194–201.
8. British Committee for Standards in Haematology General Haematology Task Force. Guidelines for the investigation and management of Idiopathic Thrombocytopenic Purpura in adults, children and in pregnancy. Br J Haematol. 2003;120:574–96.
9. Burrows RF. Platelet disorders in pregnancy. Curr Opin Obstet Gynecol. 2001;13:115–9.
10. Burrows RF, Kelton JG. Incidentally detected thrombocytopenia in healthy mothers and their infants. N Engl J Med. 1988;319:142–5.
11. Burrows RF, Kelton JG. Thrombocytopenia at delivery: a prospective survey of 6715 deliveries. Am J Obstet Gynecol. 1990;162:731–4.
12. Burrows RF, Kelton JG. Fetal thrombocytopenia and its relation to maternal thrombocytopenia. N Engl J Med. 1993;329:1463–6.
13. Bussel JB, Sola-Visner M. Current approaches to the evaluation and management of the fetus and neonate with immune thrombocytopenia. Semin Perinatol. 2009;33:35–42.
14. Chow L, Aslam R, Speck E, Kim M, Criland N, Webster ML, Chen P, Sanib K, Ni H, Lazarus AH, Garvey B, Freedman J, Semple JW. A murine model of severe immune thrombocytopenia is induced by antibody and CD8+ T cell mediated responses that are differentially sensitive to therapy. Blood. 2010;115(6):1247–53.
15. Cines DB, Millan M. Pathogenesis of chronic immune thrombocytopenic purpura. Curr Opin Hematol. 2007;14(5):511–4.
16. Clark AL, Gall SA. Clinical uses of intravenous immunoglobulin in pregnancy. Am J Obstet Gynecol. 1997;176:241–53.
17. Cook RL, Miller RC, Katz VL, Cefalo RC. Immune thrombocytopenic purpura in pregnancy: a reappraisal of management. Obstet Gynecol. 1991;78:578–83.
18. Cooper N. Intravenous immunoglobulin and intravenous anti RhD therapy in the management of idiopathic thrombocytopenic purpura. Hematol Oncol Clin North Am. 2009;23:1317–27.
19. Cooper N, Bussel J. The pathogenesis of immune thrombocytopaenic purpura. Br J Haematol. 2006;133:364–74.
20. Cooper N, Heddle NM, Haas M, Reid ME, Lesser ML, Fleit ME, Woloski BMR, Bussel JB. Intravenous immunoglobulin and intravenous anti RhD achieve acute platelet increases by different mechanisms: modulation of cytokine and platelet responses to IV anti-D by FcγRIIa and FcγRIIa polymorphisms. Br J Haematol. 2004;124:511–8.
21. Cooper N, Arnold DM. The effect of rituximab on humoral and cell mediated immunity and infection in the treatment of autoimmune diseases. Br J Haematol. 2010;149(1):3–13.
22. Cromwell C, Tarantino M, Aledort LM. Safety of anti-D during pregnancy. Am J Hematol. 2009;84:261–2.
23. Crow AR, Lazarus AH. Role of Fcgamma receptors in the pathogenesis and treatment of ITP. J Pediatr Hematol Oncol. 2003;25(S1):S14–8.
24. Frederiksen H, Schmidt K. The incidence of idiopathic thrombocytopenic purpura increases with age. Blood. 1999;94(3):909–13.
25. Fujimura K, Harada Y, Fujimoto T, Ikeda Y, Kuramoto A, Akatsua J, Kazuo D, Mitsuhiro O, Mizoguchi H. Nationwide study of Idiopathic Thrombocytopenic Purpura in pregnant women and clinical influence on neonates. Intern J Hematol. 2002;75:426–33.
26. George JN, Woolf SH, Raskob GE, Wasser JS, Aledort LM, Balem PJ, Blanchette VS, Bussel JB, Cines DB, Kelton JG, Lichtin AE, Mc Millan R, Okerbloom JA, Regan DH, Warrier I. Idiopathic thrombocytopenic purpura: a practice guideline developed by methods for the American Society of Hematology. Blood. 1996;88:3–40.
27. Gernsheimer T, Mc Crae KR. Immune thrombocytopenic purpura in pregnancy. Curr Opin Hematol. 2007;14:574–80.
28. Gernsheimer T, Stratton J, Ballem PJ, Sluchter SJ. Mechanisms of response to treatment in ITP. N Engl J Med. 1989;320:974–8.
29. Houwerzijl EJ, Blom NR, Want JJL, Esselink MT, Koornstra JJ, Smit JW, Louwes H, Vellenga E, Wolf JTM. Ultrastructural study shows morphologic features of apoptosis and para-apoptosis in megakaryocytes from patients with idiopathic thrombocytopenic purpura. Blood. 2004;103:500–6.

30. Houwerzijl EJ, Blom NR, Want JJL, Esselink MT, Koornstra JJ, Smit JW, Louwes H, Vellenga E, Wolf JTM. Increased peripheral platelet destruction and caspase -3 independent programmed cell death of bone marrow megakaryocytes in myelodysplastic patients. Blood. 2005;105:3472–9.

31. Klink DT, van Elburg RM, Schreurs MWJ, van Well GTJ. Rituximab administration in third trimester of pregnancy suppresses neonatal B-cell development. Clin Dev Immunol. 2008;51:1–6.

32. Kosugi S, Kurata Y, Tomiyama Y. Circulating thrombopoietin levels in chronic idiopathic thrombocytopenic purpura. Br J Haematol. 1996;93:704–6.

33. Kwon JY, Shin JC, Lee JW, Lee JK, Kim SP, Rha JG. Predictors of idiopathic thrombocytopenic purpura in pregnant women presenting with thrombocytopenia. Int J Gynecol Obstet. 2006;96:85–8.

34. Marti-Carvajal AJ, Pena-Marti GE, Comunian-Carrasco G. Medical treatments for idiopathic thrombocytopenic purpura during pregnancy. Cochrane Libr. 2009;4:1–25.

35. Mc Crae KR, Samuels P, Schreiber AD. Pregnancy-associated thrombocytopenia: pathogenesis and management. Blood. 1992;80:2697–714.

36. Mc Millan R, Wang L, Tomer A, Nichola J, Pistillo J. Suppression of in vitro megakaryocyte production by antiplatelet antibodies from adult patients with chronic ITP. Blood. 2004;103:1364–9.

37. Michel M, Novoa MV, Bussel JB. Imtravenous anti-D as a treatment for immune thrombocytopenic purpura (ITP) during pregnancy. Br J Haematol. 2003;123: 142–6.

38. Neunert C, Lim W, Crowther M, Cohen A, Solberg L, Crowther MA. The American Society of Hematology 2011 evidence-based practice guideline for immune thrombocytopenia. Blood. 2011;117:4190–207.

39. Olson B, Anderson PO, Jernas M, Jacobson S, Carlson B, Carlson LMS, Wadenvik H. T-cell-mediated cytotoxicity toward platelets in chronic idiopathic thrombocytopenic purpura. Nat Med. 2003;9:1123–4.

40. Parnas M, Sheiner E, Shoham-Vardi I, Burnstein E, Yermiahu T, Levi I, Holcberg G, Yerushalmi R. Moderate to severe thrombocytopenia during pregnancy. Eur J Obstet Gynecol Reprod Biol. 2006;128:163–8.

41. Provan D, Stasi R, Newland AC, Blanchette VS, Bolton-Maggs P, Bussel JB, Chong BH, Cines DB, Gernsheimer T, Godeau B, Grainger J, Greer I, Hunt B, Imbach PA, Lyons G, Mc Millan G, Rodeghiero F, Sanz MA, Tarantino M, Watson S, Young J, Kuter DJ. International consensus report on the investigation and management of primary thrombocytopenia. Blood. 2010;115:168–86.

42. Psaila B, Bussel JB. Fc receptors in immune thrombocytopenias: a target for immunomodulation? J Clin Invest. 2008;118:2677–81.

43. Rodeghiero F, Stasi R, Gernsheimer T, Michel M, Provan D, Arnold D, Bussel J, Cines D, Chong B, Cooper N, Godeau B, Lechner K, Mazzucconi MG, Mc Millan R, Sanz M, Imbach P, Blanchette V, Kuhne T, Ruggeri M, George JN. Standardization of termi-nology, definitions and outcome criteria in immune thrombocytopenic purpura of adults and children: report from an international working group. Blood. 2009;113:2386–93.

44. Sainio S, Joutsi L, Jarvenpaa AL, Kekomaki R, Koistinen E, Riikonen S, Teramo K. Idiopathic thrombocytopenic purpura in pregnancy. Acta Obstet Gynecol Scand. 1998;77:272–7.

45. Sainio S, Kekomaki R, Riikonen S, Teramo K. Maternal thrombocytopenia at term: a population based study. Acta Obstet Gynecol Scand. 2000;79:744–9.

46. Samuels P, Bussel JB, Braitman LE, Tomaski A, Druzin ML, Mennuti MT, Cines DB. Estimation of the risk of thrombocytopenia in the offspring of pregnant women with presumed immune thrombocytopenic purpura. N Engl J Med. 1990;323:229–35.

47. Schoonen WM, Kucera G, Coalson J, Li L, Rutstein M, Mowat F. Epidemiology of immune thrombocytopenic purpura in the General Practice Research Database. Br J Haematol. 2009;145:235–44.

48. Semple JW, Freedman J. Increased antiplatelet T helper lymphocyte reactivity in patients with immune thrombocytopenia. Blood. 1991;78:2619–25.

49. Semple JW, Milev Y, Cosgrave D, Mody M, Hornstein A, Blanchette V, Freedman J. Differences in serum cytokine levels in acute and chronic ITP: relationship to platelet phenotype and antiplatelet T-cell reactivity. Blood. 1996;87:4245–54.

50. Sieunarine K, Shapiro S, Obaidi MJ, Girling J. Intravenous anti-D immunoglobulin in the treatment of resistant immune thrombocytopenic purpura in pregnancy. BJOG. 2007;114:505–7.

51. Siragam V, Crow AR, Brinc D, Song S, Freedman J, Lazarus AH. Intravenous immunoglobulin ameliorates ITP activating Fc gamma receptors on dendritic cells. Nat Med. 2006;12:688–92.

52. Solanila A, Pasquet JM, Viallard JF, Contin C, Grosset C, Dechanet-Merville J. Platelet associated CD 154 in idiopathic thrombocytopenic purpura. Blood. 2005;105:215–8.

53. Song S, Crow AR, Siragam V, Freedman J, Lazarus AH. Monocloal antibodies that mimic the action of anti-D in the amelioration of murine ITP act by a mechanism distinct from that of IVIG. Blood. 2005;105:1546–8.

54. Stasi R, Stipa E, Masi M, Cecconi M, Scimo MT, Oliva F, Sciarra A, Perroti AP, Adomo G, Amadori S, Papa G. Long-term observation of 208 adults with chronic idiopathic thrombocytopenic purpura. Am J Med. 1995;98:436–42.

55. Stasi R, Amadori S, Osborn J, Newland AC, Provan D. Long term outcome of otherwise healthy individuals with incidentally discovered thrombocytopenia. PLoS Med. 2006;3:e24.

56. Stasi R, Poeta G, Stipa E, Evangelista ML, Trawinska M, Cooper N, Amadori S. Response to B-cell depleting therapy with rituximab reverts the abnormalities of T-cell subsets in patients with idiopathic thrombocytopenic purpura. Blood. 2007;110: 2924–30.

57. Stasi R, Cooper N, Poeta G, Stipa E, Evangelista ML, Abruzzese E, Amadori S. Analysis of regulatory T-cell changes in patients with idiopathic thrombocytopenic purpura receiving B-cell depleting therapy with rituximab. Blood. 2008;112: 1147–50.

58. Stasi R, Sarpatwari A, Segal JB, Osborn J, Evangelista ML, Cooper N, Provan D, Newland A, Amadori S, Bussel JB. Effects of eradication of helicobacter pylori infection in patients with immune thrombocytopenic purpura: a systematic review. Blood. 2009;113:1231–40.

59. Sulkenik-Halevy R, Ellis HH, Fejgin MD. Management of immune thrombocytopenic purpura in pregnancy. Obstet Gynecol Surv. 2008;63:182–8.

60. The American Society of Hematology ITP Practice Guideline Panel. Diagnosis and treatment of idiopathic thrombocytopenic purpura: recommendations of the American Society of Hematology. Ann Intern Med. 1997;126:319–26.

61. Veneri D, Franchini M, Raffaeli R, Musola M, Memmo A, Franchi M, Pizzolo G. Idiopathic thrombocytopenic purpura in pregnancy: analysis of 43 consecutive cases followed at a single Italian institution. Ann Hematol. 2006;85:552–4.

62. Webert KE, Mittal R, Sigouin C, Heddle N, Kelton JG. A retrospective 11 year analysis of obstetric patients with idiopathic thrombocytopenic purpura. Blood. 2003;102:4306–11.

63. Win N, Rowley M, Pollard C, Beard J, Hambley H, Booker M. Severe gestational (incidental) thrombocytopenia: to treat or not to treat. Hematology. 2005;10: 69–72.

64. Won YW, Moon W, Yun YS, Oh HS, Choi JH, Lee YY, Kim IS, Choi IY, Ahn MJ. Clinical aspects of pregnancy and delivery in patients with chronic idiopathic thrombocytopenic purpura (ITP). Kor J Intern Med. 2005;20:129–34.

65. Yu J, Heck S, Patel V, Levan J, Yu Y, Bussel J, Yazdanbakhsh N. Defective circulating CD25 regulatory T cells in patients with chronic ITP. Blood. 2008;112:1325–8.

66. Zandecki M, Genevieve F, Gerard J, Gordon A. Spurious counts and spurious results on haematology analysers: a review. Part I: platelets. Int J Lab Hematol. 2007;29(1):4–20.

Thrombocytopenia in Pregnancy: Fetal and Neonatal Alloimmune Thrombocytopenia

12

Sukrutha Veerareddy and Pranav Pandya

Abstract

Fetal/neonatal alloimmune thrombocytopenia (FNAIT) results from the formation of antibodies by the mother which are directed against a fetal platelet alloantigen inherited from the father. The maternal alloantibodies cross the placenta and destroy the baby's platelets, and the resulting fetal thrombocytopenia may cause bleeding, particularly into the brain, before or shortly after birth. Approximately 10–20 % of affected fetuses have intracranial hemorrhages, one quarter to one half of which occur *in utero*. There are considerable controversies regarding the optimal management of FNAIT-affected pregnancies. There is no clear approach to the antenatal management of first affected pregnancies, and several questions remain in the approaches to the management of second and subsequent affected pregnancies. Currently, antenatal management of FNAIT consists of weekly maternal intravenous immunoglobulin (IVIg) infusions, with or without oral steroid therapy – the optimal steroid dosages and protocols remain to be stratified. Some centers continue to offer serial intrauterine platelet transfusions as first-line therapy, but the multiple cordocenteses that would be required to administer the platelets carry substantial risk of fetal demise. Possibilities for antenatal screening of first pregnancies are being developed. Postnatal screening does not prevent neonatal morbidity and mortality.

S. Veerareddy, MRCOG
Consultant in Obstetrics and Gynaecology,
Queen Elizabeth Hospital, South London Healthcare Trust,
Stadium Road, Woolwich, SE18 4QH, London
e-mail: sukrutha.veerareddy@nhs.net

P. Pandya, MD, FRCOG (✉)
Consultant in Fetal Medicine,
University College London Hospitals,
250 Euston Road, London, NW1 2PG, UK
e-mail: pranav.pandya@uclh.nhs.uk

H. Cohen, P. O'Brien (eds.), *Disorders of Thrombosis and Hemostasis in Pregnancy*,
DOI 10.1007/978-1-4471-4411-3_12, © Springer-Verlag London 2012

Abbreviations

FBS	Fetal blood sampling
FNAIT	Fetal neonatal alloimmune thrombocytopenia
HPA	Human platelet antigen
ICH	Intracranial hemorrhage
ITP	Idiopathic thrombocytopenia
IUPT	Intrauterine platelet transfusion
IVIg	Intravenous immunoglobulin
NIPD	Noninvasive prenatal diagnosis
NOICH	Study: no intracranial hemorrhage study

12.1 Introduction

Fetal and neonatal alloimmune thrombocytopenia (FNAIT) occurs when the mother produces antibodies against a platelet alloantigen that the fetus has inherited from the father [68, 99]. The maternal alloantibodies against fetal platelet-specific antigens cross the placenta and destroy the baby's platelets, and this may result in internal bleeding, particular into the brain [13, 49]. As a result, babies may die *in utero* or have long-lasting disability. FNAIT is usually diagnosed following the birth of a thrombocytopenic baby, or less commonly, it may be suspected following the antenatal detection of an fetal intracranial hemorrhage (ICH).

12.2 Nature and Incidence of Fetal and Neonatal Autoimmune Thrombocytopenia (FNAIT)

Platelet-specific alloantigens or human platelet alloantigens (HPAs) are expressed predominantly on platelets. If the fetus has inherited a HPA type from the father that is incompatible with the HPA type of the mother, antibodies against that specific HPA type may be produced by the mother [48, 75, 85, 95]. These IgG antibodies can easily cross the placenta as early as the 14th week of gestation and cause fetal thrombocytopenia by prompting the fetal reticuloendothelial system to

remove antibody-coated platelets from the fetal circulation [48, 51, 74]. The severity of thrombocytopenia depends on several variables, such as (a) the concentration and subclass of maternal IgG alloantibodies, (b) the density of the target antigens on the fetal platelets, (c) the activity of phagocytes in the fetal reticuloendothelial system, and (d) the ability of the fetal bone marrow to compensate for the accelerated destruction of antibody-sensitized platelets [13]. Transfer of antibodies increases as gestation progresses, until a maximum level is attained in the late third trimester [102]. The first case of FNAIT within a family is usually detected at or shortly after birth. The newborn usually presents with skin bleeding or, in a small percentage of cases, is found to have a low platelet count. However, in severe cases, ICH may occur *in utero* or during labor or shortly after birth.

The incidence of FNAIT in Caucasian populations is between 1 in 1,000 and 1 in 1,500 live births [12, 41, 61, 69, 75]. The incidence of severe thrombocytopenia ($<50 \times 10^9$/L) is 1 in 1,695 live births [107]. However, the true incidence is likely to be higher. In the study by Turner et al., only 37 % of cases with severe FNAIT were detected [107].

In the Caucasian population, 98 % of people are HPA-1a positive; consequently, 2 % of pregnant women are HPA-1a negative (HPA1bb) and are most likely to carry a HPA-1a-positive fetus and are therefore at risk of being immunized. Interestingly, only 6–12 % of HPA1bb pregnant women develop anti-HPA1a antibodies [61]. This is because the mother's immunogenetic background plays a major role [25, 71, 75]. Several studies have shown that anti-HPA-1a sensitization occurs only if the mother is HLA type DR52a, and anti-HPA-5b sensitization occurs only with HLA type DRw6 [25, 27, 40, 107, 109].

In Caucasians, antibodies to HPA-1a are the major cause of FNAIT (75 %), followed by HPA-5b (15 %) and HPA-3a (5 %), whereas in the Japanese population most cases involve antibodies to HPA-4b (Table 12.1). The diagnosis of FNAIT is made by identifying maternal HPA antibodies and documenting parental incompatibility for the HPA allele in question.

Table 12.1 HPA antibodies involved in FNAIT in Caucasians and their prevalences, literature review

Author and year	HPA-1a (%)	HPA-1b (%)	HPA-3a (%)	HPA-5a (%)	HPA-5b (%)	HPA-15 (%)	HPA-1a &HPA-5b	Other (%)
Reznikoff-Etievant (1988) [94]	90							
Mueller-Eckhardt et al. (1989) [70]	90				8			2
Kornfeld et al. (1996) [57]	90				10			
Letsky and Greaves (1996) [63]	80–90				5–15			
Khouzami et al. (1996) [52]	75							
Kanhai et al. (1996) [42]	79		5	11				
Uhrynowska et al. (1997) [108]	91	4			4			
Spencer and Burrows (2001) [102]	78		4		4			
Davoren et al. (2002) [23]	94		3		3			
Davoren et al. (2004) [24]	79	4	2	1	9		2	
Rayment et al. (2003) [92]	85				10	5		
Mandelbaum et al. (2005) [66]					2			
Ertel et al. (2005) [29]					1			
Kroll et al. (2005) [59]	75		2		18		2	
Porcelijn et al. (2006) [84]	73	1	5	1	15			

Table 12.2 Differences between Rh disease and FNAIT

	Rh	FNAIT
Incidence	1/100	1/1,000
First child affected	No	Yes
Routine screening in place	Yes	No
Testing readily available	Yes	No
Prophylaxis available	Yes	No
Severe clinical phenotype	Hydrops	ICH
Management of next pregnancy	Red cell transfusions *in utero*	IVI ± prednisolone ± platelet transfusions

12.3 Differences Between NAIT and Rhesus D Hemolytic Disease of the Newborn

Unlike in hemolytic disease of the newborn caused by maternal sensitization to fetal Rhesus D (RhD) inherited from the father, its red cell equivalent, FNAIT often occurs in the first pregnancy. However, there is currently no consensus regarding the utility of screening in previously unaffected women for antiplatelet antibodies and thus identifying women early in gestation that could be affected by FNAIT (discussed in

Sect 12.11 below). Active antenatal management of this disease is confined to those women who have had a previously affected fetus [75]. There are important differences between RhD isoimmunization and FNAIT (Table 12.2).

12.4 Diagnosis

The diagnosis of FNAIT is based on clinical and serologic findings. The typical picture is that of a neonate presenting with purpura within minutes to hours after birth, born to a healthy mother with no history of a bleeding disorder, after an uneventful pregnancy with a normal maternal platelet count [1, 11, 46, 104]. The first step in the diagnosis of FNAIT is confirmation of neonatal thrombocytopenia, followed by exclusion of the most frequent causes of neonatal thrombocytopenia such as infection, disseminated intravascular coagulation, and maternal immune thrombocytopenia (ITP) [46, 74]. The platelet count is low at birth and tends to decrease during the first 24–48 h of life. Laboratory diagnosis involves the detection of maternal circulating alloantibodies against a HPA type shared by neonatal and paternal platelets. This is accomplished using the monoclonal antibody-specific immobilization of platelet antigen (MAIPA) test [53], the platelet immunofluorescence test, or a novel antigen-specific particle assay [8, 35, 50, 54, 63, 67, 74]. The diagnosis of FNAIT is unequivocal when a parental incompatibility with corresponding maternal alloantibody is present [13, 19, 46, 51].

Recognition of FNAIT and appropriate therapy are important both for the affected neonate and for the management of subsequent pregnancies [96]. Indications for testing for FNAIT prenatally include any fetus with ICH, selected cases of ventriculomegaly (e.g., moderate to severe unilateral), neonates with thrombocytopenia of unclear etiology, neonatal ICH with significant thrombocytopenia, and familial transient neonatal thrombocytopenia [6, 16, 60, 103]. A number of FNAIT cases (10 %) have been reported in which no HPA antibody could be detected [18, 44, 76, 112]. The diagnosis is then based on maternal-fetal or maternal-paternal HPA incompatibility and exclusion of other causes of thrombocytopenia [15, 44, 79]. In some cases, antibodies may become detectable in the weeks or months after delivery or during/after a subsequent pregnancy [46, 55, 104, 114]. In unconfirmed FNAIT cases, antibodies detected before 20 weeks in a subsequent pregnancy require confirmation by a later specimen, because early transient antibodies may exist and do not seem to be of clinical significance [114]. Some studies have demonstrated significant correlation between high anti-HPA-1a antibody titers (>1:32) and fetal platelet counts below 50×10^9/L [40, 55, 114], whereas others have not [10, 84, 107]. This discrepancy may be due to differences in the size of the series, parity of the women, timing of blood sampling, or the method of antibody titration [10].

HPA typing of mother, father and fetus/neonate is important, not only for (a) the diagnosis of FNAIT but also (b) providing HPA-matched blood components to neonates with FNAIT and (c) genetic counseling and (d) estimation of the recurrence risk [65]. Conventional serologic immunophenotyping for HPA is limited by the unavailability of certain rare but well-characterized typing antisera, such as anti-HPA-1b and anti-HPA-4b [65]. Even when nonpaternity has been ruled out, it is not always possible to demonstrate parental incompatibility of platelet-specific alloantigens in the presence of corresponding maternal alloantibodies, especially if the mother is sensitized to a rare paternal antigen, making the diagnosis more difficult [83]. If there is a strong suspicion of FNAIT, testing the maternal serum against the paternal platelets (using a blood sample from the father or the fetus/neonate) may confirm incompatibility.

12.5   Fetal/Neonatal Risks

FNAIT may affect the fetus as early as the beginning of the second trimester and usually remits spontaneously within 1–3 weeks after delivery, depending on the rate of removal of maternal platelet antibodies from the neonatal circulation. Thrombocytopenia can be severe and can cause antenatal ICH in about 10–30 % of severe cases. ICH is associated with death in 10 % and neurologic sequelae in 10–20 % of cases [16, 46, 69, 74]. Chaoying et al. [21] found that FNAIT is the most important cause of ICH and poor outcome in neonates. About 25–50 % of cases of FNAIT-related ICH occur *in utero*. The majority occur between 30 and 35 weeks gestation [16, 75], but have been reported to occur in earlier gestation. Without treatment, the risk of ICH exists as long as severe thrombocytopenia persists [94]. Thrombocytopenia is most severe in the presence of HPA-1a incompatibility, which accounts for most cases of *in utero* ICH. Because no circulating antibodies can be detected in about 10 % of FNAIT-affected women, the maternal antibody level has limited use in predicting the severity of fetal/neonatal thrombocytopenia [40, 114]. Furthermore, neonatal thrombocytopenia as the result of FNAIT usually becomes progressively more severe and occurs earlier in subsequent pregnancies [11, 50, 51]. Following severe neonatal thrombocytopenia (i.e., $<50 \times 10^9$/L), a cerebral ultrasound or nuclear magnetic resonance scan is advised to detect clinically silent ICH [74, 75]. A few cases of ICH resulting from incompatibility for HPA-3a, HPA-4b, HPA-5b, or HPA-9b alloantigens have been reported [39, 86].

12.6 Antenatal Management and Outcomes

The goal of antenatal management is to prevent severe thrombocytopenia and thus ICH which may result in death, either *in utero* or after birth, or long-lasting disability. A balance must be found between the inherent risks of the condition itself and the risks of diagnostic testing and therapy. The antenatal treatment of FNAIT has evolved over the past 25 years, largely based on published case series, detailing outcomes with differing regimens. They include (a) fetal blood sampling (FBS) and serial intrauterine platelet transfusions (IUT) [44, 72], (b) weekly intravenous immunoglobulins (IVIg), and (c) immunosuppression with corticosteroids [15, 49, 73]. Over the last 15 years, there has been a gradual change from an invasive management protocol to a less invasive management protocol to a completely noninvasive approach. However, controversy still exists over the optimal antenatal management strategy.

12.6.1 Diagnostic Fetal Blood Sampling (FBS) and Intrauterine Platelet Transfusions (IUPT)

Fetal blood sampling involves the insertion of a needle into the umbilical or intrahepatic vein to sample fetal blood in order to ascertain the platelet count. The procedure is usually complemented by the transfusion of a specially selected very concentrated platelet suspension that is both HPA and ABO and RhD blood group compatible, to reduce the risk of bleeding associated with individual procedures [72, 81, 101]. With reports of a fetal loss rate of around 6 % per pregnancy [80], serial (weekly) intrauterine platelet transfusions are considered for the management of affected fetuses that do not respond to medical management alone. An important unresolved issue in the management of at-risk pregnancies is how to safely minimize or eliminate fetal blood sampling [7, 89]. FBS, with its associated risks of bleeding, boosting of antibody levels, fetal bradycardia requiring emergency (preterm) Caesarean section, and fetal loss, may not be necessary before medical therapy for FNAIT is instituted, but may be required subsequently to determine the fetal response to treatment and IUPT in selected cases [78, 90, 91, 112].

12.6.2 Intravenous Immunoglobulin

After empirical observation by Bussel et al. [16] that antenatal maternal treatment with high-dose IVIg seemed to prevent ICH in high-risk pregnancies, IVIg became increasingly popular in the treatment of FNAIT [116]. IVIg is often given to the mother on a weekly basis, using various regimens, until delivery. After birth, the neonatal platelet count and the presence of ICH provide measures for IVIg efficacy.

The mechanism of action of IVIg in FNAIT is still unclear. Four possible explanations are cited in the literature. Firstly, in the maternal circulation, the IVIg will dilute the anti-HPA antibodies, resulting in a lower proportion of anti-HPA antibodies within the IgG transferred via the Fc-receptors in the placenta. Secondly, in the placenta, IVIg may block the placenta receptor (Fc-R) and decrease the placental transmission of maternal antibodies including anti-HPA antibodies. Thirdly, in the fetus, IVIg can block the Fc-receptors on the macrophages and thereby prevent the destruction of antibody-covered cells [89]. Another possible mechanism could be that IVIg may also enhance the expression of inhibitory receptors on splenic macrophages [98] and, as a result, suppress maternal antibody production and reduce placental transfer of the antibodies [22]. So far, evidence for only the first mechanism exists.

Short-term mild side-effects that have been associated with IVIg therapy include headaches, febrile reactions, nausea, malaise, and myalgia, but these are more common with rapid infusion and can be minimized by slowing the infusion rate. Several rare but serious side-effects such as aseptic meningitis, acute renal failure, thrombosis, transmission of blood-borne diseases, reactions including severe headaches and febrile reactions, and anaphylaxis have also been reported.

The long-term side-effects of IVIg for mother and child are still unclear, but it is generally considered safe. A possible increase of IgE in children after maternal IVIg administration compared to the normal population has been suggested. However, no clinically apparent adverse effects in early childhood could be demonstrated [89]. Since IVIg is known for its immunomodulating characteristics, there is always a possibility of long-time side-effects for the mother and child. Further more, weekly IVIg administration is expensive.

Weekly maternal IVIg is the most commonly used therapy today. The IgG level after IVIg infusion decreases by 30 % after 24 h and by 50 % after 72 h [21]. Maternal administration of IVIg has been reported to increase the fetal platelet count and/or prevent ICH in 55–85 % of FNAIT [11, 17, 31, 64]; IVIg treatment seems to reduce the risk of ICH even if the fetal platelet count is not altered [7, 87]. The mechanism of the latter effect is unclear. There is conflicting evidence on the efficacy of IVIg in preventing ICH, with most reports documenting favorable results [17, 18, 64] while others report failure of IVIg in prevent ICH [58, 73, 96]. However, in the latter reports, only IVIg 1.0 g/kg/week was utilized.

Results from the study reported by Bussel at al. [17] suggested substantial elevation in fetal platelet count following treatment with IVIg 1.0 g/kg/week. The reported response rate in the literature varies from 30 to 85 %. Results from a randomized placebo-controlled trial [17] suggest no beneficial effect of adding dexamethasone to the administered IVIg. The dose of IVIg of 1.0 g/kg/week has been commonly used ever since the first publication of Bussel et al. [15]. However, the optimal treatment dose regimen of IVIg has not been formally evaluated. In treating chronic ITP, the standard dose is 400 mg/kg daily for 5 days, although 1 g/kg/day for 2 days may be more effective. Placental antibody transfer does not appear to be further increased despite high IgG concentrations in the mother as a result from IVIg treatment. This suggests a limitation of the placental Fc receptor [89].

Significant correlation between the antibody level detected by different methods in the mother and the severity of thrombocytopenia in the newborn has been observed [40, 89]. In cases of low maternal titers of anti-HPA antibodies, a lower dose of IVIg may be sufficient to reduce transmission of pathogenic HPA antibodies leading to thrombocytopenia.

Van den Akker et al. (2006) conducted a randomized international multicenter trial to compare the effectiveness of a low dose of IVIg (0.5 g/kg/week) with the commonly used dose (1.0 g/kg). Survival was 100 %; none of the neonates had an ICH; however, unfortunately, this trial ended prematurely because of a lack of patient recruitment [111]. This study might be regarded as a successful pilot study, and the use of 0.5 g/kg/week IVIg in pregnant women with FNAIT and a previous child without ICH is still an option. However, this should be restricted to patients that participate in a formal prospective study. The NOICH (no intracranial hemorrhage) 2 study is aimed at providing evidence for the effectiveness of 0.5 g/kg/week IVI in the prevention of fetal ICH in pregnancies complicated by FNAIT (www.medscinet.com/noich). Van den Akker et al. (2007) also recommend noninvasive treatment without recourse to invasive strategies, which is both safe and effective in the antenatal management of FNAIT [112].

12.6.3 Corticosteroids

The administration of steroids as the sole treatment for FNAIT is controversial, as their efficacy is variable and chronic steroid therapy has been associated with adverse effects [15]. Corticosteroids have been administered in a selection of studies alongside IVIg as a means of supporting the action of IVIg. A study in which very high-risk patients (initial fetal platelet count $<20 \times 10^9$/L or a sibling with perinatal ICH) received weekly IVIg infusions along with daily corticosteroid therapy showed that the combination was more effective than IVIg alone in eliciting a satisfactory fetal platelet response (82 % vs. 18 %) [6, 7]. Both IVIg alone and IVIg combined with any corticosteroids resulted in an improved clinical outcome in treated FNAIT fetuses compared to their untreated siblings [113]. At present, prednisone seems to be the corticosteroid of choice for treatment of FNAIT [6, 7].

Dexamethasone is now avoided as it may cross the fetal blood–brain barrier. In addition, it has been associated with oligohydramnios at higher doses [15] and a lack of efficacy at lower doses [17]. Although mothers may experience side-effects of systemic corticosteroids, clinical experience suggests no abnormalities in children of mothers treated with usual doses of prednisone throughout pregnancy.

In summary, IVIg is the mainstay of antenatal management of FNAIT. It is recommended that treatment be started 4–6 weeks before the estimated gestational age at which the ICH occurred or severe thrombocytopenia was detected in the previous affected fetus. If this information about the previous pregnancy is unavailable or if the previous sibling did not suffer ICH, IVIg therapy can be instituted at 26–28 weeks gestation because intrauterine ICH has generally been reported from 30 weeks onward [86, 87].

The role of concomitant steroids alongside IVIg needs more clarity. Bussel et al. (2010) [20] treated women with a history of previous early ICH at various gestations. Treatment comprised initial IVIg 1 or 2 g/kg/week infusion at 12 weeks, with the addition of prednisone later on only if the fetal platelet counts were $<30 \times 10^9$/L in non-responders to IVIg therapy alone. Clinical outcomes in this study were favorable. Similarly, Berkowitz et al. (2007) have proposed that 1 g/kg/week of IVI alone is clearly insufficient in siblings of fetuses with a previous ICH *in utero*. If the initial fetal platelet count is $<20 \times 10^9$/L at 20 weeks of gestation, IVIg alone 1 g/kg/week has a substantially lesser effect than IVIg and prednisone and a low response rate [6, 7]. Furthermore, they also claim that prednisone in low doses is almost as good as 1 g/kg/week of IVIg in the least affected fetuses (those with a sibling without an ICH and with a pretreatment fetal platelet count of $<20 \times 10^9$/L) [7].

Since there are substantial risks associated with FBS [78, 90, 91] and noninvasive treatment is effective, therapy for FNAIT can be instituted without invasive procedures [11, 82, 87].

A Cochrane review in 2010 [93] concluded that there are insufficient data from randomized controlled trials to determine the optimal antenatal management of FNAIT and that future trials should consider the dose of IVIg, the timing of initial treatment, monitoring of response to treatment, laboratory measures to define pregnancies with a high risk of ICH, management of nonresponders, and long-term follow-up of children.

12.6.4 Implications for Practice

1. IVIg can be used as first-line treatment for standard-risk FNAIT, where there was no peripartum ICH in an affected sibling and the pretreatment fetal platelet count (if performed) is $>20 \times 10^9$/L. However, the optimal dose of IVIg has not been established and further guidance based on the results of the NOICH 2 study is awaited.
2. IVIg in combination with prednisone has been suggested to be more effective in raising the fetal platelet count than IVIg alone in high-risk pregnancies, where the pretreatment fetal platelet count $<20 \times 10^9$/L or the affected sibling sustained a peripartum ICH. The optimal timing of administration and the dose of prednisone and IVIg is unclear, but studies demonstrating efficacy initiated treatment at 20–26 weeks.

12.7 Suggested Antenatal Management of a Subsequent Affected Fetus

Following the affected pregnancy, the father should be tested for the presence of the relevant HPA. The risk of recurrence in subsequent pregnancies is virtually 100 % if the father is homozygous for the responsible HPA and 50 % if he is heterozygous. In the latter case, it is possible to determine the fetal platelet type by 16 weeks gestation via PCR amplification of DNA obtained from amniocytes. If the fetus is found to be negative for the HPA allele, no further testing is indicated [3, 97, 102]. Preimplantation diagnosis can be considered [2]. Noninvasive prenatal diagnosis using free fetal nucleic acids obtained from maternal plasma and serum is now a clinical reality, particularly in the management of RhD hemolytic disease, and many investigators are evaluating

NIPD in FNAIT that may in the future form part of national antenatal screening programs.

The severity of FNAIT usually increases with each pregnancy. Attempts have been made to predict a fetus at risk from severe thrombocytopenia by the use of serial antibody titers in order to determine which fetus needs treatment. Although an increasing antibody titer may correlate with the severity of thrombocytopenia, occasionally the antibody may be undetectable or of low titer in severely affected cases [9, 33, 92]. Therefore, the antibody titer measurements are not useful in the clinical management of FNAIT. The clinical history of an affected sibling is currently the best indicator of risk in a current pregnancy [1, 11, 88]. The recurrence rate of ICH in the subsequent pregnancies of women with FNAIT was 72 % (of previous pregnancies without fetal deaths) and 79 % (of previous pregnancies including fetal death) [88]. Conversely, the risk of ICH in those with a history of FNAIT but without ICH was estimated to be 7 %.

It is presumed that in fetuses with early severe fetal thrombocytopenia, ICH will be seen in a second pregnancy even though this did not occur in the first sibling. In a study by Bussel and Kaplan 2007 [19], 50 % of 98 affected fetuses already had platelet counts of $<20 \times 10^9/L$ by 25 weeks, indicating early severity. Forty percent had lower fetal platelet counts at that time than their previously affected siblings had at birth, indicating increasing severity in subsequent pregnancies. They concluded that FNAIT when it occurs early in gestation is severe and is more severe in fetuses with an older affected sibling who had had an antenatal ICH. This suggests that fetuses may require different management strategies depending upon the history of their previous sibling. There has been a trend and a strong recommendation to utilize noninvasive strategies (IVIg) in the management of FNAIT at high risk of *in utero* or postnatal ICH [26, 43].

For platelet antigen incompatibilities other than HPA-1a, much less data exist regarding antenatal management and clinical course. Incompatibility of HPA-3a, while infrequent, is as severe as that of HPA-1 [34], while incompatibilities of HPA-5b and HPA-9b are less severe [45]. HPA-4 incompatibility seems also to be severe [30], and most rare antigens are identified because of a severe case of neonatal FNAIT.

12.8 Timing and Mode of Birth

The delivery plan should be based on the patient's risk category, the response to treatment, and the most recent fetal platelet count if pertinent [36]. The appropriate gestational age for delivery has not been established. The risk of prematurity and the costs of neonatal intensive care unit admission should be weighed against the risk of continued exposure of the fetus to the harmful antibodies and the cost of IVIg therapy. Different units recommend delivery between 35 weeks and term. Vaginal delivery is reasonable if fetal platelet counts exceed $50 \times 10^9/L$ [17]. With platelet counts below $50 \times 10^9/L$, IUPT have been performed before vaginal delivery for protection against bleeding at the time of delivery, with associated risks. There is no evidence that vaginal delivery of a fetus with a platelet count $<50 \times 10^9/L$ increases the risk of ICH. In a Dutch study of 32 pregnancies complicated by FNAIT in which the thrombocytopenic sibling did not have an ICH, vaginal delivery was not associated with neonatal intracranial bleeding, even though the platelet count was $<50 \times 10^9/L$ in four neonates [110]. Caesarean delivery alone is not considered to be effective in preventing antenatal or perinatal hemorrhage [74, 100]. Instrumental vaginal delivery, ventouse, fetal scalp electrodes, and fetal scalp blood samples should be avoided. The neonatologist on duty during delivery should be informed in advance, as should a consultant in haematology/transfusion medicine and the blood transfusion laboratory should also be asked in advance to obtain HPA compatible platelets.

12.9 Treatment of the Neonate

Treatment of the neonate is dictated by the condition of the newborn. If there are no signs of bleeding and the thrombocytopenia is mild or moderate, no therapy is necessary. In cases of neonatal bleeding or a platelet count $<30 \times 10^9/L$, therapy is needed and must be rapid and effective. First-line therapy is prompt transfusion of ideally HPA-compatible platelets which will not be destroyed by maternal antibodies in the neonate's circulation. Blood centres should be able to supply platelets, which should be HPA-1a and 5b negative. If these are not available, an amendment to the British Committee in Standards for Haematology (BCSH) guidelines recommends using platelets that are not selected for HPA status [114]. Treatment of neonatal FNAIT with IVIg and/or steroids is advised when severe thrombocytopenia and/or hemorrhage persist despite transfusion of HPA-compatible platelets. Platelet transfusion thresholds of $20–30 \times 10^9$/L and 50×10^9/L are recommended for neonates depending on the clinical situation [114]. The effectiveness of IVIg in the neonate has not been shown in some studies [106]. The therapeutic effect on the platelet count, however, is delayed for 24–48 h, when the neonate remains at risk of ICH.

12.10 Preconception Counseling

Pregnant women are at risk for FNAIT if they have a history of a previous neonate with FNAIT or are known to have circulating alloantibodies [13]. Before a subsequent pregnancy, these women should be referred to a tertiary center which specializes in the treatment of FNAIT. The risks of ICH in a subsequent pregnancy and the diagnosis and treatment strategies that might be of benefit should be discussed, as addressed above. If the previously affected child had an ICH, there is a 70–80 % chance that the next affected child will have an ICH. However, if the pregnancy complicated by FNAIT did not involve ICH, the risk of ICH in a subsequent pregnancy is less than 10 % [5, 11, 88]. Counseling is most effective after HPA typing of the father. If the father is homozygous for the HPA allele, the risk of recurrence of FNAIT is 100 %, whereas the risk of recurrence is 50 % if the father is heterozygous.

12.11 Screening for FNAIT in the First Pregnancy

The implementation of an antenatal screening program for FNAIT depends on cost-effectiveness and is currently under debate. Several studies provided calculations and reached the conclusion that screening is likely to be cost-effective [11, 32, 56, 62, 76], although this was not a universal view [28]. Antenatal screening for FNAIT might identify alloimmunized women during their first pregnancy, allowing antenatal intervention to prevent ICH. Even if no antenatal intervention was undertaken, delivery could be planned so that compatible platelets would be available [75].

The major determinants of the costs are the initial HPA typing, antibody detection in those at risk, and costs of interventions. Although these costs are considerable, even in the most expensive strategy (e.g., offering IVIg to all immunized women), they are easily outweighed by the savings made in preventing most cases of lifelong severe neurological morbidity.

Three large studies of antenatal screening for HPA-1a incompatibility have been performed [61, 107, 115]. Two, from East Anglia [115] and Scotland [107] in the UK, were performed in approximately 25,000 cases each. The largest study in Norway encompassed more than 100,000 pregnancies [61]. Another study from Norway concluded that without a screening programme, the detection rate of NAIT in Norway is only 14% of expected [105]. Key findings from these studies suggest that the incidence of FNAIT in the neonate was approximately 1:5,000, but on antenatal screening, a higher incidence of 1:1,000 using HPA-1a incompatibility only was noted. A systematic review suggests screening for HPA-1a alloimmunization detects about two cases in 1,000 pregnancies and that severe FNAIT occurs in about 40 per 1,000,000 pregnancies. Despite several antenatal interventions, severe ICH occurred in three to four children per 1,000,000 pregnancies screened. Furthermore, the review highlighted that the incidence of ICH in non-screened populations is likely to be higher. Screening of all pregnancies together with effective antenatal treatment such as IVIg may reduce the mortality and morbidity associated with FNAIT without known risks for the mother or child [41, 47, 90, 91]. These data indeed indicate that large-scale screening studies including comparison of intervention strategies are warranted [37, 38].

Conclusions

The most serious complication of FNAIT is ICH, which occurs in 10–30 % of severe cases, causing death (10 %) and neurologic sequelae (10–20 %). In the majority of cases, fetal thrombocytopenia is more severe and occurs successively earlier in subsequent pregnancies [16]. There is a 70–80 % risk of antenatal ICH in a subsequent pregnancy complicated by FNAIT if a previous child had ICH [11, 87]. Most cases of *in utero* ICH involve HPA-1a incompatibility with severe thrombocytopenia, although a few cases have resulted from incompatibility for HPA-3a, HPA-4b, HPA-5b, or HPA-9b alloantigens.

Antenatal management of FNAIT includes weekly maternal IVIg infusions which is very effective. Concomitant usage of steroids alongside IVIg has been suggested to show favorable results in high-risk fetuses that have not responded to IVIg alone [4–6, 20]. Treatment should start 4–6 weeks before the estimated gestational age at which ICH or severe thrombocytopenia occurred in the previous pregnancy or at approximately 28 weeks gestation [86, 87].

FBS with its significant associated risks may not be necessary before therapy for FNAIT is instituted, but may become necessary to determine the fetal response to treatment [112]. Spontaneous vaginal delivery is preferred in FNAIT cases while avoiding procedures that might increase the risk of fetal hemorrhage (no scalp electrodes, no fetal scalp blood samples, and no instrumental vaginal delivery or ventouse) [110]. Caesarean section may be performed in high-risk fetuses selectively.

At present, there is no approved method of antenatal screening to detect the first affected pregnancy [55, 77, 115]. Postnatal screening, although simple, cannot prevent neonatal morbidity and mortality [76].

The aim of current research must be to develop reliable predictors of disease severity in affected infants and increase the effectiveness of noninvasive treatment strategies for FNAIT. Prospective trials (such as NOICH 2, www.medscinet.com/noich) are necessary to evaluate different treatment strategies and to acquire additional data on optimal prevention programs.

Learning Points

1. All cases of FNAIT should be managed by maternal-fetal medicine specialists in tertiary referral centers, with appropriate liaison with specialists in neonatology and haematology/transfusion medicine.
2. If the previously affected sibling had an ICH, the next affected fetus is highly likely to have early, severe thrombocytopenia and *in utero* ICH, in the absence of effective treatment.
3. Effective noninvasive antenatal treatment (IVIg) exists for cases recognized as a result of a previously affected sibling.
4. Invasive treatment (intrauterine platelet transfusions) appears to be required only in nonresponders.

References

1. Ahya R, Turner ML, Urbaniak SJ. Fetomaternal alloimmunethrombocytopenia. Transfus Apher Sci. 2001;25:139–45.
2. Bennett PR, Vaughan J, Handyside A. Potential for pre-implantation determination of human platelet antigen type using DNA amplification: a strategy for prevention of allo-immune thrombocytopenia. Fetal Diagn Ther. 1994;9:229–32.
3. Bennett PR, Warwick R, Vaughan J. Prenatal determination of human platelet antigen type using DNA amplification following amniocentesis. Br J Obstet Gynaecol. 1994;101:246–9.
4. Berkowitz RL, Bussel JB, Mc Farland JG. Alloimmune thrombocytopenia: state of the art. Am J Obstet Gynecol. 2006;195:907–13.
5. Berkowitz R, Bussel JB, Hung C, Wissert M. A randomised prospective treatment trial for patients with "standard risk" alloimmune thrombocytopenia (AIT). Am J Obstet Gynecol. 2006;195 Suppl 1:S23.
6. Berkowitz RL, Kolb A, Mcfarland JG. Parallel randomized trials of risk-based therapy for fetal alloimmune thrombocytopenia. Obstet Gynecol. 2006;107:91–6.
7. Berkowitz RL, Lesser ML, McFarland JG, Wissert M, Primiani A, Hung C. Antepartum treatment without early cordocentesis for standard-risk alloimmune thrombocytopenia: a randomised controlled trial. Obstet Gynecol. 2007;110(2 Pt 1):249–55.
8. Bertrand G, Jallu V, Gouet M. Quantification of human platelet antigen-1a antibodies with monoclonal antibody immobilization of platelet antigens procedure. Transfusion. 2005;45:1319–23.

9. Bertrand G, Martageix C, Jallu V. Predictive value of sequential maternal anti-HPA-1a antibody concentrations for the severity of fetal allo immune thrombocytopenia. J Thromb Haemost. 2006;4:628–37.

10. Bessos H, Turner M, Urbaniak SJ. Is there a relationship between anti-HPA-1a concentration and severity of neonatal alloimmune thrombocytopenia? Immunohematology. 2005;21:102–8.

11. Birchall J, Murphy MF, Kaplan C. European collaborative study of the antenatal management of feto-maternal alloimmune thrombocytopenia. Br J Haematol. 2003; 122:275–88.

12. Blanchette VS, Chen L, de Friedberg ZS. Alloimmunisation to the PlA1 platelet antigen: results of a prospective study. Br J Haematol. 1990;74:209–15.

13. Blanchette VS, Johnson J, Rand M. The management of alloimmune neonatal thrombocytopenia. Baillieres Best Pract Res Clin Haematol. 2000;13:365–90.

14. Burrows RF, Kelton JG. Fetal thrombocytopenia and its relation to maternal thrombocytopenia. N Engl J Med. 1993;329:1463–6.

15. Bussel JB, Berkowitz RL, McFarland JG. Antenatal treatment of neonatal alloimmune thrombocytopenia. N Engl J Med. 1988;319:1374–8.

16. Bussel JB, Skupski DW, Mcfarland JG. Fetal alloimmune thrombocytopenia: consensus and controversy. J Matern Fetal Med. 1996;5:281–92.

17. Bussel JB, Berkowitz RL, Lynch L, Lesser ML, Paidas MJ, Huang CL. Antenatal management of alloimmune thrombocytopenia with intravenous gamma-globulin: a randomized trial of the addition of low dose steroid to intravenous gamma-globulin. Am J Obstet Gynecol. 1996;174(5):1414–23.

18. Bussel JB. Immune thrombocytopenia in pregnancy: autoimmune and allo-immune. J Reprod Immunol. 1997;37:35–61.

19. Bussel JB, Kaplan C. The fetal and neonatal consequences of maternal alloimmune thrombocytopenia. Baillieres Clin Hematol. 2007;11:391–408.

20. Bussel JB, Berkowitz RL, Hung C, Kolb EA, Wissert M, Primiani A, Tsaur FW, Macfarland JG. Intracranial hemorrhage in alloimmune thrombocytopenia: stratified management to prevent recurrence in the subsequent affected fetus. Am J Obstet Gynecol. 2010;203(2):135. e1–14.

21. Chaoying M, Junwu G, Chituwo BM. Intraventricular haemorrhage and its prognosis, prevention and treatment in term infants. J Trop Pediatr. 1999;45:237–9.

22. Clark AL, Gall SA. Clinical uses of intravenous immunoglobulin in pregnancy. Am J Obstet Gynecol. 1998;176:241–53.

23. Davoren A, McParland P, Barnes CA. Neonatal alloimmune thrombocytopenia in the Irish population: a discrepancy between observed and expected cases. J Clin Pathol. 2002;55:289–92.

24. Davoren A, Curtis BR, Aster RH. Human platelet antigen-specific alloantibodies implicated in 1162 cases of neonatal alloimmune thrombocytopenia. Immunohematol. 2004;44:1220–5.

25. Decary F, L'Abbe D, Tremblay L. The immune response to the HPA-1a antigen: association with HLA-DRw52a. Transfus Med. 1991;1:55–62.

26. Deruelle P, Wibaut B, Manessier L, Subtil D, Vaast P, Puech F, Valat AS. Is a non-invasive management allowed for maternofetal alloimmune thrombocytopenia? Experience over a 10-year period. Gynecol Obstet Fertil. 2007;35(3):199–204.

27. Doughty HA, Murphy MF, Metcalfe P. Antenatal screening for fetal alloimmune thrombocytopenia: the results of a pilot study. Br J Haematol. 1995;90:321–5.

28. Durand-Zaleski I, Schlegel N, Blum-Boisgard C, Uzan S, Dreyfus M, Kaplan C. Screening primiparous women and newborns for fetal/neonatal alloimmune thrombocytopenia: a prospective comparison of effectiveness and costs. Am J Perinatol. 1996;13:423–31.

29. Ertel K, Al-Tawil M, Santoso S. Relevance of the HPA-15 (Gov) polymorphism on CD109 in alloimmune thrombocytopenic syndromes. Transfusion. 2005;45:366–73.

30. Friedman JM, Aster RH. Neonatal alloimmune thrombocytopenic purpura and congenital porencephaly in two siblings associated with a "new" maternal antiplatelet antibody. Blood. 1985;65:1412–5.

31. Gaddipati S, Berkowitz RL, Lembet AA. Initial fetal platelet counts predict the response to intravenous gammaglobulin therapy in fetuses that are affected by PLA1 incompatibility. Am J Obstet Gynecol. 2001; 185:976–80.

32. Gafni A, Blanchette VS. Screening for alloimmune thrombocytopenia: an economic perspective. Curr Stud Hematol Blood Transfus. 1988;54:140–7.

33. Ghevaert C, Campbell K, Stafford P, Metcalfe P, Casbard A, Smith GA, Allen D, Ranasinghe E, Williamson LM, Ouwehand WH. HPA-1a antibody potency and bioactivity do not predict severity of feto-maternal alloimmune thrombocytopenia. Transfusion. 2007;7:1296–305.

34. Glade-Bender J, McFarland JG, Kaplan C, Porcelijn L, Bussel JB. Anti-HPA-3A induces severe neonatal alloimmune thrombocytopenia. J Pediatr. 2001;138: 862–7.

35. Goldman M, Trudel E, Richard L. Report on the eleventh international society of blood transfusion platelet genotyping and serology workshop. Vox Sang. 2003;85:149–55.

36. Gyamfi C, Eddleman KA. Alloimmune thrombocytopenia. Clin Obstet Gynecol. 2005;48:897–909.

37. Husebekk A, Killie MK, Kjeldsen-Kragh J. General overview over screening programs. Vox Sang. 2006; 91:15. Abstract 49.

38. Husebekk A, Killie MK, Kjeldsen-Kragh J, Skogen B. Is it time to implement HPA-1 screening in pregnancy? Curr Opin Hematol. 2009;16(6):497–502.

39. Ino H, Torigoe K, Numata O. A case of neonatal alloimmune thrombocytopenic purpura by anti-HPA-4b with intracranial hemorrhage. J Jpn Pediatr Soc. 2000;104:682–5.

40. Jaegtvik S, Husebekk A, Aune B. Neonatal alloimmune thrombocytopenia due to anti-HPA-1a antibod-

ies; the level of maternal antibodies predicts the severity of thrombocytopenia in the newborn. Br J Obstet Gynaecol. 2000;107:691–4.

41. Kamphuis MM, Paridaans N, Porcelijn L, De Haas M, van der Schoot CE, Brand A, Bonsel GJ, Oepkes D. Screening in pregnancy for fetal or neonatal alloimmune thrombocytopenia: systematic review. BJOG. 2010;117(11):1335–43.

42. Kanhai HHH, Porcelijn L, van Zoeren D. Antenatal care in pregnancies at risk of alloimmune thrombocytopenia: report of 19 cases in 16 families. Eur J Obstet Gynecol Reprod Biol. 1996;68:67–73.

43. Kanhai HH, van den Akker ES, Walther FJ, Brand A. Intravenous immunoglobulins without initial and follow-up cordocentesis in alloimmune fetal and neonatal thrombocytopenia at high risk for intracranial hemorrhage. Fetal Diagn Ther. 2006;21(1):55–60.

44. Kaplan C, Daffos F, Forestier F. Management of alloimmune thrombocytopenia: antenatal diagnosis and *in utero* transfusion of maternal platelets. Blood. 1988;72:340–3.

45. Kaplan C, Morel-Kopp MC, Kroll H, Kiefel V, Sohlege N, Chesnel N, Mueller-Eckhardt C. HPA-5b (Br(a)) neonatal alloimmune thrombocytopenia: clinical and immunological analysis of 39 cases. Br J Haematol. 1991;78:425–9.

46. Kaplan C, Morel-Kopp MC, Clemenceau S. Fetal and neonatal alloimmune thrombocytopenia: current trends in diagnosis and therapy. Transfus Med. 1992; 2:265–71.

47. Kaplan C. Alloimmune thrombocytopenia of the fetus and neonate: prospective antenatal screening. Third European symposium on platelet and granulocyte immunobiology. Cambridge. 26–29 June 1994.

48. Kaplan C, Forestier F, Daffos F. Management of fetal and neonatal alloimmune thrombocytopenia. Transfus Med Rev. 1996;10:233–40.

49. Kaplan C, Murphy MF. Feto-maternal alloimmune thrombocytopenia: antenatal therapy with IvIgG and steroids – more questions than answers. European Working Group on FMAIT. Br J Haematol. 1998; 100(1):62–5.

50. Kaplan C. Alloimmune thrombocytopenia of the fetus and the newborn. Blood Rev. 2002;16:69–72.

51. Kaplan C. Platelet alloimmunity: the fetal/neonatal alloimmune thrombocytopenia. Vox Sang. 2002;83 Suppl 1:289–91.

52. Khouzami AN, Kickler TS, Callan NA. Devastating sequelae of alloimmune thrombocytopenia: an entity that deserves more attention. J Matern Fetal Med. 1996;5:137–41.

53. Kiefel V. The MAIPA assay and its applications in immunohaematology. Transfus Med. 1992;2:181–8.

54. Killie MK, Kjeldsen-Kragh J, Skogen B. Maternal anti-HPA1a antibody level as predictive value in neonatal alloimmune thrombocytopenic purpura (NAITP). Blood. 2004;104:Abstract 2072.

55. Killie MK, Husebekk A, Kjeldsen-Kragh J. Significance of antibody quantification. Vox Sang. 2006;91:15. Abstract 51.

56. Killie MK, Kjeldsen-Kragh J, Husebekk A, Skogen B, Olsen JA, Kristiansen IS. Cost-effectiveness of antenatal screening for neonatal alloimmune thrombocytopenia. BJOG. 2007;114:588–95.

57. Kornfeld I, Wilson RD, Ballem P. Antenatal invasive and noninvasive management of alloimmune thrombocytopenia. Fetal Diagn Ther. 1996;11:210–7.

58. Kroll H, Kiefel V, Giers G, Bald R, Hoch J, Hanfland P. Maternal intravenous immunoglobulin treatment does not prevent intracranial haemorrhage in fetal alloimmune thrombocytopenia. Transfus Med. 1994;4(4): 293–6.

59. Kroll H, Yates J, Santoso S. Immunization against a low-frequency human platelet alloantigen in fetal alloimmune thrombocytopenia is not a single event: characterization by the combined use of reference DNA and novel allele-specific cell lines expressing recombinant antigens. Transfusion. 2005;45:353–8.

60. Kuhn MJ, Couch SM, Binstadt DH. Prenatal recognition of central nervous system complications of alloimmune thrombocytopenia. Comput Med Imaging Graph. 1992;16:137–42.

61. Kjeldsen-Kragh J, Killie MK, Tomter G, Golebiowska E, Randen I, Hauge R. A screening and intervention program aimed to reduce mortality and serious morbidity associated with severe neonatal alloimmune thrombocytopenia. Blood. 2007; 110:833.

62. Kjedsen-Kragh J, Husebekk A, Kjaer Killie M, Skogen B. Is it time to include screening for neonatal alloimmune thrombocytopenia in the general antenatal health program? Transfus Apher Sci. 2008;38: 183–8.

63. Letsky EA, Greaves M. Guidelines on the investigation and management of thrombocytopenia in pregnancy and neonatal alloimmune thrombocytopenia. Br J Haematol. 1996;95:21–6.

64. Lynch L, Bussel JB, McFarland JG, Chitkara U, Berkowitz RL. Antenatal treatment of alloimmune thrombocytopenia. Obstet Gynecol. 1992;80:67–71.

65. Lyou JY, Chen YJ, Hu HY. PCR with sequence-specific primer-based simultaneous genotyping of human platelet antigen-1 to -13w. Transfusion. 2002; 42:1089–95.

66. Mandelbaum M, Koren D, Eichelberger B. Frequencies of maternal platelet alloantibodies and autoantibodies in suspected fetal/neonatal alloimmune thrombocytopenia, with emphasis on human platelet antigen-15 alloimmunization. Vox Sang. 2005;89:39–43.

67. Meyer O, Agaylan A, Borchert H. A simple and practical assay for the antigen-specific detection of platelet antibodies. Transfusion. 2006;46:1226–31.

68. Moulinier J. Alloimmunisation maternelle antiplaquettaire duzo. In: Proceedings of the 6th congress of the European society of haematology. Paris: European Society of Hematology; 1953. p. 817–20.

69. Mueller-Eckhardt C, Mueller-Eckhardt G, Willen-Ohff H, Horz A, Kuenzlen E, O'Neill GJ. Immunogenicity of and immune response to the human platelet antigen Zwa is strongly associated

with HLAB8 and DR3. Tissue Antigens. 1985; 26:71–6.

70. Mueller-Eckhardt C, Grubert A, Weisheit M. 348 cases of suspected neonatal alloimmune thrombocytopenia. Lancet. 1989;1:363–6.

71. Mueller-Eckhardt C, Santoso S, Kiefel V. Platelet alloantigens molecular, genetic, and clinical aspects. Vox Sang. 1994;67S3:89–93.

72. Murphy MF, Pullon HWH, Metcalfe P, Chapman JF, Jenkins E, Waters AH. Management of fetal alloimmune thrombocytopenia by weekly in utero platelet transfusions. Vox Sang. 1990;58:45–9.

73. Murphy MF, Waters AH, Doughty HA, Hambley H, Mibashan RS, Nicolaides K. Antenatal management of fetal alloimmune thrombocytopenia. Transfus Med. 1994;4:281–92.

74. Murphy MF, Manley R, Roberts D. Neonatal alloimmune thrombocytopenia. Haematologica. 1999;84:110–4.

75. Murphy MF, Williamson LM. Antenatal screening for fetomaternal alloimmune thrombocytopenia: an evaluation using the criteria of the UK National Screening Committee. Br J Haematol. 2000;111:726–32.

76. Murphy MF, Williamson LM, Urbaniak SJ. Antenatal screening for fetomaternal alloimmune thrombocytopenia: should we be doing it? Vox Sang. 2002;83 Suppl 1:409–16.

77. Murphy MF, Bussel JB. Advances in the management of alloimmune thrombocytopenia. Br J Haematol. 2007;136:366–78.

78. Nicolini U, Kochenour NK, Greco P, Letsky EA, Johnson RD, Contreras M. Consequences of fetomaternal haemorrhage after intrauterine transfusion. BMJ. 1988;297:1379–81.

79. Ohto H, Yamaguchi T, Takeuchi C. Anti-HPA-5b-induced neonatal alloimmune thrombocytopenia: antibody titre as predictor. Br J Haematol. 2000;110:223–7.

80. Overton TG, Duncan KR, Jolly M, Letsky E, Fisk NM. Serial aggressive platelet transfusion for fetal alloimmune thrombocytopenia: platelet dynamics and perinatal outcome. Am J Obstet Gynecol. 2002;186(4):826–31.

81. Paidas MJ, Berkowitz RL, Lynch L, Lockwood CJ, Lapinski R, McFarland JG. Alloimmune thrombocytopenia: fetal and neonatal losses related to cordocentesis. Am J Obstet Gynecol. 1995;172:475–9.

82. Paternoster DM, Cester M, Memmo A. The management of feto-maternal alloimmune thrombocytopenia: report of three cases. J Matern Fetal Neonatal Med. 2006;19:517–20.

83. Peterson JA, Balthazor SM, Curtis BR. Maternal alloimmunization against the rare platelet-specific antigen HPA-9b (Max-a) is an important cause of neonatal alloimmune thrombocytopenia. Transfusion. 2005;45:1487–95.

84. Porcelijn L, Huiskes E, Overbeeke M. Rare anti HPA-5a NAIT cases. Vox Sang. 2006;91S2:Abstract 55.

85. Proulx C, Filion M, Goldman M. Analysis of immunoglobulin class, IgG subclass and titre of HPA-1a antibodies in alloimmunized mothers giving birth to

babies with or without neonatal alloimmune thrombocytopenia. Br J Haematol. 1994;87:813–7.

86. Radder CM, Kanhai HH, de Beaufort AJ. Evaluation of gradual conversion to a less invasive therapeutic strategy for pregnant women with alloimmune thrombocytopenia in the fetus for prevention of intracranial hemorrhage. Ned Tijdschr Geneeskd. 2000;144:2015–8.

87. Radder CM, Brand A, Kanhai HH. A less invasive treatment strategy to prevent intracranial hemorrhage in fetal and neonatal alloimmune thrombocytopenia. Am J Obstet Gynecol. 2001;185:683–8.

88. Radder CM, Brand A, Kanhai HHH. Will it ever be possible to balance the risk of intracranial haemorrhage in fetal or neonatal alloimmune thrombocytopenia against the risk of treatment strategies to prevent it? Vox Sang. 2003;84:318–25.

89. Radder CM, Kanhai HH, Brand A. On the mechanism of high dose maternal intravenous immunoglobulin (IVIG) in alloimmune thrombocytopenia. In: Management of fetal alloimmune thrombocytopenia. Amsterdam: Print Partners Ipskamp; 2004. p. 69–81.

90. Radder CM, Roelen DL, Van de Meer-Prins EM, Claas FHJ, Kanhai HHH, Brand A. The immunologic profile of infants born after maternal immunoglobulin treatment and intrauterine platelet transfusions for fetal/neonatal alloimmune thrombocytopenia. Am J Obstet Gynecol. 2004;191:815–20.

91. Radder CM, de Haan MJJ, Brand A, Stoelhorst GMSJ, Veen S, Kanhai HHH. Follow up of children after antenatal treatment for alloimmune thrombocytopenia. Early Hum Dev. 2004;80:65–76.

92. Rayment R, Birchall J, Yarranton H, Hewertson J, Allen D, Murphy MF. Neonatal alloimmune thrombocytopenia. BMJ. 2003;327:331–2.

93. Rayment R, Brunskill SJ, Soothill PW, Roberts DJ, Bussel JB, Murphy MF. Antenatal interventions for fetomaternal alloimmune thrombocytopenia. Cochrane Database Syst Rev. 2011;(5):CD004226. DOI: 10.1002/14651858.CD004226.pub3.

94. Reznikoff-Etievant MF. Management of alloimmune neonatal and antenatal thrombocytopenia. Vox Sang. 1988;55:193–201.

95. Rothenberger S. Neonatal alloimmunethrombocytopenia. Ther Apher. 2002;6:3235.

96. Sainio S, Teramo K, Kekomaki R. Prenatal treatment of severe fetomaternal alloimmune thrombocytopenia. Transfus Med. 1999;9:321–30.

97. Sainio S, Jarvenpaa AL, Renlund M. Thrombocytopenia in term infants: a population-based study. Obstet Gynecol. 2000;95:441–6.

98. Samuelsson A, Towers TL, Ravetch JV. Anti-inflammatory activity of IVIG mediated through the inhibitory Fc receptor. Science. 2001;291:484–6.

99. Shulman NR, Marder VJ, et al. Platelet and leukocyte isoantigens and their antibodies: serologic physiologic and clinical studies. Prog Hematol. 1964;4:222–304.

100. Sia CG, Amigo NC, Harper RG. Failure of cesarean section to prevent intracranial hemorrhage in sib-

lings with isoimmune neonatal thrombocytopenia. Am J Obstet Gynecol. 1985;153:79–81.

101. Simsek S, Christiaens GCLM, Kanhai HHH. Human platelet antigen-1 (Zw) typing of fetuses by analysis of polymerase chain reaction-amplified genomic DNA from amniocytes. Transfus Med. 1994;4: 15–9.

102. Spencer JA, Burrows RF. Feto-maternal alloimmune thrombocytopenia: a literature review and statistical analysis. Aust N Z J Obstet Gynaecol. 2001;41: 45–55.

103. Stanworth SJ, Hackett G, Williamson LM. Feto-maternal alloimmune thrombocytopenia presenting antenatally as hydrops fetalis. Prenat Diagn. 2001; 21:418–24.

104. Taaning E. HLA antibodies and fetomaternal alloimmune thrombocytopenia: myth or meaningful? Transfus Med Rev. 2000;14:275–80.

105. Tiller H, Killie MK, Skogen B, Øian P, Husebekk A. Neonatal alloimmune thrombocytopenia in Norway: poor detection rate with nonscreening versus a general screening programme. BJOG. 2009;116(4): 594–8.

106. te Pas AB, Lopriore E, van den Akker ES, Oepkes D, Kanhai HH, Brand A, Walther FJ. Postnatal management of fetal and neonatal alloimmune thrombocytopenia: the role of matched platelet transfusion and IVIG. Eur J Pediatr. 2007;166(10): 1057–63.

107. Turner ML, Bessos H, Fagge T. Prospective epidemiologic study of the outcome and cost-effectiveness of antenatal screening to detect neonatal alloimmune thrombocytopenia due to anti-HPA-1a. Transfusion. 2005;45:1945–56.

108. Uhrynowska M, Maslanka K, Zupanska B. Neonatal thrombocytopenia: incidence, serological and clinical observations. Am J Perinatol. 1997;14:415–8.

109. Valentin N, Vergracht A, Bignon JD. HLA-DRw52a is involved in alloimmunization against PL-A1 antigen. Hum Immunol. 1990;27:73–9.

110. Van den Akker E, Oepkes D, Brand A, Kanhai HH. Vaginal delivery for fetuses at risk of alloimmune thrombocytopenia? BJOG. 2006;113(7):781–3.

111. Van den Akker ESA, Westgren M, Husbekk A, Kanhai HHH, Oepkes D. Fetal or neonatal alloimmune thrombocytopenia: a new randomized controlled trial and international multicenter data collection [abstract]. J Obstet Gynaecol. 2006;26 Suppl 1:S63.

112. Van den Akker ES, Oepkes D, Lopriore E, Brand A, Kanhai HH. Noninvasive antenatal management of fetal and neonatal alloimmune thrombocytopenia: safe and effective. BJOG. 2007;114(4):469–73.

113. Ward MJ, Pauliny J, Lipper EG, Bussel JB. Long-term effects of fetal and neonatal alloimmune thrombocytopenia and its antenatal treatment on the medical and developmental outcomes of affected children. Am J Perinatol. 2006;23(8):487–92.

114. BCSH guidelines, Gibson BES, Bolton-Maggs PHB, Pamphilon D, et al. Transfusion guidelines for neonates and older children. Br J Haematol. 2004; 124:433–53;2005 amendment to these guidelines: www.bcshguidelines.com.

115. Williamson LM, Hackett G, Rennie J. The natural history of fetomaternal alloimmunization to the platelet-specific antigen hpa-1a (pi-a1, zw-a) as determined by antenatal screening. Blood. 1998;92: 2280–7.

116. Zimmermann R, Huch A. In utero therapy with immunoglobulin for alloimmune thrombocytopenia. Lancet. 1992;340:1034–5.

The Management and Outcome of Pregnancy in Patients with Myeloproliferative Neoplasms

Susan E. Robinson and Claire N. Harrison

Abstract

The myeloproliferative neoplasms are rare blood cancers which are characterised by increased risks of thrombosis, haemorrhage and also risk of transformation to acute myeloid leukaemia. These conditions are common in older adults but they do occur in children and young adults and as a consequence fertility and management of pregnancy is an issue for patients with these conditions. In this chapter we shall briefly review the pathogenesis of MPN before describing what is known about pregnancy outcomes for these patients and presenting an algorithm for pregnancy management.

13.1 Introduction

The myeloproliferative disorders are clonal, generally indolent stem cell malignancies which are characterized by clinical features of thrombosis, hemorrhage, and transformation to myelofibrosis or acute myeloid leukemia. The World Health Organization classification of hemato-oncology [28] has renamed these conditions myeloproliferative neoplasms (MPN), and currently this category includes the following disorders: essential thrombocythemia (ET), polycythemia vera (PV), primary myelofibrosis (PMF), MPN unclassified, MPN syndromes overlapping with myelodysplasia, mast cell disorders, chronic neutrophilic leukemia, and hypereosinophilic syndrome. These are all rare myeloid malignancies, and in this chapter we focus on the management of pregnancy in the commoner MPNs – ET, PV, and PMF.

These conditions are rare (e.g., the incidence of ET is 1–1.5/100,000 per annum) and are usually diagnosed in patients who are in their sixth or seventh decade. However, for ET in particular, there is another peak in women of reproductive age, and 15 % of patients with PV are aged less than 40 years at the time of diagnosis. These diseases are therefore encountered in patients with reproductive potential and may indeed be first diagnosed in pregnancy. Furthermore, pregnancy in these conditions may be complicated, and current data suggest that a proportion of patients with MPN will require disease-specific intervention in pregnancy, without which they risk significant complications for themselves and their pregnancy.

S.E. Robinson, BMBCh, M.Sc., MRCP, FRCPath
C.N. Harrison, DM, FRCP, FRCPath (✉)
Department of Haematology,
Guy's and St Thomas' NHS Foundation Trust,
Guy's Hospital, London, UK
e-mail: claire.harrison@gstt.nhs.uk

H. Cohen, P. O'Brien (eds.), *Disorders of Thrombosis and Hemostasis in Pregnancy*, 185
DOI 10.1007/978-1-4471-4411-3_13, © Springer-Verlag London 2012

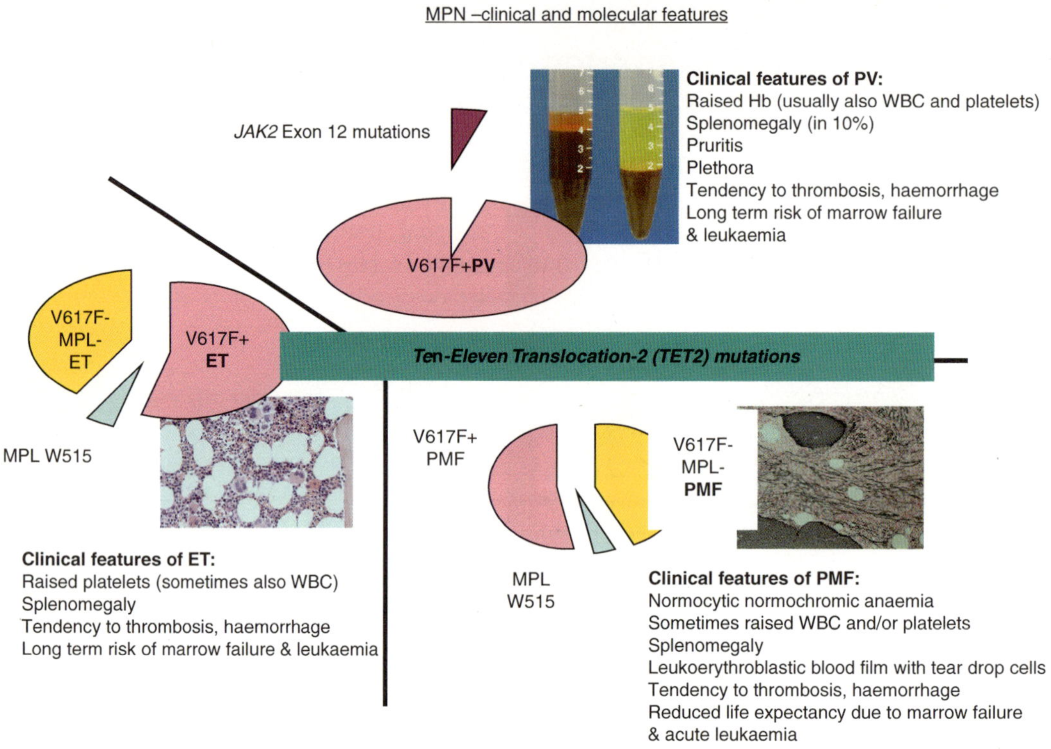

MPN −clinical and molecular features

JAK2 Exon 12 mutations

Clinical features of PV:
Raised Hb (usually also WBC and platelets)
Splenomegaly (in 10%)
Pruritis
Plethora
Tendency to thrombosis, haemorrhage
Long term risk of marrow failure
& leukaemia

V617F+**PV**

V617F-
MPL-
ET

V617F+
ET

Ten-Eleven Translocation-2 (TET2) mutations

MPL W515

V617F+
PMF

V617F-
MPL-
PMF

Clinical features of ET:
Raised platelets (sometimes also WBC)
Splenomegaly
Tendency to thrombosis, haemorrhage
Long term risk of marrow failure & leukaemia

MPL
W515

Clinical features of PMF:
Normocytic normochromic anaemia
Sometimes raised WBC and/or platelets
Splenomegaly
Leukoerythroblastic blood film with tear drop cells
Tendency to thrombosis, haemorrhage
Reduced life expectancy due to marrow failure
& acute leukaemia

Fig. 13.1 Summary of clinical and molecular features in MPN

13.2 Pathogenesis of MPN

Our understanding of the molecular pathogenesis of these conditions was revolutionized in 2005 when four groups simultaneously reported the discovery of a point mutation in exon 14 of Janus kinase 2 (JAK2V617F) [2, 12, 17, 20]. Here, a bulky phenylalanine is substituted by valine which causes constitutive activation of JAK2. Both wild-type and mutant JAK2 are bound to the intracytoplasmic tail of many common hemopoietic cytokine receptors including those for erythropoietin, thrombopoietin, and granulocyte colony-stimulating factor. When the ligand binds to one of these cognate receptors, phosphorylation of JAK2 and the receptor itself occurs, leading to signaling via JAK-STAT, MAPK, and PI3K pathways. This process occurs independent of ligand receptor interaction in the presence of JAK2V617F. Strikingly, the JAK2V617F mutation is highly prevalent in these patients, affecting 95 % of patients with PV (most of the

remaining PV patients have a mutation in exon 12 of JAK2 [27]) and 50 % of patients with ET or PMF. In patients with ET or PMF, a proportion have one of several mutations of the transmembrane domain of the thrombopoietin receptor cMPL which also causes constitutive activation of the receptors [25]. All these mutations produce the phenotype of MPN in a mouse transplantation model. The clinical and molecular features of PV, ET, and PMF are shown in Fig. 13.1.

13.3 Diagnosis and Natural History of MPN

13.3.1 Diagnosis

The discovery of the JAK2V617F mutation has also had a major impact on the diagnostic process for these patients. In the past, these diagnoses were made by exclusion and frequently involved

Table 13.1 Diagnostic algorithm for MPNs

Careful clinical assessment to evaluate for secondary cause and additional risk factors	
Screen for *V617F JAK2 ± CMPLW515L/K*	
POSITIVE *V617F JAK2*	NEGATIVE *V617F JAK2*
PV: if *V617F JAK2 and all of:*	PV: *if 1 +2 and either one A or two B criteria*:
1. PCV > 0.51 in M and > 0.48 in F or raised red cell mass	1. PCV > 0.60 in M and > 0.56 F or raised red cell mass
2. No secondary cause of high PCV	2. No secondary cause of high PCV and normal erythropoietin
3. Normal/low serum erythropoietin	A Palpable splenomegaly
	A Presence of acquired cytogenetic abnormality
	B Neutrophilia (>10×10^9/L; or >12.5×10^9/L in smokers
	B Splenomegaly on imaging
	B Endogenous erythroid colonies or low erythropoietin
	B Thrombocytosis (plts> 400×10^9/L)
ET: *if V617F JAK2 and all of*:	ET: *if all of*:
Platelet count > upper limit normal range	Platelet count >600×10^9/L
No other myeloid disease (includes PV, MDS, MF)	No other myeloid disease (includes CML, PV, MDS, MF)
	No reactive cause and normal iron status
MF: if *V617F JAK2* and:	MF: if all of:
Reticulin > grade three-fourths or presence of collagen	Reticulin > grade three-fourths or presence of collagen
	Absence of *V617F JAK2* and *BCR/ABL*
And any two of:	And any two of:
Palpable splenomegaly	Palpable splenomegaly
Unexplained anemia	Unexplained anemia
Teardrop red cells	Teardrop red cells
Leucoerythroblastic film	Leucoerythroblastic film
Systemic symptoms (night sweats, >10% weight loss, bone pain)	Systemic symptoms (night sweats, >10% weight loss, bone pain)
Biopsy proven extramedullary hematopoiesis	Biopsy proven extramedullary hematopoiesis

multiple tests to exclude other potential disorders such as an underlying malignancy for isolated thrombocytosis. The current diagnostic criteria are shown in Table 13.1. It is apparent that any patients with sustained elevation of hemoglobin (i.e., a hematocrit or packed cell volume of more than 0.51 for men and 0.48 for women), elevated platelet count (in excess of 450×10^9/L), and splenomegaly should be investigated. These disorders should also be suspected in patients presenting with thrombosis in an unusual site; for example, 60 % of patients with no clear cause for a splanchnic vein thrombosis have been reported to have a JAK2V617F-positive MPN [24]. In the context of pregnancy, it is important to consider this diagnosis in a patient with adverse pregnancy outcome, even if the blood count is normal; this is because the expanded plasma volume dur-

ing the second and third trimesters may cause blood counts to completely normalize in these conditions.

13.3.2 Natural History

The patient with MPN has an enhanced risk of thrombotic complications. This increased risk is thought to be due to platelet-platelet and platelet-leukocyte interaction, possibly directly related to the pathological activation of JAK2, although other as yet unclear factors are likely to contribute, for example, perturbation of the bone marrow microenvironment. Yet, not all patients will suffer from this complication, and thus risk assessment has been developed to tailor treatment strategies appropriately. It is well recognized that the risk of thrombosis latent to MPN is increased by age and history of a prior thrombotic event [10]. Interestingly, there is poor correlation between the degree of elevation of blood counts and thrombosis. However, patients with a platelet count in excess of $1,500 \times 10^9$/L are considered as a high-risk group because of their predisposition to hemorrhage (see below). Many clinicians would also include patients currently receiving antihypertensives and hypoglycemic agents as high-risk candidates. Hemorrhage, usually characterized by mucocutaneous bleeding, is less common and may be due to a reduction in the number of high molecular weight von Willebrand factor molecules which are thought to bind to the megakaryocyte and platelet membranes. This causes an acquired von Willebrand's disease, but the presence of these laboratory features may not necessarily indicate risk of future clinically significant acquired von Willebrand's disease. These and other factors should be considered to assess risk in the context of the current or indeed planned pregnancy; this is discussed in further detail below.

13.4 The Potential for Genetic Susceptibility to MPN

Patients diagnosed with MPN in their youth pose particular management problems over and above those faced by older patients. These include the potential for enhanced risk of long-term treatment toxicity, as well as management of fertility and pregnancy, including consideration of potential heritability of the disease. An inherited tendency to develop MPN was previously assumed to be uncommon. However, during the 1990s, studies of large kindreds with an apparent predisposition to an MPN phenotype (i.e., thrombocytosis) allowed the identification of mutations in 5'untranslated [30] region of the thrombopoietin (TPO) gene and in *cMpl*, the cognate receptor for TPO [4]. Interest in a potential genetic predisposition to MPNs was rekindled following the discovery of the JAK2V617F mutation in 2005, as previously described. However, this

mutation has not been reported in constitutional DNA, and families have been reported in which members affected with MPN are discordant for the *JAK2*V617F mutation. In addition, epidemiological studies indicate that inherited factors may predispose to the development of many MPNs. The largest study assessed the risk of MPN in 24,577 first-degree relatives of 11,039 MPN patients in Sweden. The results suggest that these relatives have a significantly increased risk of developing an MPN. For example, a first-degree relative of a subject with PV has a relative risk (RR) of 5.7 (95 % confidence interval 3.5–9.1); for ET, the RR is 7.4 (3.7–14.8). For all of these cases, there was no evidence of anticipation of the age at presentation [19]. In Spring 2009, three papers appeared in the same edition of the journal Nature Genetics describing a common haplotype (single-nucleotide polymorphism) designated 46/1 conferring susceptibility to JAK2V617F-positive MPNs [13, 16, 22]. The exact mechanism of this predisposition remains uncertain, but one hypothesis suggests the "fertile ground" idea, that is, that the presence of 46/1 increases the probability of the V617F mutation occurring downstream. Despite this evidence of genetic susceptibility, routine testing of the offspring of MPN patients would not at present be recommended.

13.5 Management of MPN

Patients with MPN are generally treated according to an assessment of their risk of thrombotic or hemorrhagic potential. Agents such as low-dose aspirin (LDA), hydroxycarbamide, anagrelide, or interferon alpha are used to reduce the risk of thrombotic events; patients with PV may require venesection and aspirin, either alone or in addition to the cytoreductive agents listed. LDA and low molecular weight heparin (LMWH) are variably used in pregnancy, which is clearly a time of transient increased thrombotic risk. However, of the cytoreductive agents, only interferon alpha would generally be recommended for the management of high-risk patients in pregnancy. Hydroxycarbamide and anagrelide both have potential to harm the fetus [11] and should ideally be stopped prior to conception (see below); for male patients wishing to father a child, both anagrelide and interferon are appropriate, but hydroxycarbamide should be stopped for 3 months prior to trying to conceive and substituted with another agent where appropriate. There is increasing interest in the utility of a pegylated interferon as a better-tolerated agent with the potential to induce complete remission at a clinical and molecular level in a cohort of patients [15]. However, the safety of this agent in pregnancy has yet to be established. JAK2 inhibitors are currently the subject of clinical trials, largely in patients with PMF, and are not yet licensed or considered standard of care. Only a very small proportion of patients with MPN will undergo bone marrow transplantation when the severity of their disease merits this high-risk approach; the management of fertility and pregnancy in this cohort of patients is beyond the scope of this text.

The development of long-term complications of ET and PV, such as transformation to acute leukemia and the more aggressive disorder myelofibrosis, appears to be dependent upon time. These complications are an inherent tendency of these conditions, possibly related to genetic instability which has been described in association with the JAK2V617F mutation. Leukemic transformation may also be related to the use of drugs such as alkylating agents. However, current therapeutic options are not thought to significantly increase the risk of leukemic transformation although there is ongoing debate with regard to the leukemogenic potential of hydroxycarbamide [10]. Whether treatment strategies can influence the risk of myelofibrotic transformation is currently the subject of debate. Pregnancy does not affect the risk of either leukemic or myelofibrotic transformation.

13.6   Pregnancy Outcomes

ET is the commonest MPN in women of childbearing age, and a significant number of pregnancies have been described in the literature, but these data do not enable confident management guidelines to be drawn up. A number of factors have variably been used to identify high-risk pregnancies in patients with MPN, and these are shown in Table 13.2. Analysis of pregnancy outcomes in women with ET suggests that the presence of JAK2V617F may increase the risk of pregnancy loss [23]. However, the strength of this association is not sufficient to recommend adjusting management strategy on this basis. It should be noted that thrombophilia screening, unless in specific situations (e.g., a strong personal or family history of thrombotic events), does not contribute to risk assessment for pregnancy in MPNs. The current literature for pregnancy outcome in MPN is relatively sparse, and it is important to recognize that it is likely to be subject to reporting bias; the details are summarized as follows:

ET: As ET has a second peak in incidence in women of reproductive age, the medical literature for these patients is much more abundant than for the other MPNs. A meta-analysis reported data from 461 pregnancies in women with ET whose median age was 29 years and platelet count at the outset of pregnancy of $1,000 \times 10^9/L$, declining to $599 \times 10^9/L$ in the second trimester. The live birthrate ranged from 50 to 70 %; first trimester loss affected 25–40 % and late pregnancy loss 10 %; the rate of placental abruption was 3.6 % and intrauterine growth restriction (IUGR) 4.5 % [1]. Maternal morbidity is rare in ET, but stroke has been reported [31].

PV: The reported outcomes of 18 pregnancies combined with a literature review of an additional 20 cases is available in the literature outcomes were concordant with those for ET [26]. First trimester loss was most prevalent 21 % and late pregnancy loss 18 %; IUGR was reported in 15 % and preterm delivery in 13 %, associated with three neonatal deaths. The overall successful pregnancy rate was 50 %. Maternal morbidity was significant including one maternal death due to thrombosis and disseminated intravascular coagulation. It should be noted, however, that the literature review included cases reported in the 1960s, at which time treatment had not yet been standardized.

ALGORITHM FOR MPN MANAGEMENT IN PREGNANCY

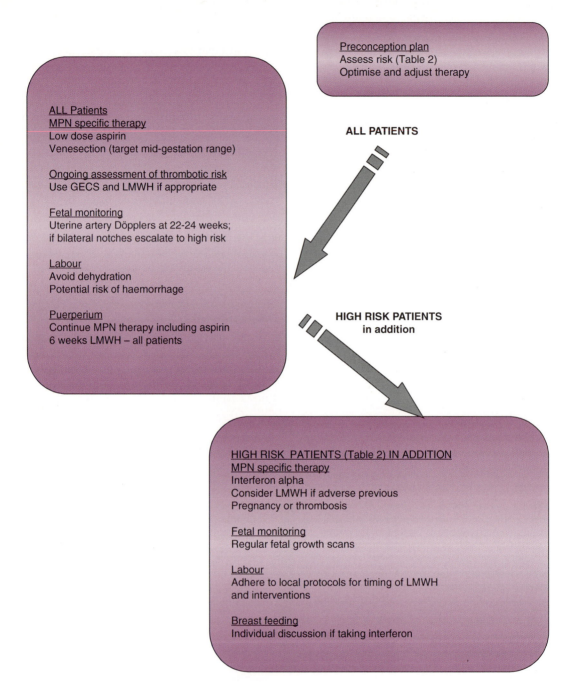

Fig. 13.2 Algorithm for MPN Management in Pregnancy

PMF: A report of four pregnancies in PMF combined with four historical cases suggests a 50 % risk of fetal loss but no evidence of maternal complications [29].

The literature in this area, particularly that relating to PV and PMF, is too small to permit conclusions about the current risks and makes a strong case for international collaboration to document pregnancy outcomes.

13.7 Therapeutic Strategies for Pregnancy in MPN

Therapeutic strategies for MPN in pregnancy are influenced by the patients' disease status and prior obstetric history. For this reason, it is useful to discuss pregnancy with young MPN patients. It is of course integral to consenting patients for cytoreductive agents that the implications of unplanned pregnancy while taking these agents are discussed. The majority of patients can and should be managed in local obstetric units under the combined care of obstetric and hematology teams. However, detailed discussion of pregnancy would ideally be provided in the form of preconception counseling when a formal risk assessment and management strategy can be developed. The key components of such a meeting would include:

- Risk assessment for pregnancy
- Discussion of therapeutic options
- Need for additional monitoring during pregnancy
- A comprehensive delivery and postpartum plan
- Discussion about breast-feeding
- Options to optimize disease control if fertility is an issue
- Informed multidisciplinary care and education

13.7.1 Fertility Treatment and Contraception

There is currently insufficient evidence to either support or refute an association between estrogen-based hormone treatment and thrombosis risk in ET and no evidence with regard to PV or

PMF. A retrospective review of thrombotic events in a total of 305 women with ET followed for a median of 133 months suggested that combined oral contraceptive pill use might be associated with an increased risk of deep vein thrombosis, but other estrogen-based hormone therapies may be safe in ET [7]. Therefore, the use of combined oral contraceptives is discouraged for women for MPN. There are no data with regard to ovarian stimulation therapy in MPN. However, ovarian hyperstimulation increases the risk of thrombosis, so each case should be assessed individually and offered thromboprophylaxis when appropriate. This would include, for example, patients with previous arterial or venous thrombotic events.

13.7.2 Standard Pregnancy Management

Low-dose aspirin is safe in pregnancy and seems advantageous in ET [6] and probably PV [26]. We would therefore recommend that, in the absence of a clear contraindication, all patients should receive LDA (75 mg once daily) throughout pregnancy. For patients with PV, venesection can be continued to maintain the hematocrit within a target range which will alter through the course of pregnancy due to the expansion of the plasma volume relative to the red cell mass. Venesection may be associated with a risk of syncope, particularly for patients in the third trimester; this is due to reduced venous return, and formal intravenous fluid replacement may be required in this context.

13.7.3 High-Risk Pregnancies

A pregnancy is likely to be at high risk of maternal or fetal complications if one or more of a number of factors are either present at the outset or develop during the pregnancy (Table 13.2). In addition to the standard measures described above, cytoreductive therapy and low molecular weight heparin (LMWH) should be considered for patients with any such factors present at the outset or developing during pregnancy.

Table 13.2 Risk factors for complications in pregnancy

Marked sustained rise in platelet count rising to above 1,500 × 10⁹/L[a]

Previous venous or arterial thrombosis in mother (whether pregnant or not)

Previous hemorrhage[a] attributed to ET (whether pregnant or not)

Development of persistent notching of uterine artery Dopplers

Previous pregnancy complication that may have been caused by ET, for example:

    Unexplained recurrent first trimester loss (three unexplained first trimester losses)

    Intrauterine growth restriction (birthweight <5th centile for gestation)

    Intrauterine death or stillbirth (with no obvious other cause, evidence of placental dysfunction, and growth restricted fetus)

    Severe preeclampsia (necessitating preterm delivery <34 weeks) or development of any such complication in the index pregnancy

    Placental abruption

    Significant ante- or postpartum hemorrhage (requiring red cell transfusion)

[a]These would represent indications for interferon only rather than interferon plus low molecular weight heparin

If cytoreductive treatment is deemed necessary (see Table 13.2), interferon alpha is the drug of choice, for there have been no reports of teratogenic effects with this agent in animals or adverse effects in the small numbers of reported human pregnancies exposed to this drug, with the exception of one case of neonatal lupus possibly related to this agent [5]. However, interferon alpha may impair fertility [9] so may be better avoided in women who have difficulty in conceiving. A few pregnancies have been reported in patients treated with hydroxycarbamide [11, 21], most without fetal complications. However, hydroxycarbamide is probably contraindicated around the time of conception (this also applies to male patients) and during pregnancy due to the risk of teratogenicity. Anagrelide is not recommended because there are insufficient data regarding its use in pregnancy and the molecule is small enough to cross the placenta. Thus, hydroxycarbamide and/or anagrelide should ideally be gradually withdrawn 3–6 months prior to planned conception and substituted by interferon alpha if necessary. The dose of interferon alpha

should be titrated against the blood count with a target platelet count of 400×10^9/L and hematocrit within the gestation appropriate normal range.

LMWH is safe in pregnancy; heparin-induced thrombocytopenia has not been described with LMWH in pregnancy, and the risk of osteopenia is extremely low [8]. It has been used anecdotally in women with MPN and previous thrombosis and/or fetal morbidity, when an empirical dose of LMWH (e.g., enoxaparin 40 mg) has been used throughout pregnancy. This dose may be altered at extremes of body weight (e.g., <50 kg or BMI >30 kg/m²). If the patient has had a previous venous thromboembolism, thromboprophylaxis is indicated during pregnancy, with unmonitored intermediate dose LMWH being widely used (e.g., for venous thromboprophylaxis, enoxaparin 40 mg o.d. initially, increasing to 40 mg twice daily from 16 weeks' gestation and dropping to 40 mg o.d. for 6 weeks postpartum). Patients with previous or current arterial or recurrent thrombosis may require higher doses of LMWH and should be discussed on an individual basis with a hematologist. Persistence of bilateral uterine artery Döppler notching at 22–24 weeks' gestation (see below) is a predictor of potential placental dysfunction, and some consider this an additional indication for LMWH, although its benefit is uncertain when started at this late gestation.

13.7.4 Thromboprophylaxis

The Royal College of Obstetricians and Gynaecologists' guideline [32] for thromboprophylaxis in pregnancy recommends continual reassessment of the venous thrombotic risk during pregnancy and that all women with previous VTE should be encouraged to wear graded elastic compression stockings (GECS) throughout pregnancy and for 6–12 weeks after delivery. The use of GECS is also recommended for pregnant women traveling by air [14], while patients with two additional risk factors (one of which would be ET) should receive one dose of LMWH prior to the flight.

13.7.5 Fetal Assessment

During pregnancy, regular fetal monitoring is imperative. Standard care includes ultrasound scans at 12 and 20 weeks, with assessment of uterine artery Döppler at 22–24 weeks. If the uterine artery Döppler is abnormal, it should be repeated at 24 weeks, and if notching (indicating increased resistance to flow) persists at this stage, options for escalating therapy should be explored. These options include the addition, or increasing the dose, of either LMWH or interferon alpha. Regular growth scans should also be performed throughout pregnancy.

13.7.6 Intrapartum

It is important to discuss the implications of the use of thromboprophylaxis with the obstetrician and obstetric anesthetist and plan for eventualities including instrumental delivery, Caesarean section, and epidural or spinal anesthesia. Local protocols with regard to interruption of LMWH should be adhered to during labor, and dehydration should be avoided (see Chap. 3).

13.7.7 Postpartum

In the puerperium, we recommend thromboprophylaxis with 6 weeks of LMWH for all mothers with MPN, in addition to ongoing management of their MPN. It is important to note that changes due to increased plasma volume and the well-described tendency for the platelet count to fall during the third trimester will reverse during the puerperium, and this is a time when thrombotic events have been described [31].

13.7.8 Breast-feeding

Breast-feeding is safe with heparin and warfarin (providing the baby receives adequate vitamin K) but is traditionally contraindicated with the cytoreductive agents. However, the recommendation to avoid breast-feeding during maternal interferon-alpha therapy is based on reports that this agent is variably excreted in breast milk and may be active orally [3, 18]. In essence, this represents an absence of evidence of safety, rather than any evidence of harm to the neonate. The substantial benefits of breast-feeding are well documented and include a reduced risk of infection and gastroenteritis. Any decision about breast-feeding should therefore be made on an individual basis, after discussion of the possible risks and benefits.

Conclusions

The current literature suggests that pregnancy in women with MPN is associated with increased morbidity and mortality to both mother and child. The retrospective nature of reports, case study reporting bias, and lack of standardized management historically limits interpretation regarding the current epidemiology and outcome of these pregnancies. This is particularly true in the light of the recent revival of interest in MPNs and their modern-day management.

A prospective UK-based survey of pregnancy in women with MPN is being run in association with the UK Obstetric Surveillance System (UKOSS). This will enable an up-to-date review of the epidemiology and outcome of pregnancy in women with this diagnosis and an assessment of variation in current practice. This survey should provide more robust evidence on which to base management of these pregnancies.

As outlined in this chapter, all women with MPN should have a detailed plan of management for pregnancy, which should encompass preconceptual planning, individual risk assessment, and a treatment strategy agreed in a multidisciplinary setting.

References

1. Barbui T, Finazzi G. Myeloproliferative disease in pregnancy and other management issues. Hematology Am Soc Hematol Educ Program. 2006;246–52.
2. Baxter EJ, Scott LM, Campbell PJ, East C, Fourouclas N, Swanton S, Vassiliou GS, Bench AJ, Boyd EM, Curtin N, Scott MA, Erber WN, Green AR. Acquired mutation of the tyrosine kinase JAK2 in human myeloproliferative disorders. Lancet. 2005;365:1054–61.

3. Bayley D, Temple C, Clay V, Steward A, Lowther N. The transmucosal absorption of recombinant human interferon-alpha B/D hybrid in the rat and rabbit. J Pharm Pharmacol. 1995;47:721–4.

4. Ding J, Komatsu H, Wakita A, Kato-Uranishi M, Ito M, Satoh A, Tsuboi K, Nitta M, Miyazaki H, Iida S, Ueda R. Familial essential thrombocythemia associated with a dominant-positive activating mutation of the c-MPL gene, which encodes for the receptor for thrombopoietin. Blood. 2004;103:4198–200.

5. Fritz M, Vats K, Goyal RK. Neonatal lupus and IUGR following alpha-interferon therapy during pregnancy. J Perinatol. 2005;25:552–4.

6. Gangat N, Wolanskyj AP, Schwager S, Tefferi A. Predictors of pregnancy outcome in essential thrombocythemia: a single institution study of 63 pregnancies. Eur J Haematol. 2009;82:350–3.

7. Gangat N, Wolanskyj AP, Schwager SM, Mesa RA, Tefferi A. Estrogen-based hormone therapy and thrombosis risk in women with essential thrombocythemia. Cancer. 2006;106:2406–11.

8. Greer IA, Nelson-Piercy C. Low-molecular-weight heparins for thromboprophylaxis and treatment of venous thromboembolism in pregnancy: a systematic review of safety and efficacy. Blood. 2005;106:401–7.

9. Griesshammer M, Bergmann L, Pearson T. Fertility, pregnancy and the management of myeloproliferative disorders. Baillieres Clin Haematol. 1998;11:859–74.

10. Harrison CN. Essential thrombocythaemia: challenges and evidence-based management. Br J Haematol. 2005;130:153–65.

11. Harrison C. Pregnancy and its management in the Philadelphia negative myeloproliferative diseases. Br J Haematol. 2005;129:293–306.

12. James C, Ugo V, Le Couedic JP, Staerk J, Delhommeau F, Lacout C, Garcon L, Raslova H, Berger R, Bennaceur-Griscelli A, Villeval JL, Constantinescu SN, Casadevall N, Vainchenker W. A unique clonal JAK2 mutation leading to constitutive signalling causes polycythaemia vera. Nature. 2005; 434:1144–8.

13. Jones AV, Chase A, Silver RT, Oscier D, Zoi K, Wang YL, Cario H, Pahl HL, Collins A, Reiter A, Grand F, Cross NC. JAK2 haplotype is a major risk factor for the development of myeloproliferative neoplasms. Nat Genet. 2009;41:446–9.

14. Royal College of Obstetricians and Gynaecologists. Air travel and pregnancy. Scientific Advisory Committee Opinion Paper 1. London: RCOG Press; 2008.

15. Kiladjian JJ, Cassinat B, Chevret S, Turlure P, Cambier N, Roussel M, Bellucci S, Grandchamp B, Chomienne C, Fenaux P. Pegylated interferon-alfa-2a induces complete hematologic and molecular responses with low toxicity in polycythemia vera. Blood. 2008;112:3065–72.

16. Kilpivaara O, Mukherjee S, Schram AM, Wadleigh M, Mullally A, Ebert BL, Bass A, Marubayashi S, Heguy A, Garcia-Manero G, Kantarjian H, Offit K, Stone RM, Gilliland DG, Klein RJ, Levine RL. A germline JAK2 SNP is associated with predisposition to the development of JAK2(V617F)-positive myeloproliferative neoplasms. Nat Genet. 2009;41:455–9.

17. Kralovics R, Passamonti F, Buser AS, Teo SS, Tiedt R, Passweg JR, Tichelli A, Cazzola M, Skoda RC. A gain-of-function mutation of JAK2 in myeloproliferative disorders. N Engl J Med. 2005;352: 1779–90.

18. Kumar AR, Hale TW, Mock RE. Transfer of interferon alfa into human breast milk. J Hum Lact. 2000;16:226–8.

19. Landgren O, Goldin LR, Kristinsson SY, Helgadottir EA, Samuelsson J, Bjorkholm M. Increased risks of polycythemia vera, essential thrombocythemia, and myelofibrosis among 24,577 first-degree relatives of 11,039 patients with myeloproliferative neoplasms in Sweden. Blood. 2008;112:2199–204.

20. Levine RL, Wadleigh M, Cools J, Ebert BL, Wernig G, Huntly BJ, Boggon TJ, Wlodarska I, Clark JJ, Moore S, Adelsperger J, Koo S, Lee JC, Gabriel S, Mercher T, D'Andrea A, Frohling S, Dohner K, Marynen P, Vandenberghe P, Mesa RA, Tefferi A, Griffin JD, Eck MJ, Sellers WR, Meyerson M, Golub TR, Lee SJ, Gilliland DG. Activating mutation in the tyrosine kinase JAK2 in polycythemia vera, essential thrombocythemia, and myeloid metaplasia with myelofibrosis. Cancer Cell. 2005;7:387–97.

21. Liebelt EL, Balk SJ, Faber W, Fisher JW, Hughes CL, Lanzkron SM, Lewis KM, Marchetti F, Mehendale HM, Rogers JM, Shad AT, Skalko RG, Stanek EJ. NTP-CERHR expert panel report on the reproductive and developmental toxicity of hydroxyurea. Birth Defects Res B Dev Reprod Toxicol. 2007;80:259–366.

22. Olcaydu D, Harutyunyan A, Jager R, Berg T, Gisslinger B, Pabinger I, Gisslinger H, Kralovics R. A common JAK2 haplotype confers susceptibility to myeloproliferative neoplasms. Nat Genet. 2009;41:450–4.

23. Passamonti F, Randi ML, Rumi E, Pungolino E, Elena C, Pietra D, Scapin M, Arcaini L, Tezza F, Moratti R, Pascutto C, Fabris F, Morra E, Cazzola M, Lazzarino M. Increased risk of pregnancy complications in patients with essential thrombocythemia carrying the JAK2 (617V>F) mutation. Blood. 2007; 110:485–9.

24. Patel RK, Lea NC, Heneghan MA, Westwood NB, Milojkovic D, Thanigaikumar M, Yallop D, Arya R, Pagliuca A, Gaken J, Wendon J, Heaton ND, Mufti GJ. Prevalence of the activating JAK2 tyrosine kinase mutation V617F in the Budd-Chiari syndrome. Gastroenterology. 2006;130:2031–8.

25. Pikman Y, Lee BH, Mercher T, McDowell E, Ebert BL, Gozo M, Cuker A, Wernig G, Moore S, Galinsky I, DeAngelo DJ, Clark JJ, Lee SJ, Golub TR, Wadleigh M, Gilliland DG, Levine RL. MPLW515L Is a novel somatic activating mutation in myelofibrosis with myeloid metaplasia. PLoS Med. 2006;3:e270.

26. Robinson S, Bewley S, Hunt BJ, Radia DH, Harrison CN. The management and outcome of 18 pregnancies in women with polycythemia vera. Haematologica. 2005;90:1477–83.

27. Scott LM, Tong W, Levine RL, Scott MA, Beer PA, Stratton MR, Futreal PA, Erber WN, McMullin MF, Harrison CN, Warren AJ, Gilliland DG, Lodish HF, Green AR. JAK2 exon 12 mutations in polycythemia vera and idiopathic erythrocytosis. N Engl J Med. 2007;356:459–68.
28. Swerdlow SH. WHO classification of tumours of haematopoietic and lymphoid tissues – IARC WHO classification of tumours v. 2. 2nd ed. Geneva: World Health Organization; 2008.
29. Tulpule S, Bewley S, Robinson SE, Radia D, Nelson-Piercy C, Harrison CN. The management and outcome of four pregnancies in women with idiopathic myelofibrosis. Br J Haematol. 2008;142:480–2.
30. Wiestner A, Schlemper RJ, van der Maas AP, Skoda RC. An activating splice donor mutation in the thrombopoietin gene causes hereditary thrombocythaemia. Nat Genet. 1998;18:49–52.
31. Willoughby SJ, Fairhead S, Woodcock BE, Pearson TC. Postpartum thrombosis in primary thrombocythaemia. Eur J Haematol. 1997;59:121–3.
32. Royal College of Obstetricians and Gynaecologists. Green-top guideline no. 37. Thrombosis and embolism during pregnancy and the puerperium, Reducing the risk. 2009.

Hemoglobinopathies in Pregnancy   14

Joanna Howard, Susan Tuck, Asma Eissa,
and John Porter

Abstract

Pregnancies in women with both sickle and thalassemia disorders are seen increasingly worldwide, but outside a small number of specialist centers, most obstetricians and hematologists will see only a few affected pregnancies. Prospective trials addressing the challenges of managing these disorders in pregnancy remain limited so that current management often differs between centers. Both sickle and thalassemia disorders share increased thromboembolic and infection risks, but other complications differ. The UK and international data on maternal and fetal morbidity and mortality in pregnancies complicated by maternal sickle cell disease and thalassaemia disorders are described here in order to assist both obstetricians and haematologists in arriving at informed decisions.

14.1   Introduction

Pregnancies in women with both sickle and thalassemia disorders are seen increasingly worldwide,

J. Howard MA, MRCP, MRCPath
St. Thomas' Hospital, Westminster Bridge Road,
London SE1 7EH, UK
e-mail: joanna.howard@gstt.nhs.uk

S. Tuck MD, FRCOG, DCH, MRCGP
Consultant in Obstetrics & Gynaecology,
Royal Free Hospital, Pond Street, London NW3 2QG, UK
e-mail: susan.tuck@nhs.net

A. Eissa, MRCOG
Royal Free Hospital, Pond Street,
London NW3 2QG, UK
e-mail: asma.eissa@nhs.net

J. Porter MA, MD, FRCP, FRCPath (✉)
University College London Hospitals NHS Foundation
Trust, 250 Euston Road, London NW1 2PJ, UK
e-mail: j.porter@ucl.ac.uk

but outside a small number of specialist centers, most obstetricians and hematologists will see only a few. Prospective trials addressing the challenges of managing these disorders in pregnancy remain limited so that current management often differs between centers. Both sickle and thalassemia disorders share increased thromboembolic and infection risks, but other complications differ. For example, in sickle syndromes, the risk of exacerbating the underlying condition with vasoocclusive crisis and sickle chest syndrome needs to be considered, whereas in thalassemia syndromes, the risks of exacerbating iron-mediated complications such as cardiomyopathy or diabetes need careful consideration. Women with hemoglobinopathy traits have few complications in pregnancy, other than the difficulty of distinguishing concurrent iron deficiency and the increased incidence of urinary tract infections in women with sickle cell trait. The UK and international data on

H. Cohen, P. O'Brien (eds.), *Disorders of Thrombosis and Hemostasis in Pregnancy*,
DOI 10.1007/978-1-4471-4411-3_14, © Springer-Verlag London 2012

maternal and fetal morbidity and mortality in pregnancies complicated by maternal sickle cell disease and thalassaemia disorders are described here in order to assist both obstetricians and haematologists in arriving at informed decisions.

14.2 Sickle Cell Disease

14.2.1 Key Issues

Sickle cell disease (SCD) is the most common inherited condition worldwide, and in the UK, there are over 12,000 affected individuals with over 300 affected babies born each year. The term SCD refers to both homozygous sickle cell disease (HbSS) and compound heterozygotes with a clinically significant phenotype, such as those with HbSC, HbS-beta thalassemia, HbSD, and HbSO-Arab. SCD is associated with lifelong hemolytic anemia, intermittent episodes of severe pain from vasoocclusion and tissue ischemia, and chronic complications including stroke, pulmonary hypertension, renal disease, and retinal damage. Previously, SCD was associated with early mortality, but the majority of children born in the UK now survive to adulthood [85] with median survival to at least to the sixth decade [104]. Increased birth rates with SCD and improved survival have led to increasing numbers of women of childbearing age with SCD.

Pregnancy with SCD is associated with increased maternal and fetal morbidy and mortality, although these can be improved with comprehensive multidisciplinary care. Even if the clinical phenotype is mild before pregnancy, affected women should be treated as high risk and offered antenatal, intrapartum, and postnatal care by a team with appropriate experience. Multidisciplinary care by a team which includes a hematologist, is essential. Prophylactic blood transfusion throughout pregnancy is not necessary for all women, but should be discussed in the multidisciplinary setting, and is advisable in higher-risk situations. Women with SCD often face practical difficulties in receiving appropriate advice on safe and effective contraception, which would enable their pregnancies to be planned. Such advice would allow women to aim for pregnancy when their SCD and related health issues were in an optimal state which would be associated with improved outcomes.

14.2.2 Maternal Mortality Data

The Confidential Enquiries into Maternal Deaths in England and Wales show small numbers of maternal deaths in most trienna. Between 1973 and 1981 there were eight deaths [28, 29]. If one estimates 30 sickle cell disease pregnancies per year in the UK, this would equate to a mortality rate of 3 %. This is 200 times higher than the contemporaneous overall maternal UK mortality rate of 15 per 100,000 births. However, an almost contemporaneous survey of 125 pregnancies in women with SCD in the UK from 1975 to 1981 which only surveyed centers with ten or more adult SCD patients [94] included no maternal deaths. The Confidential Enquiries looking at the 16 years between 1982 and 1996 show four maternal deaths due to SCD, despite an increase in numbers of pregnancies in women with SCD over this time. The most recent Confidential Enquiries reports indicate similar rates of maternal mortality, with three deaths in the 2000–2002 triennium (two with HbSS and one with HbSC), two deaths in the 2003–2005 triennium (one with HbSS and one with HbSC) and one death in the 2006 to 2008 triennium (in a woman with HbSC) [48, 49] despite increasing numbers of pregnancies in women with SCD. However, contemporaneous series from three centers in London, with well-established specialist services, reported no maternal deaths in series of 25, 62, and 71 pregnancies, respectively, between 2000 and 2007 [19, 80, 105]. Taken together, these data raise concern that there is an increased risk of maternal mortality in hospitals without regular experience of patients with SCD. Indeed, this is a general concern raised in the National Confidential Enquiry into Deaths in sickle cell disease in the United Kingdom covering the years 2005 and 2006 [59].

The UK data are echoed in the published international data. Mortality rates from the 1980s and 1990s vary from 0.4 % (2 deaths in 445 pregnancies) in the US cooperative study of 19 hospitals [79] to 9.2 % (7 deaths in 76 pregnancies) in a 1980–1988 series from a hospital in Ile-Ife, Nigeria [23]. Figures from Benin (in West Africa), Lagos (Nigeria), Guadeloupe (in the French Antilles), and Bahrain fall between these extremes [2, 30, 46, 69]. The women with SCD in the Benin study were provided with information and education about SCD and were advised on nutrition, malarial prevention, and early detection of bacterial infections. While maternal mortality was 1.8 %, it was not markedly higher than the 1.2 % maternal mortality in their maternity unit [69]. Some of the more recent data have shown improvement in maternal mortality. The USA's Nationwide Inpatient Sample for 2000–2003, which included nearly 18,000 pregnant women with SCD, found a mortality rate of 72 per 100,000 deliveries (0.07 %), which is sixfold higher than their rate of 12.7 per 100,000 deliveries in women without SCD [98]. In Saudi Arabia, one maternal death (0.4 %) was reported in a series of 255 pregnancies between 2000 and 2007 although this may reflect the more benign natural history of the prevailing mutation in that country [3]. Figures from Bahrain [71] reported four maternal deaths in 351 pregnancies between 1998 and 2002 (1.1 % maternal mortality). Evidence from the Jamaican cohort study showed 2 deaths in 94 pregnancies in women with HbSS (a mortality rate of 2.1 %) [77] but no maternal deaths in 95 pregnancies in women with HbSC.

14.2.3 Perinatal Mortality Data

Perinatal mortality data (i.e., stillbirths and deaths in the first week after live birth) show a similar variability, although the absolute numbers are not so much higher than the prevailing rates in the general population. In the UK, the perinatal mortality rate (PMR) in the 1975–1981 series was 48 per 1,000 births (four times the national PMR) {Tuck, 1983} and in the 1991–1993 series was 60 per 1,000 (six times the contemporary national rate) [36]. International data show similar outcomes, with perinatal mortality varying from 44 per 1,000 in Guadeloupe [46] to 78.2 per 1000 deliveries in Saudi Arabia [3] and 134–187 per 1,000 in Nigeria [2, 69]. Several reports support the impression that outcomes can be better in hospitals where there is expertise with the condition, with one perinatal loss in the three UK series, among a total of 158 pregnancies [19, 80, 105].

14.2.4 Maternal Morbidity

Maternal morbidity is also increased in SCD pregnancies. The US Nationwide Inpatient Sample showed increased antenatal hospital admissions in women with SCD [18], partly as a result of increased painful crises, and other studies have shown a rate of antenatal painful crisis, which occur most commonly in the third trimester, varying from 20 to 56 % [37, 44, 70, 75, 79, 105]. Painful crises also occurred postnatally in 7.7 % of SCD pregnancies [37], and were also seen in women with HbSC [75].

Infection is also more common, especially urinary tract infections (seen in 16–23 % of pregnancies) [4, 36, 68, 105]. Pulmonary complications have an incidence of 11–17 % [4, 36, 66, 105] and include the acute chest syndrome. This is a serious potentially life-threatening complication of SCD, caused by sequestration of sickle cells in the pulmonary vasculature, and characterized by signs and symptoms of chest consolidation with decreased oxygen saturation and new infiltrates on chest X-ray.

Patients with SCD show laboratory evidence of hypercoagulability, with increased thrombin generation, tissue factor [16], and expression of procoagulants on sickle cells and microparticles [102], as well as decreased markers of fibrinolysis. However, linking these prothrombotic changes to an increased risk of venous thromboembolism (VTE) in a given individual is not usually possible unless independent additional prothrombotic risk factors are identified or there is a previous history of VTE, which has been reported at increased frequency in some SCD pregnancies in some studies, but not in others. These differences are probably due in part to the small size of studies and because the differential diagnosis of pulmonary embolism (PE) and pneumonia or acute chest syndrome can be difficult without modern imaging techniques. Therefore, data may not be accurate in older studies or in centers without imaging techniques that allow differentiation between chest syndrome and VTE. VTE is 40 % more common in black Americans than white controls, and this can be a confounding factor in the interpretation of incidence data [34]. The Nationwide Inpatient Sample in the USA, which is the largest reported series and analyzed the inpatient admissions in nearly 18,000 pregnant women with SCD, showed a significant increase in deep venous thrombosis (DVT) and cerebral vein thrombosis, but a nonsignificant increase in PE [100]. Deaths due to VTE are well described, however, and are often associated with prolonged immobilization or admission for painful crisis [30].

An increased incidence of preeclampsia and pregnancy-induced hypertension has been reported in some studies [3, 79, 93, 94] but not in others [2, 65, 70], but a significant increase was seen in large US inpatient data surveys, implying that severe hypertension, requiring hospital admission, was more common in women with SCD [18, 100]. This link may be related to the endothelial damage resulting from the altered shape and increased rigidity of sickled red blood cells.

14.2.5 Fetal and Neonatal Morbidity

These are nonspecific and are as would be expected from a suboptimal intrauterine environment. They include intrauterine fetal growth restriction (IUGR), (in 10–44 %), increased preterm delivery (in 16–33 %), and fetal distress during labor [2, 18, 19, 36, 70, 75, 79, 80, 105].

14.2.6 Pre-pregnancy Care

A survey of 149 sexually active women with SCD in north London [35] indicated that 64 % of pregnancies had been unplanned, suggesting a lack of practical help with optimal planning and effective contraception. Only 28 % had a correct understanding of the relevant genetics of their condition, although 60 % had heard of the concept of prenatal testing of fetuses. This information should ideally be clarified before pregnancy, so that the relevant options can be considered without the pressure of time. Partner screening should be encouraged preconceptually, and if the partner is a hemoglobinopathy carrier, the couple should be counseled accordingly about the availability of prenatal diagnosis and of preimplantation genetic screening (if in vitro fertilization is used), or prenatal diagnosis. Preconceptual advice to the woman should include screening for hepatitis B and C, HIV, and rubella, and pneumococcal and hepatitis vaccination should be administered if not already done. Screening investigations such as protein-creatinine ratio, echocardiography, and ophthalmology screening should be performed if not done in the recent past. A specific assessment of any additional thrombotic conditions should be made, so that appropriate prophylaxis during pregnancy can be planned.

Medications should be reviewed, and the woman should be advised to take folic acid supplements 5 mg daily and penicillin prophylaxis (because of functional hyposplenism) [94]. Any other medication should be reviewed in the context of possible teratogenicity and stopped or changed to alternatives, as appropriate. Hydroxycarbamide (hydroxyurea) is used to decrease the incidence of painful crisis and acute chest syndrome, but it is teratogenic in animals, and current UK advice is that women should stop taking hydroxycarbamide for three months before they conceive. There are anecdotal reports of women who have received hydroxycarbamide in pregnancy without adverse effects; therefore, if a woman conceives while taking it, they should not automatically be advised to consider termination of the pregnancy, but detailed anomaly scans are indicated. Some women may be taking iron chelators, which are essential treatment to reduce the organ damage which would result from excessive iron deposition derived from multiple blood transfusions, and these should be stopped as soon as pregnancy is diagnosed, because of possible teratogenicity [24, 41, 92]. Vitamin C which is usually given with desferrioxamine to enhance efficacy, should also be stopped when the chelators are stopped. Some women will be taking ACE inhibitors or angiotensin receptor blockers for the treatment of proteinuria, and these should be stopped preconceptually. There may also be general health issues that need to be addressed before pregnancy, such as advising on smoking cessation, alcohol intake, or blood pressure control. Women should be made aware of local arrangements for pregnancy care and whom to inform when they become pregnant.

14.2.7 Pregnancy Care

The level of care and attention in pregnancy and the puerperium should be the same for women with all types of SCD including those with infrequent complications prior to their pregnancy, as it is not possible to predict which individuals will have complications during pregnancy. Care should be provided by a multidisciplinary team including obstetricians and midwives, haematologists and obstetric anaesthetists who are all experienced in the care of high-risk pregnancies. It is also helpful to have access to a health psychology team as there are often psychosocial issues involved with coming to terms with chronic health problems and motherhood [86]. There should be a clearly coordinated plan of care, with effective communication between all those involved, including a clear system for enabling the patient to seek emergency help without delay. This needs to continue into the puerperium, when the patient is still at risk of sickle cell crises and other serious complications.

Women should be encouraged to come to hospital promptly if they experience pain which does not rapidly settle with simple analgesia at home. Treatment should include rapid assessment and analgesia with opiates, if required, which can be given orally, by intermittent subcutaneous injection or via a patient-controlled analgesia device.

Pethidine should be avoided, because it is less effective, its metabolites have longer-lasting depressant effects and it is associated with an increased risk of seizures. Nonsteroidal anti-inflammatory drugs should be avoided from 28 weeks' gestation because they can cause premature closure of the ductus arteriosus in the fetus. Further supportive care should include hydration, infection screening, and early recourse to antibiotics for any infection, which may have been the trigger for the crisis. This particularly includes urinary and chest infections, endometritis in the puerperium, and malaria in those who have undertaken recent foreign travel. Oxygen saturations on air should be measured and oxygen therapy given if saturations are less than 97 %. Oxygen saturations which fall to below 94 or 3 % below baseline may indicate pulmonary complications such as PE, pneumonia, or acute chest syndrome, and the patient should have an immediate medical review and appropriate treatment with oxygen or other respiratory support, intravenous antibiotics, thromboprophylaxis, and exchange transfusion. There should be a low threshold for transfer to a high dependency unit or intensive care unit.

Planned antenatal care should be tailored to the individual patient and should include a review at least at 2- to 4-week intervals throughout pregnancy. The hemoglobin concentration, hematocrit, platelet count, bilirubin, transaminase, and lactate dehydrogenase levels should be checked at least every 4 weeks. Blood pressure checks and urine checks for infection, hematuria, and proteinuria should be made at least every 4 weeks. Fetal growth should be monitored at least four weekly from 24 weeks with serial ultrasound scans.

A thromboprophylactic plan should be made both antenatally and postpartum, which, as a minimum, should include daily injections of low molecular weight heparin while an inpatient and for at least 7 days postpartum. Additional risk factors (e.g., age, obesity, operative delivery) should be considered using the recommendations in the RCOG guidelines [72]. The timing and mode of delivery should depend on the individual pregnancy, along standard obstetric lines.

Vigilance and care should be sustained into the postnatal period, when there is also an increased incidence of painful crises and thromboembolic events.

14.2.8 The Use of Blood Transfusion

During pregnancy, blood transfusions can be given either on an "as required basis" for the treatment of acute complications or on a prophylactic basis. Two *Cochrane Database Systematic Reviews* [51] concluded that there is "not enough evidence to draw conclusions" on the extent to which prophylactic blood transfusions help pregnancy outcomes. Both a randomized controlled trial [44] and the retrospective studies [37, 61] have shown that prophylactic transfusion decreased maternal painful crises but did not show other measurable differences in fetal or maternal outcome. However, the randomized study was small, and the number of units ultimately transfused during pregnancy in those randomized to "no blood transfusion" did not differ significantly from those randomized to "transfusion" because many in the "no transfusion" arm received emergency blood transfusion for vasoocclusive crises. Many centers still advise prophylactic top-up or exchange transfusion for SCD during pregnancy, particularly for high-risk cases or where potential organizational delays in providing timely emergency transfusions would increase the maternal and fetal risks. There are significant risks of transfusion, however, that include alloimmunization, delayed hemolytic transfusion reactions [91, 37], hemolytic disease of the newborn, and infection transmission. Iron overload from repeated transfusions in SCD rarely deposits in organs other than the liver [101], but if patients receive prophylactic top-up transfusions in several pregnancies, iron loading of the liver may require treatment in the longer term. The need for prophylactic transfusion throughout pregnancy should therefore be discussed in the multidisciplinary clinic and considered if the woman has a poor obstetric or previous sickle history, if there are the increased demands of a twin pregnancy or if the woman has stopped hydroxycarbamide in order to conceive. Most clinicians will have a greater readiness to give blood transfusions during the third trimester of pregnancy.

Ad hoc top-up blood transfusions for correction of anemia are indicated where the hematocrit has dropped below 0.26 and/or significantly below the patient's normal steady-state values. An emergency exchange transfusion, either by the manual or automated route, is indicated when a patient presents with an acute chest syndrome or a stroke and should be considered when persistent or recurrent acute pain develops. Once a patient has required a blood transfusion during pregnancy, prophylactic transfusions should be continued to maintain the hematocrit and suppress the HbS level below 30 %. The resulting hematocrit needs to be a compromise between sufficient red blood cells to provide adequate oxygen delivery, without increasing the viscosity of the blood to a level which may precipitate vasoocclusion. To reduce alloimmunization (the formation of antibodies to red cell antigens), patients with SCD should have an extended red cell phenotype performed at presentation, and all transfusions should be matched for C, E, and Kell antigens [99]. If red cell antibodies are already present, extended red cell matching may be required.

14.2.9 Contraception in SCD

As many as two-thirds of pregnancies are unplanned, with the attendant lost opportunity to optimize the health of the woman and the potential outcome of her pregnancy [35]. Barrier methods of contraception are safe and effective. There is limited evidence about the efficacy and safety of hormonal contraception. A Cochrane review [52] identified only one randomized controlled trial which included 25 women with HbSS studied over a 2-year period in a single-blind crossover design of depot medroxyprogesterone acetate. A reduction in acute sickling and hemolysis was found in those receiving the active injections [26]. A further study randomly assigned women to intramuscular depo-medroxyprogesterone (DMPA) or Microgynon (combined oral contraceptive pill) and showed a decrease of painful episodes in both groups, more in the DMPA group [25]. Thus, progestogen-containing contraceptives appear to be safe and effective, and there is a suggestion that they may decrease painful episodes. Women who take oral contraceptive pills may have "pill failures" when treatment is interrupted by an emergency admission to hospital. Also, the efficacy of the contraceptive pill may be compromised by the use of broad-spectrum antibiotics, which are frequently prescribed. Clinicians are often reluctant to advise use of the intrauterine contraceptive device, because of the potential complications of menorrhagia, exacerbating anemia and infection, provoking acute sickling crises. Both these concerns would, in principle, be avoided by use of the progestogen-releasing intrauterine system (Mirena). Some clinicians have concerns about using the combined oral contraceptive pill in women with SCD because of the risk of venous thromboembolism, but there is no evidence to confirm this.

SCD is listed by the British National Formulary and by manufacturers' literature as a contraindication to the prescription of combined oral contraceptive pills. The UK Medical Eligibility Criteria (UKMEC) which is based on the World Health Organization criteria to classify contraceptive use classifies the combined oral contraceptive pill and the copper intrauterine device as category 2, which means the advantages outweigh the disadvantages. However, other methods of contraception, including the progestogen-only pill, Depo-Provera, and the levonorgestrel intrauterine system (Mirena), and emergency contraception are rated as category 1, implying there is no restriction on their use. The level 2 methods should therefore be used as second line.

The outcome of this paucity of guidance is that the majority of women with SCD receive either confused advice or none at all. A survey of 149 sexually active women with SCD in north London in 1993 [36] found that 36 % had been specifically advised to avoid pregnancy. Concerns of the significant mortality risks both for the mother and the baby, as well as a consideration of the generally reduced ability of the woman to care for her child subsequently, are perhaps less likely to prevail nowadays.

14.3 Sickle Cell Trait

14.3.1 Genetic Counseling

Genetic counseling for women with sickle cell trait (HbAS) should be provided as part of the United Kingdom national antenatal hemoglobinopathy screening program, introduced in 2001. Ideally, the woman's carrier status should be identified as part of general pre-pregnancy health advice prior to planning pregnancy. Failing that, in high-prevalence areas, all women are offered hemoglobinopathy screening at the time of booking for antenatal care. In low-prevalence areas (with fewer than 1.5 per 10,000 pregnancies with sickle cell disease fetuses/babies per year), initial screening is undertaken by ascertaining ethnicity using a standardized family origin questionnaire, followed by laboratory testing, when relevant. Currently 1 in 35 pregnant women in the UK are identified by the national screening program as carrying a hemoglobinopathy.

If the screening of a woman by full blood count and Hb electrophoresis suggests she is a carrier of a sickle hemoglobin (or of thalassemia or another significant haemoglobin variant, see below), her partner's hemoglobinopathy carrier status should be ascertained as a matter of urgency. If he also carries a significant hemoglobinopathy, the expected inheritance pattern is that of an autosomal recessive condition, and genetic counseling should be given in a timely manner at an expert center that is able to provide full and balanced relevant information of the risks for the child. The possibilities of fetal testing by chorionic villus sampling (from 11 weeks of pregnancy) or amniocentesis or fetal blood sampling later in pregnancy should be explained, together with their potential complications and the possibility of selective termination of the pregnancy if the fetus is found to be affected. As in all such counseling, it is important to give the couple full and up-to-date information on the potential health issues and care for the expected child, all of which is available through the NHS Sickle Cell and Thalassaemia Screening Programme (www.screening.nhs.uk/sickleandthal).

14.3.2 Other Pregnancy Complications

Few additional complication rates in sickle trait compared with other women of the same ethnic and obstetric backgrounds have been reported, the main issue of significance being a susceptibility to urinary tract infections. Studies in the USA and in the UK found recurrent urinary tract infections in 6 % of women during pregnancy, with 16 % showing microscopic hematuria [11, 94]. The latter finding is a reflection of microinfarcts from localized sickling in the peculiarly challenging renal microenvironment, which may be sufficient to provoke sickling of red blood cells, even when only half the hemoglobin they contain is Hb S.

14.3.3 Thromboembolism

A case-control study suggests an increased incidence of VTE [6] with a statistically significant increase in pulmonary embolism, compared with similar individuals without sickle hemoglobin, and a non-significant increase in DVT. A further study looking at hormonal contraception found a nonstatistically significant increase in VTE in the sickle trait group [7]. Published studies however have not included pregnant women, who already have an increased likelihood of VTE by virtue of the changes related to pregnancy itself. Whether this is sufficient justification for specific thromboprophylaxis with heparin preparations is debatable, but this and other standard risk reduction precautions should be considered if any further complica-

tions were to be added to the pregnancy or delivery.

14.4 β-Thalassemia Major (TM)

Pregnancy in TM was rarely seen before the 1970s, before iron chelation became available, because hypogonadotropic hypogonadism (HH) rendered patients infertile (see below) and, in any case, most died before the age of 20. There has however been a gradual increase in experience of managing pregnancies in the last two decades. Chelation therapy was introduced in the early 1970s, and despite there being only about 800 patients with TM in the UK, early experience in the management of TM was described [87]. However, the probability of most doctors in the United Kingdom encountering a pregnant woman with TM is very small, as there are only an estimated 800 patients with TM in the UK. Many of the challenges of fertility and management of pregnancy are peculiar to TM. The input of a specialist center in the planning and management of pregnancy in this condition is therefore essential.

14.4.1 Pregnancy Outcomes in TM

Prior to the 1980s, experience with pregnancy in true TM was not described, but as cohorts of patients who had been treated with DFO entered reproductive age, occasional cases of spontaneous pregnancy were reported [45, 53, 55, 84]. Later, the deliberate induction of ovulation with successful pregnancies in patients with hypogonadotropic hypogonadism (HH) also began to be reported [45, 56]. The first successful twin pregnancy following in vitro fertilization and tubal embryo transfer was described in 1994 [72]. There are now several relatively large series of pregnancies in TM described in the literature.

In a series of 29 pregnancies in 22 women cared for at the Royal Free Hospital, London, between 1989 and 2005 (personal communication, S. Tuck, 2005), 13 of these pregnancies followed ovulation induction therapy. Four women had preexisting diabetes. Five had hepatitis C and one had hepatitis B before pregnancy. Five women had significant cardiomyopathy prior to pregnancy, two of whom died during the postnatal period. Of the 29 pregnancies, two resulted in miscarriage and three had termination procedures. There were 26 live births, including two sets of twins (both following gonadotrophin stimulation of ovulation). Only four of the pregnancies were delivered before 37 weeks' gestation, and the birth weights of the 21 term babies ranged from 2,050 to 4,100 g, with a mean of 3,240 g. The rate of delivery by Caesarean section was high, involving 18 of the 24 relevant pregnancies, and in 14 cases this was because of fetomaternal cephalopelvic disproportion.

In a review of 14 pregnancies in 11 TM patients over the last 15 years at UCLH [8], there were two sets of twins and one set of triplets. One patient developed a thromboembolic episode and two had preeclampsia. The mean serum ferritin concentration increased from a pre-pregnancy value of 2,000 to 5,000 μg/L postdelivery. Although no significant cardiac complications and no mortality were encountered, the incidence of preterm labor and growth restriction was threefold higher than in the background population. None of the fetuses had congenital malformations. The mean fetal birth weight was 2.5 kg. Breast-feeding was encouraged in all cases. In high-risk cases, planned Caesarean was recommended and this was performed in 73 % of cases. In the remaining pregnancies, planned induction of labor was undertaken before full term. In high-risk cardiac cases (as currently assessed by myocardial T2*, left ventricular ejection fraction (LVEF) by MRI, and by serial echocardiography), either approach was preceded by the use of DFO at low continuous doses in the run-up to the procedure. DFO was also recommenced in the immediate postpartum period and, in high-risk cases, from the third trimester of pregnancy. No case of maternal mortality was seen, but at least one woman showed increased cardiac iron deposition during pregnancy (see case discussion) having had normal cardiac iron immediately before becoming pregnant. Rapid myocardial iron loading in a pregnant TM woman was also reported in another case [33].

In an Italian series of 58 pregnancies in 46 TM women, conception was achieved after gonadotrophin-induced ovulation in 33 of these women. 91 % of the pregnancies resulted in successful delivery of 45 singleton live-born neonates, five sets of twins, and one set of triplets. When considering only the singleton pregnancies, the proportion of babies with intrauterine growth restriction did not differ from that reported in the general Italian population [63]. Although chelation was continued in the first few weeks of pregnancy in some unplanned cases, chelation was not given in the later stages of pregnancy. Overall, left ventricular ejection fraction did not change significantly during the pregnancies, although significant increases in left ventricular end diastolic dimension were seen, which returned to pre-pregnancy levels following delivery. Longitudinal myocardial T2* data were not available except in two patients, but values fell from 16.9 to 8.4 ms in one of these, where myocardial T2* measurement was undertaken. In this series, there were five spontaneous miscarriages, one termination of pregnancy, and a high prevalence of preterm births [63].

Thus, despite some differences in obstetric management between centers, there are some consistent themes. Overall there is a good fetal outcome, although there is some evidence of increased premature labor. It is clear that cardiac risks from iron overload are not trivial and risks can be decreased by selecting patients with the lowest cardiac risk and by the use of intensive chelation pre-pregnancy, where appropriate. Where this is not possible, the maternal risks may be decreased by the use of Caesarean section and the avoidance of prolonged labor. Some centers have also used DFO in the latter weeks of pregnancy, without adverse fetal effects.

14.4.2 Fertility and Other Endocrine Complications in TM

Individuals with TM major are dependent on regular and frequent (at least monthly) blood transfusions. As each unit of blood contains about

200 mg of iron, which cannot be physiologically excreted, repeated transfusion results in the accumulation of iron in the liver and subsequently in endocrine tissues such as the anterior pituitary, the islet cells of the pancreas, the thyroid and parathyroids, and the heart, if the iron burden is not well managed with adequate chelation therapy. Ovarian function, however, is usually well preserved. Hypogonadotropic hypogonadism (HH), from iron deposition in the anterior pituitary, is one of the earliest manifestations of insufficient control of iron overload, leading to poor growth and sexual development, often with primary amenorrhea or early secondary amenorrhea [20, 78]. Once HH has developed, there is no evidence that this can be reversed with intensive chelation therapy. However, with optimal chelation therapy during childhood and adolescence, HH can be prevented in many cases and the frequency is falling. For example in 1996, a study of 97 individuals in London found 66 % of young adult thalassemics with HH, 20 % with diabetes, and 10 % with hypothyroidism [39]. A slightly later study in over 1,000 patients in Italy found hypogonadism in 55 % of patients over 12 years old [13]. Progressive birth cohorts treated from an early age with desferrioxamine (DFO) show a falling incidence of HH; at the age of 20, 65 % of patients born between 1970 and 1974 had evidence of hypogonadism, but this fell to 14 % in the 1980–1984 birth cohort [14].

Because ovarian function is usually well preserved, the effects of HH on fertility in TM women can be circumvented by induction of ovulation with gonadotrophins [21] and successful pregnancy is often achievable. The success rate in pregnancies following induction of ovulation is surprisingly high. For example, in 11 women with TM managed at University College London Hospitals (UCLH), over the last 15 years and who had HH but functionally intact ovaries, 14 healthy newborn infants were delivered [8]. Worldwide over 350 successful pregnancies have been reported with this approach.

It is important that the management of infertility includes comprehensive pre-pregnancy counseling of the couple and should include evaluation of the partner according to standard criteria as well as assessment for his hemoglobinopathy carrier status. If the partner of a patient with TM is heterozygous for beta-thalassemia, there is a 1 in 2 chance of the baby having TM. If such a couple proceeds with ovulation induction and wishes to have prenatal diagnosis, the acceptability to the couple of a 1 in 2 chance of an affected pregnancy needs to be discussed in advance. At UCLH, we have encountered two couples where both had TM but wished to conceive. The use of donor gametes, preferably using donor sperm, is an option in such circumstances, as sperm is relatively easily available from sperm banks, whereas the use of donor eggs is technically more complicated with unpredictable success rates [8]. In TM patients with severe organ damage or where both partners have TM, adoption should be considered. Preimplantation testing is also theoretically possible if in vitro fertilization techniques are used to achieve pregnancy [31], provided the couple are prepared to accept the lower overall chances of pregnancy compared with the combination of natural conception and the use of antenatal diagnostic procedures.

14.4.3 Pre-pregnancy Assessment in TM

Most but not all patients will require induction of ovulation, allowing a planned approach to the management of pregnancy [8, 27, 77]. Previous long-term treatment with iron chelation therapies such as desferrioxamine (DFO), deferasirox (DFX), and deferiprone (DFP) usually prevents the extrahepatic effects of iron overload, if used appropriately and regularly. While these therapies are offered to all patients treated in the UK, adherence is not always ideal, and they may not be available to patients treated elsewhere. The main cause of early mortality in poorly chelated patients with TM has been due to cardiac toxicity. Important decisions concerning the maternal risk with respect to cardiomyopathy during pregnancy and labor will therefore need to be made, as healthy cardiac function is essential for the increased demands of pregnancy. Indeed there have been several reported maternal deaths from cardiac failure in pregnancy (see below). A detailed assessment of cardiac function is therefore essential before a planned pregnancy. This should involve a myocardial T2*, assessment of LVEF, a detailed assessment of any history of previous heart failure and/or arrhythmias and review by a cardiologist with expertise in this area. If the myocardial T2* shows evidence of cardiac iron overload, especially in the presence of decreased left ventricular function, a course of intensive chelation therapy will be necessary before considering pregnancy. This may take over a year to achieve, so long-term planning of pregnancies is an important aspect of overall management. This decision is not always straightforward however: the development of cardiac iron overload as a result of withholding chelation during the entirety of pregnancy has been seen at UCLH (see case 2). In the same clinic, patients with evidence of moderate cardiac iron loading but with well-preserved cardiac function have been successfully managed using small doses of DFO in the final trimester (see below).

A detailed assessment for other comorbidities is required, including glucose tolerance, and bone densitometry [40, 92]. Hypothyroidism and diabetes are recognized complications of hemosiderosis in adults with transfusion-dependent thalassemias. Treatment should be optimized before pregnancy, in the same way as in the general population, with the same issues being relevant, including the risks of fetal anomalies and miscarriage, if not closely controlled. Given their lifelong dependence on transfusions with donated blood, hepatitis B, hepatitis C, and HIV status should be checked before pregnancy, although the risk of transmission from the UK blood supply is extremely low. Appropriate antiviral treatment should be given before conception if required, both for the benefit of the woman herself and in order to reduce the risk of transmission to the fetus, but this may take months or years to complete. The risk of transmission of hepatitis C and HIV to the baby is relatively low if managed appropriately. At UCLH, an adult TM patient with HIV has been successfully managed through pregnancy with anti-retroviral treatment, with the birth of a healthy unaffected child.

Osteoporosis is a significant problem, affecting about 40 % of adult patients, caused by a combination of endocrine, genetic factors, and direct effects of the dysfunctional bone marrow on the skeleton. During pregnancy, a degree of bone loss is seen physiologically, and as TM patients often start from a low baseline of bone density, this can be a particular problem. Many TM patients now routinely receive bisphosphonates to improve bone density, and a careful plan of stopping these several months before conception is required, due to the long biological half-life of these agents and their potential adverse effects on fetal skeletal development. Stopping these agents can add to bone loss during pregnancy. Prolonged heparin anticoagulation during pregnancy, which is necessary in some women, (see below) may exacerbate bone loss in this patient group. Other supportive measures, such as weight-bearing exercise and appropriate calcium and vitamin D supplements, can, however, be continued. Patients should therefore be advised of the risks of worsening osteopenia before embarking on induction of ovulation. Ideally, a TM woman who wishes to become pregnant at a future date should have the opportunity of discussing how to maximize bone mass several years before a planned pregnancy. Efforts should be made to minimize activities which may increase the risk of spinal fractures, such as heavy lifting.

The presence of atypical red cell antibodies should be reviewed prior to pregnancy and assessed for the risk of haemolytic disease of the fetus and newborn (HDFN). The likelihood of new alloantibodies forming during pregnancy in someone who has received lifetime transfusions is small.

14.4.4 Care of Thalassemia Major During Pregnancy

14.4.4.1 Transfusion

The dilutional effects of the physiological anaemia in pregnancy are also seen in TM, and blood transfusions may be needed at more frequent intervals than before pregnancy, in order to maintain the same mean hemoglobin and to minimize major fluctuations in the hemoglobin concentration and cardiac workload, particularly in the later stages of pregnancy. In the Italian study [63], blood consumption increased significantly, from 132 to 157 mL of red cells per kg per year during pregnancy.

Although there is some variation in transfusion practice worldwide, usually the aim should be to maintain the hemoglobin concentration above 10 g/dL for TM patients. Reported policy from an Italian study was to transfuse only if the hemoglobin concentration fell below 10 g/dL [63]. It has been argued that the relatively high rate of intrauterine growth restriction (IUGR) of 22 % in this study suggests that a more aggressive transfusion policy may be needed [89]. If IUGR is present despite maintaining the hemoglobin concentration above 10 g/dL, other fetoplacental and maternal factors should be considered (bearing in mind that 30 % of IUGR in the general population have no identifiable underlying cause).

14.4.4.2 Cardiac Risk and Chelation Therapy in TM Pregnancy

The physiological effects of pregnancy with an increased blood volume, hemodilution, increased stroke volume, heart rate, and cardiac output may precipitate heart failure in patients with preexisting LV dysfunction or with evidence of myocardial siderosis. Progressive changes in many body systems during pregnancy result in increased basal oxygen consumption and increased susceptibility to oxidative stress that peaks by the second trimester of pregnancy [17], but is also likely to increase during prolonged labor. Added to this risk is the common practice of withholding chelation therapy during pregnancy because of potential teratogenic risks. Indeed, some pregnancies have been terminated because of concern about DFO toxicity [24, 41, 92]. Thus, although patients with normal resting cardiac performance and adequate pregestational chelation therapy usually proceed through pregnancy and delivery without complications, a woman with marginally impaired cardiac performance or with myocardial

hemosiderosis may be at risk of developing heart failure. There have been at least four case reports of fatal heart failure during pregnancy in the literature [90, 92]. In another report of three cases, end-systolic diameters, fractional shortening, and ejection fraction were within the normal range before pregnancy, but worsened during gestation, and one patient developed incipient congestive heart failure [64]. Key aspects of avoiding such complications are careful pre-pregnancy counseling and full cardiovascular assessment, aimed at avoiding pregnancy in high-risk patients. In an Italian study, patients with impaired LV function were not given induction of ovulation or were advised not to become pregnant until intensive chelation therapy had been undertaken [63].

If a patient with preexisting myocardial siderosis or LV dysfunction becomes pregnant, the risk and benefits of chelation therapy, particularly with DFO, need to be carefully considered. When a woman with TM is actively trying for pregnancy or receiving fertility treatment, her iron chelation therapy is usually discontinued, because of possible teratogenic risks from chelation therapy, in line with the manufacturers' recommendations. This approach has not been universally adopted, however. In the Origa study [63], chelation therapy [deferoxamine ($n=31$), deferiprone ($n=2$), and deferasirox ($n=2$)] was being taken at the time of conception and was continued for the following 2–10 weeks in the spontaneous pregnancies and in ten pregnancies achieved by ovarian stimulation with no adverse fetal effects. In patients with a history of high myocardial iron load, the withholding of chelation therapy for repeated cycles of ovulation induction may pose an unacceptable risk. In such cases, some patients at UCLH have continued DFO (but not other chelators) until pregnancy has been confirmed. No fetal abnormalities have been seen. Furthermore, in the latter part of pregnancy, where teratogenic effects are theoretically less than in the first trimester, the potential benefits of DFO in high-risk cases may need to be considered. The potential teratogenic effects of DFP are well recognized [9], but with DFO, the risks may not be as great as hitherto considered. Firstly, DFO, by nature of its positive charge, its relative hydrophilic properties, and its larger molecular weight than orally absorbed chelators, transits biomembranes more slowly [66], and this would also be expected with placental transfer [22]. Although teratogenic effects and skeletal anomalies were noted in animal studies with DFO, it can be difficult to extrapolate the degree of placental transfer to humans. Furthermore, over three decades, there have been over 40 pregnancies reported in iron-overloaded subjects given DFO at various stages of pregnancy without apparent teratogenic effects [10, 15, 43, 54, 72, 76, 95, 97]. There have also been reports of DFO use throughout the second and third trimesters of pregnancy without adverse fetal effects [76, 90]. At UCLH [8], it has been recent practice to give low doses of DFO (1 g/day) in the later stages of pregnancy to patients with a high risk of heart disease, based on either a previous history of LV dysfunction or with evidence of myocardial iron deposition, either immediately before pregnancy or of progressive myocardial iron accumulation during pregnancy. Such patients are admitted for early induction of labor or Caesarean section, to avoid spontaneous (i.e. unplanned) labor, and DFO is given in the days immediately preceding induction of labor.

14.4.4.3 Thrombosis Risk in TM Pregnancy

Thalassemic patients have a chronic hypercoagulable state, with an increased incidence of thromboembolic episodes (TE). In a survey of Italian thalassemic centers, 32 TE episodes were identified in a total of 735 subjects [12], but this series also included thalassemia intermedia (TI) patients. As will be seen below, thromboembolism is generally two to four times greater in TI than TM [12, 55, 80]. Sites of TE risks included the central nervous system (with a clinical picture of headache, seizures, and hemiparesis), pulmonary, mesenteric, and portal sites [12, 80]. Deep venous thrombosis, intracardiac thrombosis, and laboratory signs of disseminated intravascular coagulation (DIC)

have also been observed during pregnancy in two patients [12].

The mechanisms for the increased thrombotic tendency include the presence of abnormal red cells that express phosphatidylserine on their cell surface [16] and that shed prothrombotic microvesicles [102]. A wide variety of laboratory changes are seen including increased urinary excretion of thromboxane A2 metabolites, enhanced expression of P-selectin in intact thalassemic platelets, elevated plasma levels of thrombin-antithrombin complexes, elevated levels of endothelial adhesion protein (ICAM-1, ELAM-1, VCAM-1, von Willebrand factor, and thrombomodulin) [16], and low plasma levels of the natural anticoagulants, protein C and protein S, and heparin cofactor II [62, 67].

Many TM and TI patients will have undergone splenectomy and this further increases the risk of thrombosis [82] and the number of PS-expressing red-cell-derived microparticles [102]. VTE appears more common in patients with associated organ dysfunction [12] such as diabetes, cardiopulmonary abnormalities, hypothyroidism, and liver function anomalies. These risks may be combined with the known effects of pregnancy such as increased levels of clotting factors II, VII, VIII, and X, increased fibrin formation, decreased fibrinolysis, decreased free-protein S levels, and acquired resistance to activated protein C. Many of these effects can be partially abrogated by hypertransfusion, which will suppress endogenous red cell production, and hence thromboses are less likely in TM than TI syndromes. It is therefore not surprising that the incidence of VTE is less common in TM than in TI, occurring in to 3.95 and 9.61 % of patients, respectively [12]. Thus, unless there is a history of VTE or additional risk factors such as antiphospholipid syndrome, routine thromboprophylaxis has not generally been used in TM pregnancies. In splenectomized patients, low-dose aspirin has been suggested, as its use does not seem to be associated with risk to the central and regional circulation of the fetus [98]. The risks of VTE postpartum are increased, and it is routine practice at UCLH to recommend subcutaneous low molecular weight heparin prophylaxis postdelivery for 6 weeks.

14.4.4.4 Endocrine Issues During TM Pregnancy

The care of diabetes and hypothyroidism is along the same principles as in all women with these conditions, recognizing that endocrine disorders are more common in TM and may manifest themselves for the first time during pregnancy. Tight glycemic control requires multidisciplinary care, and additional ultrasound scans are needed to check for fetal anomalies and to monitor the fetal growth pattern. Delivery at between 38 and 39 weeks' gestation is likely to be advised, to reduce the risk of sudden intrauterine fetal death in late pregnancy with maternal diabetes. The mother should be checked in each trimester for possible retinal and renal complications of her diabetes. For those with hypothyroidism, their dose of thyroxine replacement therapy usually needs to be increased during pregnancy, because of the physiological increase in carrier proteins, but this can be easily monitored by measurements of serum TSH and free thyroxine at intervals of approximately 6–8 weeks, as appropriate for the individual patient.

14.4.4.5 Infection Risk in TM Pregnancy

In TM patients who have undergone splenectomy, there is an increased risk of bacterial infections, particularly streptococcal infections. Pneumococcal vaccination is advised, and a booster dose should be given prior to planned pregnancy if required. Splenectomized patients are commonly maintained on prophylactic penicillin V, which should be continued prior to and during pregnancy, with an ongoing awareness of the patient's susceptibility to infections. Patients with severe iron overload are also at increased risk of infection with organisms such as *Klebsiella* and *Yersinia enterocolitica*.

14.4.4.6 Optimal Timing and Method of Delivery

A series of 58 pregnancies showed a high prevalence of preterm births (33 %) [63]. Therefore, if the mother is being managed in a specialist thalassemia center at a significant geographical distance from her home, a planned antenatal admission for induction of labor or Caesarean section may be appropriate. If a TM mother is significantly iron overloaded, the risks of prolonged labor with attendant acidosis and the risk of liberating toxic iron pools should also be taken into account. In a series from Italy, with all the women cared for in the centers at Cagliari, Genoa, and Brindisi, 67 % of women in Turin gave birth by Caesarean section [63]. In series from Greece, all were delivered by elective Caesarean section [1, 24, 41]. The fact that most patients with transfusion-dependent thalassemia are themselves of shorter than average stature means that they often require Caesarean delivery because of cephalopelvic disproportion. However, elective Caesarean section is not a universal approach, and in the absence of the confounding influences of maternal diabetes, fetal growth restriction, or high maternal cardiac risk, pregnancy often proceeds normally, allowing plans for timing and mode of delivery to be made along relatively standard obstetric principles.

14.4.4.7 Postnatal Care and Complications in TM

Because of the increased thrombotic risks described above, it is usual practice to recommend low molecular weight heparin prophylaxis in the postpartum period and in splenectomized women to continue low-dose aspirin [63]. The longer-term risks of being without chelation therapy for 9 months have not been studied systematically, but there is some evidence of significant consequences. In one study, endocrine complications developed during the 6 months following delivery, with two women developing diabetes [92]. In the same study, two developed new significant cardiomyopathy, and five women developed secondary amenorrhea. It is therefore recommended to reinstitute chelation therapy as soon as practical postnatally. If the mother wishes to breast-feed, DFO is the chelator of choice, as it is not absorbed by the oral route. In a twin pregnancy where DFO was given to the mother postnatally, normal iron levels were observed in breast milk, and no clinical or hematological abnormalities due to DFO therapy could be shown in the breast-fed newborns [81]. At UCLH, DFO has been given to some mothers while breast-feeding, and although low levels of DFO were found in the breast milk, no clinical or hematological abnormalities due to DFO have been observed in the babies.

14.5 Thalassemia Intermedia (TI)

14.5.1 Overview of Management Issues

Unlike TM, patients with TI do not usually receive regular transfusion therapy. The frequency of transfusion is highly variable between TI patients and also within individual patients during their lifetime, with a tendency to increasing transfusion requirements with advancing age. The lack of regular transfusion in TI has three major consequences relevant to pregnancy: firstly, iron overload will have previously advanced more slowly than in TM so that cardiomyopathy and other risks from iron overload are less common. Hypogonadotropic hypogonadism is therefore less common or occurs later than in TM. Thus, pregnancy can usually occur without the need for induction of ovulation. The second consequence is that previous exposure to red cell alloantigens is less in TI than in TM, so the formation of new red cell alloantibodies, if transfusion is given during pregnancy, is more likely. Thirdly, because a higher proportion of red cells are endogenous in TI and express PS on their cell surface, there is an increased risk of thrombin generation. VTE is two to three times more common in TI than TM. Rarer issues that have occasionally arisen in TI pregnancy include worsening extramedullary hematopoiesis [43] and spinal cord compression [32].

14.5.2 Pregnancy Outcome and Management of Anemia

Pregnancy outcome in TI has been described in 44 women, with 83 pregnancies from Lebanon and Italy [59]. Spontaneous miscarriages occurred in 21 % of pregnancies, with two intrauterine fetal deaths, at 26 weeks' and 36 weeks' gestation. In pregnancies progressing beyond 20 weeks' gestation, preterm delivery and IUGR were noted in 32 and 24 %, respectively. Transfusion was given in 80 % of women during

pregnancy, with 27 % receiving transfusion for the first time. Two women developed severe alloimmune hemolytic anemia, one of whom progressed to cardiac failure at 35 weeks' gestation and was delivered by Caesarean section. Thrombotic events during pregnancy were seen in 7 % of patients.

Several patient series from Asia have described pregnancy outcomes in HbE-beta thalassemia (E-β Thal), a clinical syndrome that ranges in phenotype from TI to TM. In a series of 80 pregnancies from Thailand [88], outcomes were examined retrospectively in 80 patients with E-β Thal (29 %) or HbH (65 %). (Hemoglobin H disease is a form of alpha thalassemia, in which three of the four genes responsible for the production of the alpha-globin chains for hemoglobin are defective). In general, a less aggressive transfusion policy was given in E-β Thal than is typically recommended in Europe to TM patients in pregnancy. Overall, fetal growth restriction was seen in 27 %, with preterm births in 21 % and low birth weight (<2,500 g) in 44 %. The mean gestational age at delivery was 37 weeks (range 27–42). Thirty-three percent had delivery by Caesarean section, and the remainder had successful vaginal deliveries. Baseline hemoglobin (Hb) levels and the mean birth weight of babies born to women with E-β Thal were significantly lower than in those with HbH disease. This suggests that the lower Hb level in E-β Thal may have contributed to the less desirable obstetric outcomes. This conclusion is supported by a retrospective case control cohort study from Thailand in 54 E-β Thal women with singleton pregnancies that has relevance to transfusion policy in TI phenotypes [49]. Although maternal outcomes were similar in both groups, gestational age at birth and birth weight were significantly lower in the E-β Thal women, and the Caesarean section rate was higher (relative risk 2.1). The incidences of fetal growth restriction, preterm birth, and low birth weight were also significantly higher, with relative risks of 2.8, 2.7, and 5.6, respectively. The influence of transfusion policy on these outcomes is of potential importance. The patient population consisted mainly of people with milder forms E-β Thal, and 35 % of patients had not received blood transfusions before pregnancy. The mean Hb levels during pregnancy were significantly lower in the E-β Thal than in the control group (8.1 g/dL vs. 12.8 g/dL). However, most "required" 1–5 transfusions during pregnancy (mean 2.4 transfusions), based on an intention to keep the patients' hemoglobin higher than 7.0 g/dL. This transfusion policy differs from studies of TM populations in Europe where there has typically been an intention to maintain Hb >10 g/dL [40]. There is some evidence that anemia <10 g/dL is an independent risk factor for low birth weight and preterm delivery in non-thalassemic women [47]. However, in the clinical management of TI (or E-β Thal), the potential risk of low birth weight and preterm delivery has to be balanced against the risk of alloimmunization in otherwise infrequently transfused patients.

14.5.3 Management of Thrombotic Risk

The greater inherent risks of TI compared with TM are well recognized, with VTE being two to four times more frequent [12, 82]. Thrombotic risks in TI in descending order of frequency include DVT, PE, superficial thrombophlebitis, portal vein thrombosis, and stroke [83]. Venous thrombotic events are proportionately greater in TI compared with TM, whereas arterial events are more common in TM. Splenectomy is a clear risk factor for thrombosis in TI [82] [83], as is a high nucleated red cell count ($>300 \times 10^9$L), a platelet count $>500 \times 10^9$/L, evidence of pulmonary hypertension (PHT), or being transfusion naïve [83]. The median time to thrombosis following splenectomy is 8 years in Middle Eastern and Italian TI populations [83]. The pro-thrombotic mechanisms for thalassemia syndromes have been outlined above, but transfusion appears to have a protective influence. Transfused patients have lower numbers of thrombogenic red cells and microparticles [102], and transfusion also corrects deficiency of natural anticoagulants in TI [62]. The practical implication of these findings for pregnant TI patients with identifiable risk factors, such as a previous history of thrombosis, splenectomy, high platelet and nucleated

red blood cell counts, or in whom laboratory investigations demonstrate thrombophilia risk, is that prophylactic measures need to be considered. Options are anticoagulation [59] and/or hypertransfusion. Anticoagulation alone may not protect against thrombosis in high-risk cases [5], and at UCLH, cases of intractable ongoing VTE in TI have been corrected by hypertransfusion, when anticoagulation therapy alone has failed, one of these cases occurring during pregnancy. Although transfusion may decrease the risk of VTE, as well as low birth weight deliveries, these potential advantages need to be balanced against the risk of alloimmunization [12, 58]. With the current level of evidence, clinical decisions about whether to institute transfusion and/or anticoagulation in TI pregnancies need to be made on a case-by-case basis.

14.6   α- and β-Thalassemia Traits

Antenatal counseling is a key part of the management of thalassemia traits. The identification of at-risk couples before pregnancy and/or early in pregnancy and the provision of appropriate expert counseling in a timely manner are critical but beyond the scope of this chapter.

Once genetic counseling is completed, the presence of β-thalassemia trait or α-thalassemia trait usually has little impact on the care of pregnancy. The effects of thalassaemia traits have been reported in a large study of over 2,000 thalassemia trait patients and healthy controls [101], in healthy women the Hb fell by about 7 % from the end of the first trimester associated with the increase in plasma volume, and the fall in haemoglobin in β-thalassemia trait was marginally greater at 10 %. In healthy women, the Hb fell from a mean of 12.6 g/dL in the first trimester to 11.7 g/dL in the second trimester, whereas in women with β-thalassemia trait this fell from 10.8 to 9.6 g/dL [103]. This means that some women with β-thalassemia trait will develop Hb values <10 g/dL during pregnancy without any other factors contributing to anemia. However, if values fall below 9 g/dL, some additional cause for anemia should be considered such as concomitant iron or folate deficiency. For alpha-thalassemia traits, similar or slightly smaller decrements in Hb values during pregnancy have been reported. Interestingly, patients with alpha-thalassemia traits seem to have the same incidence of iron deficiency as the normal pregnant patients, whereas in those with β trait, it was four times less common [103]. Iron supplements do not improve the erythropoietic response unless there is coexisting iron deficiency, which is best confirmed by measurement of serum ferritin levels. With maternal thalassemia traits, no abnormality of placental function as assessed by serum estriol concentration or fetal growth was found, and no increase in maternal or fetal morbidity was documented.

has a progestogen-releasing intrauterine system in place for contraception and is not planning any further pregnancies.

Learning Points
- Pregnancy in women with sickle cell disease continues to show high rates of maternal and fetal mortality and morbidity.
- Outcomes can be improved by providing care in centers with specialist expertise.
- Routine prophylactic blood transfusion may not be required in pregnant women with sickle cell disease, but has a role in selected cases.
- Ad hoc transfusions may be required during pregnancy for women experiencing complications.

Case Study 1

Case 1 has homozygous sickle cell disease (hemoglobin SS). She is of Jamaican origin and was aged 24 when she delivered her first child and 31 when she delivered her second child. A year before her first pregnancy, she had a total hip replacement on the right side, having become increasingly disabled because of avascular necrosis of the femoral head. This is a common chronic complication of sickle cell disease. She was in hospital with multiple severe painful episodes during her first pregnancy and spent most of the third trimester in hospital. Because of this, she delivered by elective Caesarean section at 36 weeks, with a healthy girl, birth weight 2.931 kg. Four weeks after delivery, she had a deep vein thrombosis in her left leg. In her second pregnancy, she was given low molecular weight heparin prophylaxis from 24 weeks' gestation. She had mild bone pains throughout, but no crisis severe enough to require hospital admission. She had a normal delivery, after spontaneous onset of labor at 38 weeks, with a healthy girl, birth weight 2.928 kg. Since then, she

Case Study 2

A 39-year-old woman with thalassemia major became pregnant following induction of ovulation. In her past history, she started transfusion when aged 2 years and desferrioxamine at the age of 14. She had primary amenorrhea, secondary hypothyroidism, secondary hypoparathyroidism, osteopenia, and had hepatitis C at the age of 21, but remained HCV-RNA negative. She currently had good compliance with desferrioxamine 2.5 g five times per week, a serum ferritin of 1,734 μg/L, and this had been consistently <2,500 μg/L for the previous 3 years. Immediately prior to induction of ovulation, the myocardial T2* was 19.9 ms, the LVEF was 82 %, and liver iron was 5 mg/g dw by MRI. DFO was stopped at the commencement of ovulation induction, and she became pregnant in the first cycle of therapy. At 12 weeks, the ferritin was 3,591 μg/L, LVEF 73 %, and the myocardial T2* 22 ms. She was admitted for induction of labor at 39 weeks and given low-dose DFO infusion during labor. Due to poor progression of cervical dilatation, Caesarean section was performed, and a healthy baby was born. Thromboprophylaxis with LMW heparin was given postdelivery. Because of the high ferritin and borderline myocardial T2* pre-pregnancy, subcutaneous DFO was given after delivery at standard doses. The baby was breast-fed and measurement of DFO in breast milk showed a very low concentration (0.18 µM). Four months postdelivery, the serum ferritin had fallen to 2,789 µg/L, but the myocardial T2* was now 11.8 ms. She continued subcutaneous DFO at standard doses, and at 7 months' postdelivery, the ferritin was 2,623 µg/L and the myocardial T2* had improved to 17.9 ms. Twelve months after delivery, the myocardial T2* was 31 ms and ferritin 2,124 µg/L.

Learning Points

- Women with TM can sometimes develop rapid myocardial iron loading during pregnancy when chelation is not used.
- If the patient has a history of myocardial iron loading, close monitoring is recommended (possibly including myocardial T2* in late pregnancy).
- If the LVEF falls or myocardial T2* falls, there is a case for giving low-dose DFO in the latter weeks of pregnancy even though chelation therapy is not officially sanctioned in drug licensing. DFO was given in this patient after delivery, but the measurement of low DFO levels in breast milk, together with its lack of oral absorption, allowed this to be given without side effects in the baby.

References

1. Aessopos A, Karabatsos F, Farmakis D, Katsantoni A, Hatziliami A, Youssef J, Karagiorga M. Pregnancy in patients with well-treated ß-thalassemia: outcome for mothers and newborn infants. Am J Obstet Gynecol. 1999;180:360–5.
2. Afolabi BB, Iwuala NC, Iwuala IC, Ogedengbe OK. Morbidity and mortality in sickle cell pregnan-cies in Lagos, Nigeria: a case control study. J Obstet Gynaecol. 2009;29:104–6.
3. Al Jama FE, Gasem T, Burshaid S, Rahman J, Al Suleiman SA, Rahman MS. Pregnancy outcome in patients with homozygous sickle cell disease in a university hospital, Eastern Saudi Arabia. Arch Gynecol Obstet. 2009;280:793–7.
4. Al-Suleiman S, Rahman M, Rahman J, Al-Najashi S. Sickle cell disease and pregnancy in Saudi Arabia. J Obstet Gynaecol. 1991;11:331–5.
5. Androutsopoulos G, Karakantza M, Decavalas G. Thalassemia intermedia, inherited thrombophilia, and intrauterine growth restriction. Int J Gynaecol Obstet. 2007;99:146.
6. Austin H, Key NS, Benson JM, Lally C, Dowling NF, Whitsett C, Hooper WC. Sickle cell trait and the risk of venous thromboembolism among blacks. Blood. 2007;110:908–12.
7. Austin H, Lally C, Benson JM, Whitsett C, Hooper WC, Key NS. Hormonal contraception, sickle cell trait, and risk for venous thromboembolism among African American women. Am J Obstet Gynecol. 2009;200(620):e621–3.
8. Bajoria R, Chatterjee R. Current perspectives of fertility and pregnancy in thalassemia. Hemoglobin. 2009;33 Suppl 1:S131–5.
9. Berdoukas V, Bentley P, Frost H, SchnEßli HP. Toxicity of oral iron chelator L1. Lancet. 1993;341:1088.
10. Blanc P, Hryhorczuk D, Danel I. Deferoxamine treatment of acute iron intoxication in pregnancy. Obstet Gynecol. 1984;64:12S–4.
11. Blank AM, Freedman WL. Sickle cell trait and pregnancy. Clin Obstet Gynecol. 1969;12(1):123–33.
12. Borgna-Pignatti C, Carnelli V, Caruso V, Dore F, De Mattia D, Di Palma A, Di Gregorio F, Romeo MA, Longhi R, Mangiagli A, Melevendi C, Pizzarelli G, Musumeci S. Thromboembolic events in ß thalassemia major: an Italian multicenter study. Acta Haematol. 1998;99:76–9.
13. Borgna-Pignatti C. Modern treatment of thalassaemia intermedia. Br J Haematol. 2007;138:291–304.
14. Borgna-Pignatti C, Rugolotto S, De Stefano P, Piga A, Di Gregorio F, Gamberini MR, Sabato V, Melevendi C, Cappellini MD, Verlato G. Survival and disease complications in thalassemia major. Ann N Y Acad Sci. 1998;850:227–31.
15. Borgna-Pignatti C, Rugolotto S, De Stefano P, Zhao H, Cappellini MD, Del Vecchio GC, Romeo MA, Forni GL, Gamberini MR, Ghilardi R, Piga A, Cnaan A. Survival and complications in patients with thalassemia major treated with transfusion and deferoxamine. Haematologica. 2004;89:1187–93.
16. Bosque MA, Domingo JL, Corbella J. Assessment of the developmental toxicity of deferoxamine in mice. Arch Toxicol. 1995;69:467–71.
17. Cappellini MD. Coagulation in the pathophysiology of hemolytic anemias. Hematology Am Soc Hematol Educ Program. 2007;2007:74–8.
18. Casanueva E, Jimenez J, Meza-Camacho C, Mares M, Simon L. Prevalence of nutritional deficiencies in

Mexican adolescent women with early and late prenatal care. Arch Latinoam Nutr. 2003;53:35–8.

19. Chakravarty EF, Khanna D, Chung L. Pregnancy outcomes in systemic sclerosis, primary pulmonary hypertension, and sickle cell disease. Obstet Gynecol. 2008;111:927–34.

20. Chase AR, Sohal M, Howard J, Laher R, McCarthy A, Layton DM, Oteng-Ntim E. Pregnancy outcomes in sickle cell disease: retrospective cohort study of two tertiary referral centres in the UK. Obstetric Medicine. 2010;3:110–12.

21. Chatterjee R, Katz M, Cox TF, Porter JB. Prospective study of the hypothalamic-pituitary axis in thalassaemic patients who developed secondary amenorrhoea. Clin Endocrinol (Oxf). 1993;39:287–96.

22. Chatterjee R, Wonke B, Porter JB, Katz M. (1995) Correction of primary and secondary amenorrhoea and induction of ovulation by pulsatile infusion of gonadotrophin releasing hormone (GnRH) in patients with ß thalassaemia major. In: Sickle cell disease and thalassaemia: new trends in therapy. Eds Beuzard Y, Lubin B, Rosa J. Colloq. Inserm.1995;234, 451–455.

23. Curry SC, Bond GR, Raschke R, Tellez D, Wiggins D. An ovine model of maternal iron poisoning in pregnancy. Ann Emerg Med. 1990;19:632–8.

24. Dare F, Makinde O, Faasuba O. The obstetric performance of sickle cell disease patients and homozygous haemoglobin C patients in Ile-Ife, Nigeria. Int J Gynaecol Obstet. 1992;37(3):163–8.

25. Daskalakis GJ, Papageorgiou IS, Antsaklis AJ, Michalas SK. Pregnancy and homozygous ß thalassaemia major. Br J Obstet Gynaecol. 1998;105:1028–32.

26. de Abood M, de Castillo Z, Guerrero F, Espino M, Austin KL. Effect of Depo-Provera or microgynon on the painful crises of sickle cell anemia patients. Contraception. 1997;56:313–6.

27. De Ceulaer K, Gruber C, Hayes R, Serjeant GR. Medroxyprogesterone acetate and homozygous sickle-cell disease. Lancet. 1982;2:229–31.

28. De Sanctis V, Vullo C, Katz M, Wonke B, Hoffbrand VA, Di Palma A, Bagni B. Endocrine complications in thalassaemia major. Prog Clin Biol Res. 1989;309:77–83.

29. DHSS, D.o.H.S.S. Report on confidential enquiries into maternal deaths in England and Wales, 1991–93. London: Her Majesty's Stationery Office; 1994.

30. DHSS, D.o.H.S.S. Reports on confidential enquiries into maternal deaths in England and Wales, 1967–69, 1970–72, 1973–75, 1976–78, 1979–81. London: Her Majesty's Stationery Office; 1976, 1979, 1982.

31. El-Shafei AM, Dhaliwal JK, Sandhu AK. Pregnancy in sickle cell disease in Bahrain. Br J Obstet Gynaecol. 1992;99:101–4.

32. El-Toukhy T, Bickerstaff H, Meller S. Preimplantation genetic diagnosis for haematologic conditions. Curr Opin Pediatr. 2010;22:28–34.

33. Esfandbod M, Malekpour M. Thalassemia and spinal cord compression in pregnancy. CMAJ. 2010; 182:E798.

34. Farmaki K, Gotsis E, Tzoumari I, Berdoukas V. Rapid iron loading in a pregnant woman with transfusion-dependent thalassemia after brief cessation of iron chelation therapy. Eur J Haematol. 2008;81:157–9.

35. Heit JA, Beckman MG, Bockenstedt PL, Grant AM, Key NS, Kulkarni R, Manco-Johnson MJ, Moll S, Ortel TL, Philipp CS. Comparison of characteristics from White- and Black-Americans with venous thromboembolism: a cross-sectional study. Am J Hematol. 2010;85:467–71.

36. Howard RJ, Lillis C, Tuck SM. Contraceptives, counselling, and pregnancy in women with sickle cell disease. BMJ. 1993;306:1735–7.

37. Howard RJ, Lillis C, Tuck S. Contraception, counselling and pregnancy in women with sickle cell disease. Br Med J. 1995;306:1735–7.

38. Howard RJ, Tuck S, Pearson T. Pregnancy in sickle cell disease in the UK: results of a multicentre survey of the effect of prophylactic blood transfusion on maternal and fetal outcome. Br J Obstet Gynaecol. 1995;102:947–51.

39. Jensen CE, Tuck SM, Old J, Morris RW, Yardumian A, De Sanctis V, Hoffbrand AV, Wonke B. Incidence of endocrine complications and clinical disease severity related to genotype analysis and iron overload in patients with ß- thalassaemia. Eur J Haematol. 1997;59:76–81.

40. Jensen CE, Tuck SM, Wonke B. Fertility in ß thalassaemia major: a report of 16 pregnancies, preconceptual evaluation and a review of the literature. Br J Obstet Gynaecol. 1995;102:625–9.

41. Karagiorga-Lagana M. Fertility in thalassemia: the Greek experience. J Pediatr Endocrinol Metab. 1998;11 Suppl 3:945–51.

42. Khoury S, Odeh M, Oettinger M. Deferoxamine treatment for acute iron intoxication in pregnancy. Acta Obstet Gynecol Scand. 1995;74:756–7.

43. Konstantopoulos K, Plataniotis G, Maris T, Voskaridou E, Rekoumi L, Stratigaki M, Loukopoulos D. Extramedullary haemopoiesis in thalassaemia intermedia: an unusual case of relapsing paraparesis in pregnancy. Haematologia (Budap). 1995;27: 29–32.

44. Koshy M, Burd L, Wallace D, Moawad A, Baron J. Prophylactic red-cell transfusions in pregnant patients with sickle cell disease. A randomized cooperative study. N Engl J Med. 1988;319:1447–52.

45. Kumar RM, Rizk DE, Khuranna A. ß-thalassemia major and successful pregnancy. J Reprod Med. 1997;42:294–8.

46. LEßorgne-Samuel Y, Janky E, Venditelli F, Salin J, Daijardin JB, Couchy B, Etienne-Julan M, Berchel C. Sickle cell anemia and pregnancy: review of 68 cases in Guadeloupe. J Gynecol Obstet Biol Reprod (Paris). 2000;29:86–93.

47. Levy A, Fraser D, Katz M, Mazor M, Sheiner E. Maternal anemia during pregnancy is an independent risk factor for low birthweight and preterm delivery. Eur J Obstet Gynecol Reprod Biol. 2005;122: 182–6.

48. Lewis GE. The confidential enquiry into maternal and child health, 2000–02, 2003–05. Reports on confidential

enquiries into maternal deaths in the United Kingdom. London: CEMACH; 2004 and 2007.

49. Lewis GE. Confidential Enquiry into Maternal and Child Health. Saving mothers' lives: reviewing maternal deaths to make motherhood safer, 2006–08. The eighth report of the confidential enquiries into maternal deaths in the United Kingdom. London: CEMACH; 2011. www.cmace.org.uk/Publications/CEMACHPublications/Maternal-and-Perinatal-Health.aspx

50. Luewan S, Srisupundit K, Tongsong T. Outcomes of pregnancies complicated by ß-thalassemia/hemoglobin E disease. Int J Gynaecol Obstet. 2009; 104:203–5.

51. Mahomed K. Prophylactic versus selective blood transfusion in sickle cell disease pregnancies. Cochrane Database Syst Rev. 2000 and 2006; (2):CD000040, and update in (3), CD000040.

52. Manchikanti A, Grimes DA, Lopez LM Schulz KF. Steroid hormones for contraception in women with sickle cell disease. Cochrane Database Syst Rev. 2007;CD006261.

53. Martin K. Successful pregnancy in ß-thalassaemia major. Aust Paediatr J. 1983;19:182–3.

54. McElhatton PR, Roberts JC, Sullivan FM. The consequences of iron overdose and its treatment with desferrioxamine in pregnancy. Hum Exp Toxicol. 1991;10:251–9.

55. Meadows K. A successful pregnancy outcome in transfusion dependent thalassaemia major. Aust N Z J Obstet Gynaecol. 1984;24:43–4.

56. Moratelli S, De Sanctis V, Gemmati D, Serino ML, Mari R, Gamberini MR, Scapoli GL. Thrombotic risk in thalassemic patients. J Pediatr Endocrinol Metab. 1998;11:915–21.

57. Mordel N, Birkenfeld A, Goldfarb AN, Rachmilewitz EA. Successful full-term pregnancy in homozygous ß-thalassemia major: case report and review of the literature. Obstet Gynecol. 1989;73:837–40.

58. Nassar AH, Naja M, Cesaretti C, Eprassi B, Cappellini MD, Taher A. Pregnancy outcome in patients with ß-thalassemia intermedia at two tertiary care centers, in Beirut and Milan. Haematologica. 2008;93:1586–7.

59. Nassar AH, Usta IM, Taher AM. ß-thalassemia intermedia and pregnancy: should we anticoagulate? J Thromb Haemost. 2006;4:1413–4.

60. Lucas SB et al. A report of the National Confidential Enquiry into Patient Outcome and Death (NCEPOD): A Sickle Crisis? 2008. http://www.ncepod.org.uk/2008report1/Downloads/Sickle_report.pdf.

61. Ngo C, Kayem G, Habibi A, Benachi A, Goffiret F, Galacteros F, Haddad B. Pregnancy in sickle cell disease: maternal and fetal outcomes in a population receiving prophylactic partial exchange transfusions. Eur J Obstet Gynecol Repro Biol. 2010;152:138–42.

62. O'Driscoll A, Mackie IJ, Porter JB, Machin SJ. Low plasma heparin cofactor II levels in thalassaemia syndromes are corrected by chronic blood transfusion. Br J Haematol. 1995;90:65–70.

63. Origa R, Piga A, Quarta G, Forni GL, Longo F, Melpignano A, Galanello R. Pregnancy and ß-thalassemia: an Italian multicenter experience. Haematologica. 2010;95:376–81.

64. Perniola R, Magliari F, Rosatelli MC, De Marzi CA. High-risk pregnancy in ß-thalassemia major women. Report of three cases. Gynecol Obstet Invest. 2000;49:137–9.

65. Poddar D, Maude GH, Plant MJ, Scorer H, Serjeant GR. Pregnancy in Jamaican women with homozygous sickle cell disease. Fetal and maternal outcome. Br J Obstet Gynaecol. 1986;93:727–32.

66. Porter JB, Rafique R, Srichairatanakool S, Davis BA, Shah FT, Hair T, Evans P. Recent insights into interactions of deferoxamine with cellular and plasma iron pools: implications for clinical use. Ann N Y Acad Sci. 2005;1054:155–68.

67. Porter JB, Young L, Mackie IJ, Marshall L, Machin SJ. Sickle cell disorders and chronic intravascular haemolysis are associated with low plasma heparin cofactor II. Br J Haematol. 1993;83:459–65.

68. Powars DR, Sandhu M, Niland-Weiss J, Johnson C, Bruce S, Manning PR. Pregnancy in sickle cell disease. Obstet Gynecol. 1986;67:217–28.

69. Rahimy MC, Gangbo A, Adjou R, Deguenon C, Goussanou S, Alihonou E. Effect of active prenatal management on pregnancy outcome in sickle cell disease in an African setting. Blood. 2000;96:1685–9.

70. Rajab KE, Issa AA, Mohammed AM, Ajami AA. Sickle cell disease and pregnancy in Bahrain. Int J Gynaecol Obstet. 2006;93:171–5.

71. Rayburn WF, Donn SM, Wulf ME. Iron overdose during pregnancy: successful therapy with deferoxamine. Am J Obstet Gynecol. 1983;147:717–8.

72. Royal College of Obstetricians and Gynaecologists. Green-top guideline no. 37. Thrombosis and embolism during pregnancy and the puerperium, Reducing the risk. 2009.

73. Seracchioli R, Porcu E, Colombi C, Ciotti P, Fabbri R, De Sanctis V, Flamigni C. Transfusion-dependent homozygous ß-thalassaemia major: successful twin pregnancy following in-vitro fertilization and tubal embryo transfer. Hum Reprod. 1994;9:1964–5.

74. Serjeant GR, Hambleton I, Thame M. Fecundity and pregnancy outcome in a cohort with sickle cell-haemoglobin C disease followed from birth. BJOG. 2005;112:1308–14.

75. Serjeant GR, Loy LL, Crowther M, Hambleton IR, Thame M. Outcome of pregnancy in homozygous sickle cell disease. Obstet Gynecol. 2004;103:1278–85.

76. Singer ST, Vichinsky EP. Deferoxamine treatment during pregnancy: is it harmful? Am J Hematol. 1999;60:24–6.

77. Singh N, Deka D, Dadhwal V, Gupta N, Mittal S. Optimizing antenatal care and delivery in thalassemic mothers: single center experience. Arch Gynecol Obstet. 2008;278:101–2.

78. Skordis N, Petrikkos L, Toumba M, Hadjigavriel M, Sitarou M, Kolnakou A, Skordos G, Pangalou E, Christou S. Update on fertility in thalassaemia

major. Pediatr Endocrinol Rev. 2004;2 Suppl 2:296–302.

79. Smith J, Espeland M, Bellevue R, Bonds D, Brown A, Koshy M. Pregnancy in sickle cell disease: experience of the cooperative study of sickle cell disease. Obstet Gynecol. 1996;87:199–204.

80. Sohal M, Davies J, Howard J, Vogt K, McCarthy A, Layton D. Pregnancy in sickle cell disease (SCD): experience in a single tertiary centre. Br J Haematol. 2008;141:111.

81. Surbek DV, Glanzmann R, Holzgreve W. Pregnancy and homozygous ß thalassemia major. Br J Obstet Gynaecol. 1999;106:87.

82. Taher A, Isma'eel H, Mehio G, Bignamini D, Kattamis A, Rachmilewitz EA, Cappellini MD. Prevalence of thromboembolic events among 8,860 patients with thalassaemia major and intermedia in the Mediterranean area and Iran. Thromb Haemost. 2006; 96:488–91.

83. Taher AT, Otrock ZK, Uthman I, Cappellini MD. Thalassemia and hypercoagulability. Blood Rev. 2008;22:283–92.

84. Tampakoudis P, Tsatalas C, Mamopoulos M, Tantanassis T, Christakis JI, Sinakos Z, Mantalenakis S. Transfusion-dependent homozygous ß-thalassaemia major: successful pregnancy in five cases. Eur J Obstet Gynecol Reprod Biol. 1997;74:127–31.

85. Telfer P, Coen P, Chakravorty S, Wilkey O, Evans J, Newell H, Smalling B, Amos R, Stephens A, Rogers D, Kirkham F. Clinical outcomes in children with sickle cell disease living in England: a neonatal cohort in East London. Haematologica. 2007;92:905–12.

86. Thomas VJ, Rawle H, Howard J, Abedian M, Westerdale N, Oteng-Ntim E, Musumadi L. Psychological help for pregnant women with sickle cell disease. Prim Health Care. 2009;19:26–9.

87. Thomas RM, Skalicka AE. Successful pregnancy in transfusion-dependent thalassaemia. Arch Dis Child. 1980;55:572–4.

88. Traisrisilp K, Luewan S, Tongsong T. Pregnancy outcomes in women complicated by thalassemia syndrome at Maharaj Nakorn Chiang Mai Hospital. Arch Gynecol Obstet. 2009;279:685–9.

89. Tsironi M, Karagiorga M, Aessopos A. Iron overload, cardiac and other factors affecting pregnancy in thalassemia major. Hemoglobin. 2010;34:240–50.

90. Tsironi M, Ladis V, Margellis Z, Deftereos S, Kattamis C, Aessopos A. Impairment of cardiac function in a successful full-term pregnancy in a homozygous ß-thalassemia major: does chelation have a positive role? Eur J Obstet Gynecol Reprod Biol. 2005; 120:117–8.

91. Tuck SM, James CE, Brewster EM. Prophylactic blood transfusion in maternal sickle cell syndromes. Br J Obstet Gynaecol. 1987;94:121–5.

92. Tuck SM, Jensen CE, Wonke B, Yardumian A. Pregnancy management and outcomes in women with thalassaemia major. J Pediatr Endocrinol Metab. 1998;11 Suppl 3:923–8.

93. Tuck SM, Studd J. Sickle haemoglobin and pregnancy. Br Med J (Clin Res Ed). 1983;287:1143–4.

94. Tuck SM, Studd JW, White JM. Pregnancy in sickle cell disease in the UK. Br J Obstet Gynaecol. 1983; 90:112–7.

95. Turk J, Aks S, Ampuero F, Hryhorczuk DO. Successful therapy of iron intoxication in pregnancy with intravenous deferoxamine and whole bowel irrigation. Vet Hum Toxicol. 1993;35:441–4.

96. UK-Standards. Standards for the clinical care of adults with sickle cell disease in the UK. Sickle Cell Society publication. 2008. www.sicklecellsociety.

97. Vaskaridou E, Konstantopoulos K, Kyriakou D, Loukopoulos D. Deferoxamine treatment during early pregnancy: absence of teratogenicity in two cases. Haematologica. 1993;78:183–4.

98. Veille JC, Hanson R, Sivakoff M, Swain M, Henderson L. Effects of maternal ingestion of low-dose aspirin on the fetal cardiovascular system. Am J Obstet Gynecol. 1993;168:1430–7.

99. Vichinsky EP. Current issues with blood transfusions in sickle cell disease. Semin Hematol. 2001;38:14–22.

100. Villers MS, Jamison MG, De Castro LM, James AH. Morbidity associated with sickle cell disease in pregnancy. Am J Obstet Gynecol. 2008;199(125):e121–5.

101. Walter PB, Harmatz P, Vichinsky E. Iron metabolism and iron chelation in sickle cell disease. Acta Haematol. 2009;122:174–83.

102. Westerman M, Pizzey A, Hirschman J, Cerino M, Weil-Weiner Y, Ramotar P, Eze A, Lawrie A, Purdy G, Mackie I, Porter J. Microvesicles in haemoglobinopathies offer insights into mechanisms of hypercoagulability, haemolysis and the effects of therapy. Br J Haematol. 2008;142:126–35.

103. White JM, Richards R, Byrne M, Buchanan T, White YS, Jelenski G. Thalassaemia trait and pregnancy. J Clin Pathol. 1985;38:810–7.

104. Wierenga KJ, Serjeant BE, Serjeant GR. CerEßrovascular complications and parvovirus infection in homozygous sickle cell disease. J Pediatr. 2001;139:438–42.

105. Yu CK, Stasiowska E, Stephens A, Awogbade M, Davies A. Outcome of pregnancy in sickle cell disease patients attending a combined obstetric and haematology clinic. J Obstet Gynaecol. 2009;29:512–6.

The Neonate

15

Vidheya Venkatesh, Anna Curley, and Simon Stanworth

Abstract

The development of the hematologic system in the neonate is a complex interplay of genetic, prenatal, intrapartum, gestational age-related, and postnatally acquired factors. Increased survival of neonates at lower limits of gestational age coupled with the dynamic changes in neonatal hematologic physiology during the transition from fetus to neonate makes diagnosis and management of disorders of neonatal hemostasis and thrombosis challenging. Thrombocytopenia is one of the commonest neonatal hematological problems encountered, but thromboembolism and coagulation defects also contribute to neonatal morbidity and mortality. This chapter will discuss the principal thrombocytopenic, thrombotic, and hemostatic disorders presenting in a neonatal population.

15.1 Thrombocytopenia

The mean fetal platelet count at the end of the first trimester is 150×10^9/L achieving a high of 175×10^9/L at the end of the second trimester [1–3]. Overall, the prevalence of neonatal thrombocytopenia varies between 1 % and 5 % of all infants, and greater than 98 % of all term babies have a platelet count of 150×10^9/L or more [4–7]. Thrombocytopenia (platelet count less than 150×10^9/L) affects at least one quarter of all babies admitted to the neonatal unit [8], and 5–10 % of admitted neonates will have severe thrombocytopenia ($<50 \times 10^9$/L) [9]. In a cross-sectional observational prospective study, 20 % of neonatal admissions of babies <28 weeks, gestation had a platelet count $<60 \times 10^9$/L [10].

15.1.1 Causes of Thrombocytopenia

Thrombocytopenia can occur during the fetal or early or late postnatal period. Fetal thrombocytopenia can occur as a result of neonatal alloimmune and autoimmune conditions and is dealt with in Chap. 12 and 11 respectively. Early-onset thrombocytopenia is most frequently associated with chronic fetal hypoxia secondary

V. Venkatesh, MRCP (✉) • A. Curley, MD, MRCPI
Neonatal Unit, Cambridge University Hospitals NHS Trust, Hills Road, 226, Cambridge CB02QQ, UK
e-mail: vidheya.venkatesh@addenbrookes.nhs.uk; anna.curley@addenbrookes.nhs.uk

S. Stanworth, DPhil, MRCP, FRCPath
NHSBT Oxford Centre, John Radcliffe Hospital, Headington Road, Oxford OX3 9DU, UK
e-mail: simon.stanworth@nhsbt.nhs.uk

H. Cohen, P. O'Brien (eds.), *Disorders of Thrombosis and Hemostasis in Pregnancy*,
DOI 10.1007/978-1-4471-4411-3_15, © Springer-Verlag London 2012

to intrauterine growth restriction (IUGR) secondary to placental insufficiency, pre-eclampsia, or maternal diabetes [11, 12]. Typically, the thrombocytopenia is benign and resolves spontaneously within the first 10 days of life [10]. Other causes of fetal-onset/early thrombocytopenia include congenital infections, perinatal bacterial infections, aneuploidies, and perinatal asphyxia (Table 15.1). Inherited thrombocytopenia is rare. The most common causes of late-onset thrombocytopenia are sepsis and necrotizing enterocolitis (NEC) which account for over 80 % of cases [8, 13].

15.1.2 Clinical and Laboratory Features of Thrombocytopenia

15.1.2.1 Alloimmune

Neonatal alloimmune thrombocytopenia (NAIT) constitutes less than 5 % of cases of neonatal thrombocytopenia but is important to exclude due to the morbidity and mortality associated with this condition [13] and the requirement for specific platelet transfusion components matched for the alloantibodies. The diagnosis and management of this condition is dealt with in Chap. 12.

15.1.2.2 Congenital Infection

The toxoplasma, rubella, cytomegalovirus, herpes (TORCH) viral infections can cause thrombocytopenia although the exact mechanism is unclear. Parvovirus can also cause thrombocytopenia through suppression of bone marrow and megakaryocyte colony formation [14]. Other viruses known to cause thrombocytopenia include enterovirus, Coxsackie virus, adenovirus, Epstein-Barr virus, and dengue virus. HIV is known to infect megakaryocytes and suppress colony growth [15] and is so frequently associated with neonatal thrombocytopenia that it has been suggested as a screening tool [16].

15.1.2.3 Aneuploidies

Thrombocytopenia is common although rarely severe in the trisomies 18 (86 %), 13 (31 %), and 21 (6 %), as well as in Turner syndrome

Table 15.1 Classification of fetal and neonatal thrombocytopenias

	Condition
Fetal	Alloimmune
	Congenital infection (e.g. CMV, toxoplasma, rubella, HIV)
	Aneuploidy (e.g. trisomies 18, 13, 21)
	Autoimmune (e.g. ITP, SLE)
	Severe rhesus hemolytic disease
	Inherited (e.g. Wiskott-Aldrich syndrome)
Early-onset neonatal (<72 h)	Chronic fetal hypoxia (e.g. pre-eclampsia IUGR, diabetes)
	Perinatal asphyxia
	Perinatal infection (e.g. E. coli, GBS, Haemophilus influenzae)
	DIC
	Alloimmune
	Autoimmune (e.g. ITP, SLE)
	Congenital infection (e.g. CMV, toxoplasma, rubella, HIV)
	Thrombosis (e.g. aortic, renal vein)
	Bone marrow replacement (e.g. congenital leukemia)
	Kasabach-Merritt syndrome
	Metabolic disease (e.g. propionic and methylmalonic acidemia)
	Inherited (e.g. TAR, CAMT)
Late-onset neonatal (>72 h)	Late-onset sepsis
	NEC
	Congenital infection (e.g. CMV, toxoplasma, rubella, HIV)
	Autoimmune
	Kasabach-Merritt syndrome
	Metabolic disease (e.g. propionic and methylmalonic acidemia)
	Inherited (e.g. TAR, CAMT)

Table reproduced from Roberts et al. [9]
CMV cytomegalovirus, *HIV* human immunodeficiency virus, *ITP* idiopathic thrombocytopenic purpura, *SLE* systemic lupus erythematosus, *IUGR* intrauterine growth restriction, *E. coli* Escherichia coli, *GBS* group B Streptococcus, *TAR* thrombocytopenia with absent radius syndrome, *CAMT* congenital amegakaryocytic thrombocytopenia, *NEC* necrotizing enterocolitis

(31 %) [17]. The mechanism of thrombocytopenia in trisomies 13 and 18 is unknown although it may have its etiology in chronic fetal hypoxia.

Thrombocytopenia in trisomy 21 is similar to that seen in growth-restricted infants: neutropenia, polycythemia, and increased circulating normoblasts. Ten percent of infants with Down syndrome, however, develop a clonal preleukemic disorder showing increased myeloblasts and variable levels of thrombocytopenia, and 20–30 % of these babies will develop acute megakaryoblastic leukemia within the first 5 years of life [18]. It is thought that trisomy of chromosome 21 disturbs fetal hemopoiesis and predisposes to mutations in the GATA1 gene, a key megakaryocyte/erythroid transcription factor [19].

15.1.2.4 Autoimmune

Autoimmune conditions such as maternal idiopathic thrombocytopenic purpura, which may occur in association with systemic lupus erythematosus, can also cause thrombocytopenia in the fetus and neonate. This is dealt with in Chap. 11.

In addition to anemia, neutropenia, and reticulocytosis, thrombocytopenia is common in severe rhesus hemolytic disease especially after intrauterine or exchange transfusions; this is due to platelet-poor blood product and suppression of platelet production in favor of erythropoiesis.

15.1.2.5 Inherited Thrombocytopenias

These are due to reduced platelet production due to abnormal hemopoietic stem or progenitor cell development. Many of these disorders will be diagnosed by their associated congenital anomalies.

Bernard-Soulier Syndrome. This syndrome can lead to fetal or early thrombocytopenia although severe bleeding is not often seen in neonates. It is characterized by mild thrombocytopenia with giant megakaryocytes. It has an autosomal recessive pattern of inheritance and leads to defects in the glycoprotein 1b-IX-V complex [20, 21]. Neonates can develop alloantibodies following platelet transfusions, so transfusions should be restricted to cases of severe hemorrhage.

Wiskott-Aldrich Syndrome and X-Linked Thrombocytopenia. These syndromes form part of a spectrum of disorders caused by a mutation in the WAS protein of the X chromosome [22] which leads to disorders of platelet function and survival. X-linked thrombocytopenia can present in the neonatal period with a mild thrombocytopenia. These conditions are characterized by microthrombocytopenia, eczema, immunodeficiency, and recurrent bacterial and viral infections [23].

15.1.3 Timing of Onset of Thrombocytopenia

15.1.3.1 Early-Onset Thrombocytopenia

Chronic Fetal Hypoxia. Placental insufficiency is associated with early-onset thrombocytopenia in preterm neonates. Impaired delivery of oxygen and essential nutrients is implicated in its development. Platelets are initially produced in the fetal liver with production transferred to the bone marrow in the third trimester [11]. In hypoxia, blood flow to the liver falls. Previous studies have also demonstrated a reduction in circulating megakaryocyte progenitors, suggesting decreased platelet production as a cause [11, 12, 14]. Typically, thrombocytopenia is mild to moderate and self-limiting, resolving in the majority of cases before 10 days of age [12]. Additional hematologic abnormalities which can help confirm growth restriction and hypoxia as causative factors include transient neutropenia, increased circulating nucleated red cells, and evidence of hyposplenism (spherocytes, target cells, and Howell-Jolly bodies) [12, 24].

Perinatal Asphyxia. Thrombocytopenia can occur after perinatal asphyxia as a result of bone marrow suppression and reduced platelet production. Asphyxia-related liver dysfunction also causes decreased production of clotting factors. Increased consumption of platelets often follows severe acidosis, hypoxia, and endothelial damage and disseminated intravascular coagulation (DIC).

Perinatal Infection: Group B streptococcus (GBS) and gram-negative enteric organisms (predominantly *Escherichia coli*) account for 70 % of early-onset sepsis. Non-typeable Haemophilus influenzae sepsis has been increasingly identified in neonates, particularly those that are premature. Other gram-negative enteric bacilli such as

Klebsiella sp. and gram-positive organisms such as Listeria monocytogenes, enterococci, group D streptococci, α-hemolytic streptococci, and staphylococci have also been implicated. The thrombocytopenia in sepsis is most likely due to increased platelet destruction. Platelet levels drop quickly after onset of symptoms of infection [25, 26]. The mean duration of thrombocytopenia is 5–6 days [25, 26]. Platelet transfusions given to septic infants have a shortened life span [26].

Thrombotic Disorders. Thrombotic thrombocytopenic purpura, hemolytic-uremic syndrome, and heparin-induced thrombocytopenia have all been reported in neonates [27–29]. Thrombocytopenia may also occur secondary to thrombosis of a major vessel.

Bone Marrow Infiltration. Congenital leukemia, osteopetrosis, and histiocytoses can also cause thrombocytopenia secondary to bone marrow infiltration.

Kasabach-Merritt Syndrome. Thrombocytopenia in this condition is associated with sequestration of platelets on the endothelium of hemangiomas, either cutaneous (80 %) or visceral [30]. Thrombocytopenia may be associated with DIC and microangiopathic anemia. Treatment options include corticosteroids, antifibrinolytic agents (e-aminocaproic acid and tranexamic acid), interferon alpha-2a, cytotoxic chemotherapy, intralesional steroids, embolization, and laser therapy.

Metabolic Disease. The organic acidemias, propionic, methylmalonic, and isovaleryl academia, can also present with neonatal thrombocytopenia and neutropenia, mimicking neonatal sepsis [31]. The clinical finding is of a healthy newborn at birth who becomes rapidly ill after the first day of life. Urine organic acid analysis is diagnostic.

Lysosomal storage diseases such as Gaucher's disease can also present with thrombocytopenia [32]. These disorders are characterized by mutations in one of a series of enzymes involved in the degradation of glycosphingolipids. Patients can present with hepatosplenomegaly, cardiomyopathy, renal dysfunction, anemia, thrombocytopenia, and neurologic degeneration. Thrombocytopenia associated with splenomegaly may also be secondary to infiltrative metabolic disorders such as the mucolipidoses and mucopolysaccharidoses.

Inherited Disorders. Inherited disorders typically presenting in the early to late neonatal period with variable severity of onset include Bernard-Soulier syndrome, X-linked thrombocytopenia, thrombocytopenia-absent radius syndrome, amegakaryocytic thrombocytopenia with radioulnar synostosis, and congenital amegakaryocytic thrombocytopenia.

Fanconi anemia is characterized by short stature, skeletal anomalies, increased incidence of solid tumors and leukemias, and aplastic anemia. It is rare to present with thrombocytopenia in the neonatal period although it should be considered in the presence of dysmorphic features and unexplained thrombocytopenia. The diepoxybutane test is almost always diagnostic of this disorder [33].

Thrombocytopenia-Absent Radius (TAR) Syndrome. Thrombocytopenia-absent radius (TAR) syndrome is a rare autosomal recessive condition in which thrombocytopenia is associated with bilateral radial aplasia, although thumbs may be present and normal. It can also be associated with lower limb abnormalities (47 %), renal anomalies (27 %), and cardiac defects (15 %) [34]. Episodes of thrombocytopenia begin in the neonatal period, and around 50 % of affected infants are symptomatic (showing evidence of bleeding) in the first week of life, with a further 40 % becoming symptomatic by the age of 4 months [35]. The platelet count spontaneously improves after the first year of life. The therapy of TAR syndrome is supportive with platelet transfusions for hemorrhage, red cell transfusions for anemia, and avoidance of stressors, such as cow's milk, known to aggravate platelet levels.

Amegakaryocytic thrombocytopenia with radioulnar synostosis (ATRUS) is caused by mutations in the HOXA11 gene and characterized by severe thrombocytopenia from birth, radioulnar synostosis, clinodactyly, and shallow acetabula [36].

Congenital amegakaryocytic thrombocytopenia (CAMT) is an autosomal recessive condition which almost always presents early in the neonatal period with severe thrombocytopenia, and 50 % of affected infants will have evidence of bleeding [37]. Although there is isolated thrombocytopenia in the newborn period, 50 % will go on to develop aplastic anemia in childhood. Stem cell transplantation is curative in cases of severe disease [38].

15.1.3.2 Late-Onset Thrombocytopenia

Thrombocytopenia occurring after 72 h of age is due to sepsis or necrotizing enterocolitis (NEC) in more than 80 % of cases [14].

Late-Onset Sepsis: The vast majority of late-onset infections are caused by gram-positive organisms, with coagulase-negative staphylococci accounting for almost half of infections [39]. The rate of infection is inversely related to birth weight and gestational age. Candida species are increasingly important causes of late-onset sepsis, occurring in 12 % of very low birth weight infants [40]. Thrombocytopenia occurs in 79–100 % of these infants [41, 42]. In late-onset sepsis, thrombocytopenia is often more severe ($<30 \times 10^9$/L) and of rapid onset, and can take several weeks to resolve [8].

Necrotizing Enterocolitis: This is the most common neonatal gastrointestinal illness affecting predominantly preterm infants (90 % of cases occurring in premature infants). Surgery is required in 20–60 %, and there is a mortality rate of 20–28 % [42]. In one study, 90 % of infants with NEC had thrombocytopenia ($<150 \times 10^9$/L) with 55 % of these infants having platelet counts below 50×10^9/L [43]. Within the group with severe thrombocytopenia, 55 % had severe bleeding complications. Severe thrombocytopenia had an 89 % positive predictive value for intestinal gangrene in one study [44]. The most likely reason for low platelets is increased platelet destruction although there may be suppression of platelet production by proinflammatory cytokines.

15.1.4 Treatment of Neonatal Thrombocytopenia

Neonatal thrombocytopenia and bleeding are common and important clinical problems for preterm neonates. The main specific treatment for thrombocytopenia in the neonate is platelet transfusion, but intravenous immunoglobulin (IVIg) may be used for maternal ITP associated thrombocytopenia. Current national guidance recommends platelet transfusion thresholds of 20–30×10^9/L and 50×10^9/L for neonates depending on the clinical situation [45], but policies and protocols for neonatal platelet transfusion therapy vary widely between clinicians and institutions [46, 47], reflecting the generally broad nature of recommendations in national guidelines, which themselves are based largely on consensus rather than evidence, and often extrapolated from adult data [48, 49].

Platelet transfusions are frequently used in modern neonatal clinical practice as prophylaxis in thrombocytopenic neonates [49]. Previous studies estimate that 25 % of neonates and 50 % of extremely low birth weight neonates whose platelet counts fall below 150×10^9/L receive one or more transfusions [50, 51]. In the only randomized controlled trial to assess a threshold level for the effectiveness of neonatal prophylactic platelet transfusions, moderate thrombocytopenia (50–150×10^9/L) was not detrimental to short-term neonatal outcome. However, neonates with severe thrombocytopenia (platelet count less than 50×10^9/L) were excluded from the study because of their perceived high risk of hemorrhage [52]. Benefits of transfusion need to be weighed up against possible risks.

Conclusions

The most common cause of early thrombocytopenia in neonates is chronic hypoxia. NAIT accounts for less than 5 % of all cases of neonatal thrombocytopenias. Sepsis and NEC account for more than 80 % of the late-onset thrombocytopenias. Inherited causes of thrombocytopenia are rare. Infants with severe thrombocytopenia and evidence of bleeding should receive platelets, but the role of prophylactic platelets in the neonate with asymptomatic thrombocytopenia is unclear.

Learning Points
- The underlying cause of thrombocytopenia is predicted by the timing of onset.
- Chronic fetal hypoxia is the most common cause of early-onset thrombocytopenia and is mild and self-limiting.
- Sepsis and/or necrotizing enterocolitis is the most common cause of late-onset thrombocytopenia.

- Bleeding risk is greater in NAIT than in sepsis/NEC and greater in sepsis/NEC than in chronic fetal hypoxia.
- The role of prophylactic platelet transfusions and the optimal platelet count thresholds are not known.

Case Study

A 570-g infant was born at 26 weeks' gestation by Caesarean section. Growth restriction was noted antenatally from his 20-week ultrasound scan. By 26 weeks' gestation, fetal growth was below the fifth centile, and Doppler studies showed reversed end-diastolic flow in the umbilical artery, with maximal cerebral redistribution, prompting delivery due to the risk of intrauterine demise.

The infant developed respiratory distress syndrome and was ventilated for 5 days. He had polycythemia on full blood count, normal white cell count and platelets of 90×10^9/L. C-reactive protein was normal, and initial blood and cerebrospinal fluid cultures were negative for infection. He had no evidence of hemorrhage.

The infant was extubated on day 6 and remained stable until day 19. Feeding was commenced slowly on day 2, and he reached full feeds by day 14. On day 19, he had apneic episodes requiring re-ventilation. Associated signs were abdominal distension, bilious aspirates, and hypotension requiring dopamine. Abdominal X-ray showed dilated bowel loops but no pneumatosis intestinalis or evidence of bowel perforation. A blood profile showed a low white cell count, thrombocytopenia (platelet count 40×10^9/L), and a C-reactive protein of 70.

What is the most likely cause and duration of this infant's first and second episodes of thrombocytopenia?

Would you perform any additional investigations?

Would you transfuse this infant?

15.2 Neonatal Thromboembolism

15.2.1 Introduction

Neonatal thromboembolism is a rare but increasingly reported condition in the neonatal unit that can cause significant neonatal mortality and morbidity. Ninety percent of thromboembolism is associated with thrombosis of arterial or venous catheters and central venous lines, but stroke is also prevalent, and the incidence of perinatal stroke ranks second only to the strokes of the elderly population (1 in 2,300 to 1 in 5,000 births) [53].

15.2.2 Etiology of Neonatal Thromboembolism

Idiopathic thromboembolism occurs in less than 1 % of cases of newborn thromboembolism as compared to 40 % in the adult population [54]. Usually at least one risk factor can be identified, either maternal or fetal, including maternal diabetes or SLE with antiphospholipid syndrome, pre-eclampsia, IUGR, maternal autoimmune conditions, maternal thrombophilia, placental vasculopathy, infection, hypovolemia, dehydration, hypoxia, acidosis, and neonatal prothrombotic disorders [55–62].

The prothrombotic disorders that have been linked with neonatal thromboembolism include deficiencies in protein C, protein S, antithrombin, and plasminogen [63–66]. Homozygous disorders usually present with severe clinical symptoms and require urgent management. However, diagnosing heterozygous prothrombotic disorders can be difficult in the neonate because physiologic values are lower than in older children and adults [67]. Diagnosis can also be complicated by the coexistence of acquired disorders present in over 80 % of newborns with systemic thromboembolism [68].

The clinical presentation of homozygous protein C deficiency in the neonatal period is purpura fulminans, cerebral stroke, and/or large-vessel thrombosis. The diagnosis is confirmed in the presence of these clinical features with an undetectable protein C level and the parents testing as heterozygotes for protein C deficiency.

Heterozygous protein C deficiency does not normally present with thrombosis in early infancy [69], but cohort studies have indicated an increased prevalence of protein C heterozygosity in neonates with thromboembolism and additional risk factors [70]. Babies with homozygous protein S deficiency also present with purpura fulminans, but like protein C deficiency, the heterozygous state is uncommonly associated with thromboembolic phenomena in infancy or childhood [71]. Homozygous antithrombin (AT) deficiency is rare but can cause severe thromboembolic events, venous or arterial, and is associated with plasma concentrations of AT that are less than 10 % of normal levels [72]. Heterozygous antithrombin deficiency is associated with diverse but less severe clinical manifestations.

Factor V Leiden and the presence of the prothrombin G20210A mutation have also been linked to neonatal thromboembolism [61, 62, 73, 74]. Approximately 5 % of Caucasians are heterozygous for the factor V Leiden mutation which decreases the rate of activation of activated factor V, and 2 % for the prothrombin G20210A mutation. A homozygous polymorphism in the C677T methylene tetrahydrofolate reductase (MTHFR) gene has been linked to an increased thrombotic risk in infants with perinatal arterial stroke [75]. An elevated homocysteine level has also been associated with an increased thrombotic risk [76], but the contribution of these risk factors to neonatal thrombosis is unclear.

15.2.3 Clinical Presentation

15.2.3.1 Thrombosis Following Umbilical Catheterization

Studies have identified central venous lines as an important risk factor for neonatal thrombosis [77]. Clinical studies have shown an incidence of 13 % [78] and autopsy studies a 20–65 % incidence of venous thromboembolism in infants with an umbilical venous catheter (UVC) *in situ* [79, 80]. UVCs have been associated particularly with portal venous thrombosis. Major venous thrombosis due to umbilical artery catheters occurs in 1–3 % of all infants [81]. High position of the UAC (UAC

tip between T6–T10) may be associated with fewer complications compared to low position (UAC tip L3–L5) [82].

Many factors contribute to catheter-related thrombosis including vessel caliber, blood flow, and catheter type. Use of a heparin infusion [83] or heparin-bonded lines [84] prolongs the duration of catheter patency but has not been shown to alter the rate of catheter-related thrombi. Catheter use should be limited to that which is necessary to reduce the incidence of catheter-related thrombosis.

The majority of babies with UAC-related thromboses remain asymptomatic, but some babies can show evidence of loss of patency of the catheter, limb ischemia, necrotizing enterocolitis secondary to mesenteric artery occlusion, or hypertension secondary to renal artery occlusion. Contrast angiography is the gold standard diagnostic method but rarely available in neonates. Ultrasound may not pick up all cases of arterial obstruction [85]. Long-term morbidity can include hypertension, impaired renal function, and paraplegia.

Clinical features of venous catheter-related thromboembolism include loss of central venous line patency, venous congestion, and/or discoloration of the limbs. Superior vena caval obstruction leads to facial and venous congestion of the upper chest. Pulmonary thromboembolism presents with respiratory compromise. Long-term complications of thromboembolism include prominent collateral circulation, catheter-related sepsis, chylothorax, portal hypertension, and post-thrombotic syndrome.

15.2.3.2 Renal Vein Thrombosis

Renal vein thrombosis is the most common non-catheter-related thromboembolism in neonates and is responsible for around 10 % of all thromboembolism. It is commonest in the first week of life, and almost 80 % of all renal vein thromboses occur in the first month of life [86–88]. Reduced renal blood flow, increased blood viscosity, hyperosmolarity, hypercoagulability due to perinatal asphyxia, polycythemia, dehydration, septicemia, and maternal diabetes have been suggested as possible pathophysiological mechanisms. Newborns usually present with hematuria, proteinuria, and a flank mass. Bilateral renal vein thrombosis is present in 24 % of newborns [88]. Ultrasound is the diagnostic method of choice. There are no recent studies on long-term morbidity of this condition.

15.2.3.3 Perinatal Stroke

Perinatal ischemic stroke is defined as "a group of heterogeneous conditions in which there is a focal disruption of cerebral blood flow secondary to arterial or venous embolisation between 20 weeks of fetal life and the 28th day of postnatal life, confirmed by neuroimaging or neuropathologic studies" [89]. The incidence of ischemic perinatal stroke is 0.25–1 infants per 1,000 live births and accounts for 30 % of all children with hemiplegic cerebral palsy born at term or late preterm [53, 55, 90].

Early neonatal stroke typically presents in the first 3 days and can occur as a result of placental embolism, infection, birth trauma, or hypoxic ischemic encephalopathy. Late neonatal stroke occurs between 4 and 28 days of age and can be secondary to infection, cardiac disease, or venous thrombosis with paradoxical embolism. Neonates with stroke may present with focal or generalized neonatal seizures or with nonspecific features such as apnea, poor feeding, irritability, abnormalities in tone, or cyanosis. The differential diagnosis includes kernicterus, bacterial and viral encephalitis, mitochondrial disorders, tumors, or hypoglycemia.

Several classifications of neonatal stroke have been suggested based either on distribution of these events [91] or the proposed underlying etiological mechanism [92]. In the neonatal period, two common subtypes of stroke are arterial ischemic stroke (AIS) and cerebral sinovenous thrombosis (SVT). In AIS it is thought that emboli originating in the placenta pass through the foramen ovale and occlude the intracerebral vessel. Neonatal AIS is characterized by documented complete or incomplete occlusion of an intracerebral vessel causing a focal lesion in the brain, or a documented lesion which can only be explained by occlusion of a particular vessel [93]. Studies have shown that middle cerebral artery infarction accounted for anywhere between 50 % and 83 % of focal events [91].

Sinovenous thrombosis in neonates accounted for 45 % of all neonatal stroke cases registered in the Canadian registry, with an incidence of 41 per 100,000 births per year [53]. Risk factors such as maternal diabetes, hypertension, infection, asphyxia, complicated delivery, and congenital cardiac disorders have been commonly identified [94].

Additional forms of vaso-occlusive ischemic events unique to the perinatal period are periventricular venous infarction and presumed fetal stroke detected in later infancy. Less common types of neonatal stroke are multifocal infarctions, subcortical infarctions, and infarctions caused by meningitis, thrombophilia, and arteriopathy. Maternal cocaine abuse has also been associated with cortical infarction in up to 17 % of infants [95].

Neuroimaging remains the mainstay in the diagnosis of stroke. Cranial ultrasound may miss the cerebral ischemic lesions, especially more anterior or posterior lesions [96, 97]. Appropriately timed conventional T2-weighted magnetic resonance imaging (MRI), diffusion-weighted imaging, and magnetic resonance angiography remain the principal methods of diagnosing neonatal stroke [98, 99]. Infants presenting with stroke should be investigated for thrombophilia.

Outcome data vary but, overall, neurologic deficits or epilepsy occurs in two thirds of survivors of acute ischemic stroke, with sensorimotor deficit being the most common. Lesions involving the motor cortex, basal ganglia, and internal capsule together are more likely to be associated with motor disability than lesions limited to the cortex or basal ganglia alone [100]. Seizure disorders have been shown to occur in 15 % of long-term survivors of AIS [78]. However, fewer than 5 % of neonates with AIS have recurrent systemic or cerebral thrombosis [53]. In contrast to AIS, a follow-up study of survivors of cerebral sinovenous thrombosis showed that 77 % of survivors had no neurological sequelae [101].

15.2.4 Treatment of Neonatal Thrombosis

Treatment options for neonatal thrombosis include supportive care, anticoagulation, and thrombolysis.

In the past, clinicians have been reluctant to use anticoagulant therapy in neonates due to the possible risks of bleeding. The German registry of neonatal thrombosis has reported rates of major hemorrhage of 2 % for heparin anticoagulation and 15 % for thrombolysis [86].

Possible anticoagulants for use in neonates include unfractionated heparin (UFH), low molecular weight heparin (LMWH), and tissue plasminogen activator (t-PA). However, target therapeutic ranges are based on adult rather than neonatal ranges. Neonates often require high doses of UFH to maintain the target therapeutic range due to physiologically decreased levels of antithrombin, increased volume of distribution, rapid heparin clearance, and non-specific protein binding in plasma [102, 103]. Anti-Xa activity levels effectively monitor LMWH therapy in neonates. Neonates with acute thrombosis that is life-threatening or that could potentially lead to loss of a limb should be considered for thrombolysis. Thrombolysis should be considered for aortic, atrial, and peripheral arterial thromboses. A starting dose of 0.06 mg/kg/h of t-PA is currently recommended for local and systemic thrombolysis in neonates [104–106] The therapeutic action of t-PA requires plasminogen and therefore its effect may be improved by the administration of fresh frozen plasma. Fibrinogen, platelet count, coagulation status and D-dimers should be monitored during therapy. In addition, cranial ultrasound imaging is recommended prior to initiation of therapy and daily thereafter [106].

Supportive care is usually provided to infants with renal vein thrombosis, and anticoagulant and thrombolytic therapy are controversial in the treatment of this condition. Unilateral renal vein thrombosis with thrombus extending into the inferior vena cava may warrant treatment with LMWH. In bilateral renal vein thrombosis, thrombolysis should be considered [107].

There are no trials supporting the efficacy or safety of anticoagulant therapy for treatment of stroke in the neonate, and currently there are no recommendations for anticoagulation or aspirin for neonatal stroke. However, the American College of Chest Physicians recommends 3 months of LMWH therapy following proven cardioembolic stroke [108].

Further studies are required to define optimal antithrombotic therapy, neonatal therapeutic ranges for antithrombotic therapy, and long-term clinical outcome in infants with evidence of thrombosis.

Learning Points
- Thromboembolic events are relatively common in the perinatal period compared to later childhood.
- There is little information on the most appropriate diagnostic methods, treatment, and outcome in this age group.
- Anticoagulation should be considered in bilateral renal vein thrombosis, cardioembolic stroke, and arterial occlusive events threatening life or limb.

15.3 Disorders of Hemostasis

This section deals with the etiology, clinical presentation, diagnosis, management, and prognosis of these disorders. The majority of these are secondary to acquired conditions, but inherited coagulation disorders can present in the perinatal period.

15.3.1 Introduction

Hemostasis describes the process by which coagulation factors, platelets, naturally occurring anticoagulants, and the fibrinolytic system combine to prevent excessive bleeding or thrombosis. Coagulation factors in the fetus begin to appear at 10 weeks' gestational age. At birth, concentrations of the vitamin K-dependent factors (FII, FVII, FIX, FX) and contact factors (FXI, FXII), antithrombin, protein C, protein S, and plasminogen, are reduced and further reduced in preterm infants [109–111]. Concentrations of FV and FXIII are similar to adult values at birth, whereas in contrast levels of FVIII and von Willebrand factor (VWF) are increased at birth [109–111]. Reference ranges for a coagulation profile must therefore take into account both gestational and postnatal age. The most frequently quoted reference range data is based on work by Maureen Andrews and colleagues who used a standardized protocol, taking venous blood samples from healthy term and preterm neonates above 30 weeks' gestational age who had received vitamin K [110, 111].

Commonly used tests of coagulation status, the prothrombin time (PT) and activated partial thromboplastin time (APTT), can be prolonged in the newborn compared to the adult as they depend on the amount of coagulation factor present. As these are less than 50 % of the adult mean and have a wide range, a longer PT and APTT is a normal finding in the term and particularly the preterm neonate [112]. Although absolute values of fibrinogen in the neonate are similar to those in the adult, the fibrinogen is present in a fetal form that differs from adult fibrinogen, so the thrombin clotting time can again be prolonged in neonates, although the exact physiological significance of the fetal type of fibrinogen is not known. The anticoagulant proteins antithrombin, protein C, protein S, and plasminogen are also reduced in the neonate [112].

15.3.2 Inherited Coagulation Disorders

15.3.2.1 Hemophilia

The most common inherited coagulation disorders in the neonatal period are hemophilia A and B resulting from deficiencies of FVIII and FIX, respectively. Hemophilia occurs in 1 in 5,000 male births and the clinical presentation and severity of bleeding are variable. Eighty to eighty-five percent of cases are hemophilia A and 15–20 % hemophilia B [112]. Two thirds of cases have a positive family history. Forty to sixty percent of infants with severe hemophilia A (FVIII levels <1 %) will be clinically symptomatic as newborns; a further 40 % present by 1 year of age; and 50 % have had a major bleed by 18 months of age [112–114]. Common clinical presentations of FVIII deficiency include hematoma formation following venepuncture, intracranial hemorrhage (41 % of cases reported in the first month of life), cephalhematoma, and

bleeding from the umbilicus or post-circumcision [115–117]. Intracranial hemorrhage is usually related to trauma at delivery and is associated with a poor outcome [115]. Although rare, severe hemophilia A may occur in females and present at birth [112]. Bleeding due to severe FIX deficiency (<1 % FIX levels) presents in a similar way to FVIII deficiency in the newborn.

Isolated prolongation of the APTT in an otherwise healthy neonate is highly suggestive of hemophilia A or B. The diagnosis is confirmed by measuring levels of FVIII and FIX concentrations, respectively. The diagnosis of mild hemophilia B may be difficult due to physiologically low levels of FIX in the newborn, and there can be a delay of 3–6 months after birth before the diagnosis can be confirmed.

If available, recombinant factor VIII or FIX concentrates are the treatment of choice for hemophilia A and B, respectively. Highly purified derived factor concentrates are the next best alternative. DiMichele et al. have provided guidelines for FVIII and FIX replacement for specific acute hemorrhages [118]. There are no data to support the use of prophylactic doses of FVIII, either intrauterine or immediately after birth, to reduce bleeding complications.

15.3.2.2 von Willebrand Disease

von Willebrand disease (VWD) is a relatively common inherited bleeding disorder which results from either quantitative or qualitative abnormalities in the VWF protein. The VWF glycoprotein mediates the adhesion of platelets to the injured vascular wall and also acts as a plasma carrier and stabilizing protein for FVIII. Bleeding due to VWF deficiency is rare in the newborn period as plasma concentrations of VWF are increased at birth with an increased proportion of high molecular weight multimers.

VWF deficiency is divided into three broad subtypes: partial or complete deficiency of VWF (type I and III) and qualitative defects in VWF (type II). Type 1 VMD is the commonest and occurs as a mild clinical phenotype. Type II VMD can be associated with neonatal thrombocytopenia and may present with bleeding. Type III VMD is a rare autosomal recessive condition characterized by markedly reduced or absent VWF levels, resulting in a severe bleeding tendency especially from the mucous membranes.

Diagnosis

Type I VWF deficiency is not usually diagnosed in the neonatal period due to higher levels of VWF present at birth. Subtypes of type II may present in association with thrombocytopenia which is apparent in the neonatal period. Type III VMD usually results in an isolated prolongation of the APTT, and the diagnosis is confirmed by measuring FVIII and VWF antigen and activity levels, and VWF multimer analysis.

Treatment

Management of bleeding in type III VMD is usually with factor replacement using an intermediate purity FVIII concentrate containing the high molecular weight multimers of VWF.

15.3.3 Rare Coagulation Disorders

This group of autosomal recessive deficiencies in the homozygous or compound heterozygous state can give rise to major clinical bleeding which may manifest in the first few days of life. Severe deficiencies of fibrinogen, FVII, FX, and FXIII are the most likely conditions to present neonatally.

Afibrinogenemia/Hypofibrinogenemia: Fibrinogen deficiency is rare but may present with bleeding in the newborn period, usually in the form of bleeding from the umbilicus or soft tissue hemorrhage. Fresh frozen plasma can be used as initial treatment, but cryoprecipitate (both methylene blue-treated in the UK) or fibrinogen concentrates are preferable.

Factor VII Deficiency: This coagulation factor is a component of the extrinsic pathway of blood coagulation. Activated factor VII activates further FVIII, FIX, and FX. Severe deficiency presents similarly to severe hemophilia. The most common presentation of FVII deficiency is

intracranial hemorrhage [119]. Deficiencies in factor VII result in an abnormal baseline coagulation screen. Specific factor assays are then required to confirm the diagnosis.

Factor X Deficiency: Activated factor X converts prothrombin to thrombin in the presence of activated factor V, phospholipids, and calcium. The most common clinical presentation of FX deficiency in the neonate is intracranial hemorrhage, but bleeding from the umbilicus, heel-prick sites, and the gastrointestinal tract, and spontaneous bruising have been reported [120]. Deficiencies in factor X result in an abnormal coagulation screen, but specific factor assays are then required to confirm the diagnosis.

Management of bleeding episodes in FVII and FX deficiency should be with a specific factor concentrate where this is available. Because of the high risk of intracranial hemorrhage, regular prophylaxis should be considered for both severe FVII and FX deficiency.

Factor XIII Deficiency: Factor FXIII deficiency leads to reduced cross-linking of clot fibrin polymer and weak clot formation. FXIII deficiency is extremely rare (<1 in one million) and associated in 80 % of homozygous cases with umbilical bleeding after the umbilical cord separates [121]. It may also be associated with intracranial hemorrhage or bleeding post-circumcision. Heterozygous neonates are not clinically affected. The time taken to clot is normal, so PT and APTT will be normal in this condition. It can be diagnosed using the clot solubility test. The FXIII screening test is only sensitive to the most severe forms of the deficiency, however, and there is currently debate about optimal testing strategies (see Chap. 9). Treatment of FXIII deficiency is with plasma-derived FXIII concentrate where available, cryoprecipitate, or fresh frozen plasma.

15.3.4 Acquired Coagulation Disorders

15.3.4.1 Vitamin K-Deficiency Bleeding

Vitamin K deficiency bleeding (VKDB), previously known as hemorrhagic disease of the newborn, is now rare due to routine administration of vitamin K to neonates. Vitamin K-dependent factors (FII, FVII, FIX, and FX) are functionally inactive and reduced in the newborn period in VKDB. The classification of VKDB as early, classical and late, depending on the timing of the presentation reflects the differing risk factors associated with this condition. Early VKDB (<24 h) is rare and typically associated with antenatal ingestion of drugs which cross the placenta and interfere with vitamin K metabolism (carbamazepine, phenytoin, barbiturates, cephalosporins, rifampicin, isoniazid) and vitamin K antagonists (warfarin). Vitamin K administration in the delivery unit has not been universally protective against this condition [122]. Classical (2–7 days) and late (week 1–week 12) forms are associated with breast-feeding and malabsorption. Presentation is often with melaena, but neonates can also present with intracranial hemorrhage or internal hemorrhage.

Diagnosis

Isolated prolongation of the prothrombin time, followed by prolongation of the APTT, in association with a normal fibrinogen concentration and a normal platelet count, suggests the diagnosis of VKDB. This is confirmed by the measurement of the specific vitamin K-dependent factors (II, VII, IX, X) deficiency of which is corrected by the administration of vitamin K.

Prophylaxis and Treatment

Intramuscular (IM) administration of 1mg of vitamin K at birth provides complete protection against VKDB. Oral administration of a single dose of 1mg of vitamin K at birth protects against early and classical VKDB but may not be effective against late-onset bleeding [123, 124]. Repeated doses of oral vitamin K have been shown to be as effective as IM vitamin K but may not protect infants with cholestatic disease against late-onset VKDB [123, 125]. For treatment of established or suspected VKDB, vitamin K (1 mg IM) should be administered to correct the existing deficiency. In the presence of major bleeding, factor replacement therapy may also be required with fresh frozen plasma, prothrombin complex concentrate

(factor II, FIX, and FX ± factor VII), preferably a four-factor prothrombin complex concentrate containing all the vitamin K-dependent factors.

15.3.4.2 Disseminated Intravascular Coagulation

In the sick neonate, disseminated intravascular coagulation (DIC) is a relatively common problem. It can occur secondary to birth asphyxia, acidosis, meconium aspiration, amniotic fluid aspiration syndromes, hypothermia, respiratory distress syndrome, viral or bacterial sepsis, and necrotizing enterocolitis [126]. Once established, DIC is often associated with increased mortality.

Clinical Presentation

Clinically, both bleeding and thrombotic problems may occur, and microvascular thrombosis in particular contributes to multiorgan damage. Failure to regulate the coagulation process results in massive uncontrolled thrombin generation, with widespread fibrin deposition and consumption of coagulation proteins and platelets.

Diagnosis

Early DIC can be difficult to diagnose. The laboratory diagnosis of DIC in the neonate is often but not invariably characterized by a prolonged prothrombin time and APTT, low fibrinogen, low platelet count, and increased D-dimers (or other markers of fibrin or fibrinogen degradation) [127]. There may be difficulty distinguishing what represents an abnormal result, particularly in preterm infants due to, for example, the frequent presence of thrombocytopenia in infants without DIC, the lack of reliable normal ranges for D-dimers, and increased baseline D-dimer concentrations in the neonatal period [128]. Fibrinogen concentrations are also increased in the first few days of life and may initially be preserved.

Treatment

The management of DIC is prompt and effective treatment of sepsis, hypoxia, and acidosis, and support of oxygenation and perfusion. Treatment continues to center around the use of supportive treatment with fresh frozen plasma, cryoprecipitate and platelets to try to maintain adequate hemostasis. BCSH transfusion guidelines for neonates and older children suggest that the platelet count in a bleeding preterm or term neonate should be maintained above $50 \times 10^9/L$ by the transfusion of platelet concentrates (10–20 mL/kg) [45]. Fresh frozen plasma (10–20 mL/kg) can be used to replace coagulation factors, although cryoprecipitate (5–10 mL/kg) or fibrinogen concentrates are better sources of fibrinogen, which should be kept above 1 g/L [125].

Learning Points

- Coagulation reference ranges vary according to gestational and postnatal age. The PT and APTT can be markedly prolonged in premature neonates.
- Hemophilia A and B are the most common inherited coagulation disorders in the neonatal period: an isolated prolongation of APTT is highly suggestive of hemophilia.
- Isolated prolongation of the PT, followed by prolongation of the APTT, with a normal fibrinogen concentration and platelet count, suggests VKDB.
- The management of DIC is prompt and effective treatment of the underlying condition, and supportive treatment with blood components/products to maintain adequate hemostasis.

References

1. Holmberg L, Gustavii B, Jonsson A. A prenatal study of fetal platelet count and size with application to the fetus at risk of Wiskott Aldrich syndrome. J Pediatr. 1983;102:773–81.
2. Forestier F, Daffos F, Galacteros F. Haematological values of 163 normal fetuses between 18 and 30 weeks of gestation. Pediatr Res. 1986;20:342–6.
3. Forestier F, Daffos F, Catherine N, Renard M, Andreux JP. Developmental hematopoiesis in normal human fetal blood. Blood. 1991;77:2360–3.
4. Burrows RF, Kelton JG. Incidentally detected thrombocytopenia in healthy mothers and their infants. N Engl J Med. 1988;319:142–5.
5. Burrows RF, Kelton JG. Thrombocytopenia at delivery: a prospective survey of 6715 deliveries. Am J Obstet Gynecol. 1990;162:731–4.
6. Burrows RF, Kelton JG. Fetal thrombocytopenia and its relation to maternal thrombocytopenia. N Engl J Med. 1993;329:1463–6.
7. Sainio S, Jarvenpaa A-S, Renlund M, et al. Thrombocytopenia in term infants: a population-based study. Obstet Gynecol. 2000;95:441–6.
8. Murray NA, Howarth LJ, McCloy MP, et al. Platelet transfusion in the management of severe thrombocytopenia in neonatal intensive care unit patients. Transfus Med. 2002;12:35–41.
9. Roberts I, Stanworth S, Murray N. Thrombocytopenia in the neonate. Blood Rev. 2008;22(4):173–86.
10. Stanworth SJ, Clarke P, Watts T, Ballard S, Choo L, Morris T, Murphy MF, Roberts I, for the Platelets and Neonatal Transfusion Study Group. Prospective, observational study of outcomes in neonates with severe thrombocytopenia. Pediatrics. 2009;124(5):e826–34.
11. Murray NA, Roberts IAG. Circulating megakaryocytes and their progenitors in early thrombocytopenia in preterm neonates. Pediatr Res. 1996;40:112–9.
12. Watts TL, Roberts IAG. Haematological abnormalities in the growth-restricted infant. Semin Neonatol. 1999;4:41–54.
13. Ghevaert C, Campbell K, Walton J, et al. Management and outcome of 200 cases of fetomaternal alloimmune thrombocytopenia. Transfusion. 2007;47:901–10.
14. Srivastava A, Bruno E, Briddell R, et al. Parvovirus B19 induced perturbation of human megakaryocytopoiesis in vitro. Blood. 1990;76:1997–2004.
15. Cole JL, Marzec UM, Gunthel CJ, Karpatkin S, Worford L, Sundell IB, et al. Ineffective platelet production in thrombocytopenic human immunodeficiency virus infected patients. Blood. 1998;91:3239–46.
16. Roux W, Pieper C, Cotton M. Thrombocytopenia as marker for HIV exposure in the neonate. J Trop Pediatr. 2001;47:208–10.
17. Hohlfeld P, Forestier F, Kaplan C, Tissot JD, Daffos F. Fetal thrombocytopenia: a retrospective survey of 5,194 fetal blood samplings. Blood. 1994;84:1851–6.
18. Webb D, Roberts I, Vyas P. The haematology of Down syndrome. Arch Dis Child. 2007;92:F503–7.
19. Wechsler J, Greene M, McDevitt MA, Anastasi J, Karp JE, LeBeau MM, et al. Acquired mutations in GATA1 in the megakaryoblastic leukemia of Down syndrome. Nat Genet. 2002;32:148–52, 1013.
20. Lopez JA, Andrews RK, Afshar-Kharghan V, Berndt MC. Bernard-Soulier syndrome. Blood. 1998; 91:4397–418.
21. Kunishima S, Kamiya T, Saito H. Genetic abnormalities of Bernard-Soulier syndrome. Int J Hematol. 2002;76:319–27.
22. Villa A, Notarangelo L, Macchi P, Mantuano E, Cavagni G, Brugnoni D, et al. X-linked thrombocytopenia and Wiskott-Aldrich syndrome are allelic diseases with mutations in the WASP gene. Nat Genet. 1995;9:414–7.
23. Dupuis-Girod S, Medioni J, Haddad E, Quartier P, Cavazzana-Calvo M, Le Deist F, et al. Autoimmunity in Wiskott-Aldrich syndrome: risk factors, clinical features, and outcome in a single center cohort of 55 patients. Pediatrics. 2003;111(5):e622–7.
24. Salvesen DR, Brudenell JM, Snijders RJ, Ireland RM, Nicolaides KH. Fetal plasma erythropoietin in

pregnancies complicated by maternal diabetes mellitus. Am J Obstet Gynecol. 1993;168:88–94.

25. Mondanlou HD, Ortiz OB. Thrombocytopenia in neonatal infection. Clin Pediatr. 1981;20:402–7.

26. Zipursky A, Jaber HM. The haematology of bacterial infection in newborn infants. Clin Haematol. 1978;7:175–93.

27. Jubinsky PT, Moraille R, Tsai HM. Thrombotic thrombocytopenic purpura in a newborn. J Perinatol. 2003;23:85–7.

28. Berner R, Krause MF, Gordjani N, et al. Hemolytic uremic syndrome due to an altered factor H triggered by neonatal pertussis. Pediatr Nephrol. 2002;17: 190–2.

29. Spadone D, Clark F, James E, et al. Heparin induced thrombocytopenia in the newborn. J Vasc Surg. 1992; 15:306–11.

30. Hall GW. Kasabach Merritt syndrome: pathogenesis and management. Br J Haematol. 2001;112:851–62.

31. Burtina AB, Bonafe L, Zacchello F. Clinical and biochemical approach to the neonate with a suspected inborn error of amino acid and organic acid metabolism. Semin Perinatol. 1999;23:162–73.

32. Roth P, Sklower Brooks S, Potaznik D, et al. Neonatal Gaucher disease presenting as persistent thrombocytopenia. J Perinatol. 2005;25:356–8.

33. Faivre L, Guardiola P, Lewis C, et al. Association of complementation group and mutation type with clinical outcome in Fanconi anaemia. Blood. 2000;96: 4064–70.

34. Greenhalgh KL, Howell RT, Bottani A, et al. Thrombocytopenia-absent radius syndrome: a clinical genetic study. J Med Genet. 2002;39:876–81.

35. Hall JG, Levin J, Kuhn JP, et al. Thrombocytopenia with absent radius (TAR). Medicine. 1969;48:411–39.

36. Thompson AA, Nguyen LT. Amegakaryocytic thrombocytopenia and radio-ulnar synostosis are associated with HOXA11 mutation. Nat Genet. 2000;26: 397–8.

37. Freedman MH, Doyle JJ. Inherited bone marrow failure syndromes. In: Lilleyman JS, Hann IM, Blanchette VS, editors. Pediatric hematology. London: Churchill Livingstone; 1999. p. P23–49.

38. Lackner A, Basu O, Bierings M, et al. Haematopoietic stem cell transplantation for amegakaryocytic thrombocytopenia. Br J Haematol. 2000;109:773–5.

39. Stoll BJ, Hansen N, Fanaroff A, et al. Late onset sepsis in very low birth weight neonates: the experience of the NICHD neonatal research network. Pediatrics. 2002;110(2):285–91.

40. Warris A, Semmekrot BA, Voss A. Candidal and bacterial bloodstream infections in premature neonates: a case control study. Med Mycol. 2001;39:75–9.

41. Dyke MP, Ott K. Severe thrombocytopenia in extremely low birth weight infants with systemic candidiasis. J Paediatr Child Health. 1993;29: 298–301.

42. Hsueh W, Caplan MS, Qu XW, et al. Neonatal necrotising enterocolitis: clinical considerations and pathogenetic concepts. Pediatr Dev Pathol. 2003;6(1): 6–23.

43. Hutter JJ, Hathaway WE, Wayne ER. Hematologic abnormalities in severe neonatal necrotising enterocolitis. J Pediatr. 1976;88:1026–31.

44. Ververidis M, Kiely EM, Spitz L, et al. The clinical significance of thrombocytopenia in neonates with necrotising enterocolitis. J Pediatr Surg. 2001;36: 799–803.

45. BCSH guidelines, Gibson BES, Bolton-Maggs PHB, Pamphilon D, et al. Transfusion guidelines for neonates and older children. Br J Haematol. 2004;124: 433–53.

46. Chaudhary R, Clarke P. Current transfusion practices for platelets and fresh, frozen plasma in UK tertiary level neonatal units. Acta Paediatr. 2008;97(1):135.

47. Strauss R. How do I transfuse red blood cells and platelets to infants with the anaemia and thrombocytopenia of prematurity. Transfusion. 2008;48: 209–17.

48. Saxonhouse M, Slayton W, Sola MC. Platelet transfusions in the infant and child. In: Hillyer CD, Luban NLC, Strauss RG, editors. Pediatric handbook of transfusion medicine. San Diego: Elsevier; 2004. p. 253.

49. Josephson CD, Su LL, Christensen RD, Hillyer CD, et al. Platelet transfusion practices among neonatologists in the United States and Canada: results of a survey. Pediatrics. 2009;123:278–85.

50. Roberts IAG, Murray NA. Thrombocytopenia in the newborn. Curr Opin Pediatr. 2003;15:17–23.

51. Baer VL, Lambert DK, Henry E, et al. Do platelet transfusions in the NICU adversely affect survival? Analysis of 1600 thrombocytopenic neonates in a multihospital healthcare system. J Perinatol. 2007;27: 790–6.

52. Kenton AB, Hegemier S, Smith EO, et al. Platelet transfusions in infants with necrotizing enterocolitis do not lower mortality but may increase morbidity. J Perinatol. 2005;25:173–7.

53. De Veber G, Canadian Pediatric Ischaemic Stroke Study Group. Canadian Pediatric Ischaemic Stroke Registry: analysis of children with ischemic arterial stroke. Ann Neurol. 2000;48:526. Abstract.

54. Albisetti M, Andrew M, Monagle P. Hemostaric abnormalities. In: De Alarcon PA, Werner EJ, editors. Neonatal hematology. New York: Cambridge University Press; 2005. p. 310–48.

55. Chalmers EA. Perinatal stroke: risk factors and management. Br J Haematol. 2005;130:333–43.

56. Benders MJ, Groenendaal F, Uiterwaal CS, Nikkels PG, Bruinse HW, Nievelstein RA, et al. Maternal and infant characteristics associated with perinatal arterial stroke in the preterm infant. Stroke. 2007;38:1759–65.

57. Günther G, Junker R, Sträter R, et al. Symptomatic ischemic stroke in full-term neonates: role of acquired and genetic prothrombotic risk factors. Stroke. 2000;31:2437–41. Published correction appears in Stroke. 2001;32:279.

58. Heller C, Becker S, Scharrer I, Kreuz W. Prothrombotic risk factors in childhood stroke and venous thrombosis. Eur J Pediatr. 1999;158 Suppl 3:S117–21.

59. Kenet G, Sadetzki S, Murad H, et al. Factor V Leiden and antiphospholipid antibodies are significant risk factors for ischemic stroke in children. Stroke. 2000;31:1283–8.

60. Manco-Johnson MJ, Nuss R, Key N, et al. Lupus anticoagulant and protein S deficiency in children with postvaricella purpura fulminans or thrombosis. J Pediatr. 1996;128:319–23.

61. McColl MD, Chalmers EA, Thomas A, et al. Factor V Leiden, prothrombin 20210GA and the MTHFR C677T mutations in childhood stroke. Thromb Haemost. 1999;81:690–4.

62. Zenz W, Bodo Z, Plotho J, et al. Factor V Leiden and prothrombin gene G20210A variant in children with stroke. Thromb Haemost. 1998;80:763–6.

63. Bauer K. Rare hereditary coagulation factor abnormalities. In: Nathan DG, Oski FA, editors. Hematology of infancy and childhood. Philadelphia: WB Saunders; 1998. p. 1660–5.

64. Pegelow CH, Ledford M. Severe protein S deficiency in a newborn. Pediatrics. 1992;89:674–5.

65. Brenner B, Fishman A, Goldsher D, Schreibman D, Tavory S. Cerebral thrombosis in a newborn with congenital deficiency of antithrombin III. Am J Hematol. 1988;27:209–11.

66. Schuster V, Mingers AM, Seidenspinner S, Nussgens Z, Pukrop T, Kreth HW. Homozygous mutations in the plasminogen gene of two unrelated girls with ligneous conjunctivitis. Blood. 1997;90:958–66.

67. Andrew M, Vegh P, Johnston M, Bowker J, Ofosu F, Mitchell L. Maturation of the hemostatic system during childhood. Blood. 1992;80:1998–2005.

68. Andrew MA, Monagle P, de Weber G, Chan AKC. Thromboembolic disease and antithrombotic therapy in newborns. Hematology Am Soc Hematol Educ Program. 2001:358–74.

69. De Stefano V, Finazzi G, Mannucci PM. Inherited thrombophilia: pathogenesis, clinical syndromes and management. Blood. 1996;87:3531–44.

70. Toumi NH, Khaldi F, Ben Becheur S, et al. Thrombosis in congenital deficiencies of AT III, protein C or protein S: a study of 44 children. Hematol Cell Ther. 1997;39:295–9.

71. Blanco A, Bonduel M, Penalva L, Hepner M, Lazzari M. Deep vein thrombosis in a 13 year old boy with hereditary protein S deficiency and a review of the pediatric literature. Am J Hematol. 1994;45:330–4.

72. Olds RJ, Lane DA, Ireland H, et al. Novel point mutations leading to type 1 antithrombin deficiency and thrombosis. Br J Haematol. 1991;78:408–13.

73. Dilley A, Austin H, Hooper WC, et al. Prevalence of the prothrombin 20210G to A variant in blacks: infants, patients with venous thrombosis, patients with suspected myocardial infarction, and control subjects. J Lab Clin Med. 1998;132:452–5.

74. Pipe SW, Schmaier AH, Nichols WC, et al. Neonatal purpura fulminans in association with factor V R506Q mutation. J Pediatr. 1996;128:707–9.

75. Curry CJ, Bhullar S, Holmes J, Delozier CD, Roeder ER, Hutchinson HT. Risk factors for perinatal arterial stroke: a study of 60 mother-child pairs. Pediatr Neurol. 2007;37:99–107.

76. Ehrenforth S, Junker R, Koch HG, Kreuz W, Münchow N, Scharrer I, Nowak-Göttl U. Multicentre evaluation of combined prothrombotic defects associated with thrombophilia in childhood. Childhood Thrombophilia Study Group. Eur J Pediatr. 1999;158 Suppl 3:S97–104.

77. Hermansen MC, Hermansen MG. Intravascular catheter complications in the neonatal intensive care unit. Clin Perinatol. 2005;32:141–56.

78. Tanke RB, van Megen R, Daniels O. Thrombus detection on central venous catheters in the neonatal intensive care unit. Angiology. 1994;45:477–80.

79. Khilnani P, Goldstein B, Todres ID. Double lumen umbilical venous catheters in critically ill neonates: a randomised prospective study. Crit Care Med. 1991; 19:1348–51.

80. Roy M, Turner Gomes S, Gill G. Incidence and diagnosis of neonatal thrombosis associated with umbilical venous catheters. Thromb Haemost. 1997;78:724. Abstract.

81. Cohen RS, Ramachandran P, Kim EH, Glasscock GF. Retrospective analysis of risks associated with an umbilical artery catheter system for continuous monitoring of arterial oxygen tension. J Perinatol. 1995;15: 195–8.

82. Barrington KJ. Umbilical arterial catheters in the newborn: effect of position of the catheter tip. Cochrane Database Syst Rev. 1999;1.Art No:CD000505.

83. Barrington KJ. Umbilical artery catheters in the newborn: effects of heparin. Cochrane Database Syst Rev. 1999;1.Art No:CD000507.

84. Barrington KJ. Umbilical artery catheters in the newborn: effects of catheter materials. Cochrane Database Syst Rev. 1999;1.Art No:CD000505.

85. Vailas GN, Brouillette RT, Scott JP, Shkolnik A, Conway J, Wiringa K. Neonatal aortic thrombosis: recent experience. J Pediatr. 1986;109:101–8.

86. Nowak-gottl U, Von Kries R, Gobel U. Neonatal symptomatic thromboembolism in Germany: two year survey. Arch Dis Child Fetal Neonatal Ed. 1997;76:F163–7.

87. Mocan H, Beattie TJ, Murphy AV. Renal venous thrombosis in infancy: long term follow up. Pediatr Nephrol. 1991;5:45–9.

88. Andrew M, Monagle P, Brooker L. Thromboembolic complications in specific organ sites and pediatric diseases. In: Thromboembolic complications during infancy and childhood. Hamilton: Decker Inc; 2000. p. 231–76.

89. Raju TNK, Nelson KB, Ferriero D, Lynch JK, and the NICHD-NINDS Perinatal Stroke Workshop Participants. Ischaemic perinatal stroke: a summary of a workshop sponsored by the National Institute of Child Health and Development and the National Institute of Child Health and Human Development and the National Institute of Neurological Disorders and Stroke. Pediatrics. 2007;120:609–16.

90. Lee J, Croen LA, Backstrand KH, et al. Maternal and infant characteristics associated with perinatal arterial stroke in the infant. JAMA. 2005;292:723–9.

91. Govaert P, Dudink J, Visser G, Breukhoven P, Vanhatalo S, Lequin M. Top of the basilar artery embolic stroke and neonatal myoclonus. Dev Med Child Neurol. 2009;51:324–7.

92. Mercuri E, Cowan F. Cerebral infarction in the newborn infant: review of the literature and personal experience. Eur J Paediatr Neurol. 1999;3(6):255–63.

93. Govaert P, Ramenghi L, Taal L, de Vries L, deWeber G. Diagnosis of perinatal stroke I: definitions, differential diagnosis and registration. Acta Paediatr. 2009;98:1556–67.

94. Wu YW, Lynch JK, Nelson KB. Perinatal arterial stroke: understanding mechanisms and outcomes. Semin Neurol. 2005;25:424–34.

95. Dominguez R, Aguirre Vila-Coro A, Slopis JM, Bohan TP. Brain and ocular abnormalities in infants with in utero exposure to cocaine and other street drugs. Am J Dis Child. 1991;145:688–95.

96. Golomb MR, Dick PT, MacGregor DL, Armstrong DC, deWeber GA. Cranial ultrasonography has a low sensitivity for detecting arterial ischemic stroke in term neonates. J Child Neurol. 2003;18:98–103.

97. Cowan F, Mercuri E, Groenendaal F, et al. Does cranial ultrasound imaging identify arterial cerebral infarction in term neonates? Arch Dis Child Fetal Neonatal Ed. 2005;90:F252–6.

98. Roelants-van Rijn AM, Nikkels PG, Groenendaal F, et al. Neonatal diffusion weighted MR imaging: relation with histopathology or follow up MR examination. Neuropediatrics. 2001;32:286–94.

99. Bydder GM, Rutherford MA, Cowan FM. Diffusion weighted imaging in neonates. Childs Nerv Syst. 2001;17:190–4.

100. Mercuri E, Rutherford M, Cowan F, et al. Early prognostic indicators of outcome in infants with neonatal cerebral infarction: a clinical electroencephalogram and magnetic resonance imaging study. Pediatrics. 1999;103:39–46.

101. deWeber GA, MacGregor D, Curtis R, Mayank S. Neurologic outcome in survivors of childhood arterial ischemic stroke and sinovenous thrombosis. J Child Neurol. 2000;15:316–24.

102. McDonald MM, Jacobson LJ, Hay Jr WW, et al. Heparin clearance in the newborn. Pediatr Res. 1981;15:1015–8.

103. McDonald MM, Hathaway WE. Anticoagulant therapy by continuous heparinisation in newborn and older infants. J Pediatr. 1982;101:451–7.

104. Wang M, Hays T, Balasa V, et al. Low dose tissue plasminogen activator thrombolysis in children. J Pediatr Hematol Oncol. 2003;25:379–86.

105. Manco-Johnson MJ. How I treat venous thrombosis in children. Blood. 2006;107:21–9.

106. Saxonhouse MA, Manco-Johnson MJ. The evaluation and management of neonatal coagulation disorders. Semin Perinatol. 2009;33:52–65.

107. Vogelzang RL, Moel DI, Cohn RA, Donaldson JS, Langman CB, Nemcek AAJ. Acute renal vein thrombosis: successful treatment with intraarterial urokinase. Radiology. 1988;169:681–2.

108. Monagle P, Chan A, Massicote P, et al. Antithrombotic therapy in children. The seventh ACCP conference on antithrombotic and thrombolytic therapy. Chest. 2004;126:645S–87.

109. Andrew M, Paes B, Milner R, et al. Development of the coagulation system in the full-term infant. Blood. 1987;70:165–72.

110. Andrew M, Paes B, Milner R, et al. Development of the human coagulation system in the healthy premature infant. Blood. 1988;80:1998–2005.

111. Andrew M, Paes B, Johnston M. Development of the haemostatic system in the neonate and young infant. Am J Pediatr Hematol Oncol. 1990;12:95–104.

112. Moskowitz NP, Karpatkin M. Coagulation problems in the newborn. Curr Paediatr. 2005;15:50–6.

113. Pollman H, Richter H, Ringkamp H, Jurgens H. When are children diagnosed as having severe haemophilia and when do they start to bleed? A 10 year single centre PUP study. Eur J Pediatr. 1999;158:S166–70.

114. Kulkarni R, Lusher J. Perinatal management of neonates with haemophilia. Br J Haematol. 2001;112:264–74.

115. Yoffe G, Buchanan GR. Intracranial hemorrhage in newborn and young infants with hemophilia. J Pediatr. 1988;113:333–6.

116. Myles LM, Massicotte P, Drake J. Intracranial hemorrhage in neonates with unrecognised hemophilia A: a persisting problem. Pediatr Neurosurg. 2001;34:94–7.

117. UKHCDO. Guideline for the selection and use of therapeutic products to treat haemophilia and other hereditary bleeding disorders. Haemophilia. 2003;9:1–23.

118. DiMichele D, Neufeld EJ. Hemophilia: a new approach to an old disease. Hematol Oncol Clin North Am. 1998;12:1315–44.

119. Matthay K, Koerper M, Ablin AR. Intracranial haemorrhage in congenital factor VII deficiency. J Pediatr. 1979;94:413–5.

120. Machin S, Winter M, Davies S, Mackie I. Factor X deficiency in the neonatal period. Arch Dis Child. 1980;55:406–8.

121. Anwar R, Minford A, Gallivan L, et al. Delayed umbilical bleeding-a presenting feature for Factor XIII deficiency: clinical features, genetics and management. Pediatrics. 2002;109:E32.

122. Suzuki S, Iwata G, Sutor A. Vitamin K deficiency bleeding during the perinatal and infantile period. Semin Thromb Hemost. 2001;27:93–8.
123. Von Kries R, Gobel U. Vitamin K prophylaxis and vitamin K deficiency bleeding (VKDB) in early infancy. Acta Paediatr. 1992;81:655–7.
124. Tonz O, Schubiger G. Neonatal vitamin K prophylaxis and vitamin K deficiency haemorrhages in Switzerland 1986–1988. Schweiz Med Wochenschr. 1988;118:1747–52.
125. Cornelissen EAM, Kollee AA, van Lith TGPJ, Motohar K, Monnens LAH. Evaluation of a daily dose of 25 micrograms vitamin K to prevent vitamin K deficiency bleeding in breastfed infant. J Pediatr Gastroenterol Nutr. 1993;16:301–5.
126. Cornelissen M, von Kries R, Loughnan P, Schubiger G. Prevention of vitamin K deficiency bleeding: efficacy of different multiple oral dose schedules of vitamin K. Eur J Pediatr. 1997;156:126–30.
127. Williams MD, Chalmers EA, Gibson BES. Guideline. The investigation and management of neonatal haemostasis and thrombosis. Br J Haematol. 2002;119: 295–309.
128. Hudson IRB, Gibson BES, Brownlie J, et al. Increased concentrations of D-dimers in newborn infants. Arch Dis Child. 1990;65:383–9.

Irfana Koita-Kazi and Paul Serhal

Abstract

Assisted conception is a women's health issue of growing importance, with the number of women undergoing in vitro fertilization (IVF) increasing world-wide. IVF treatment involves ovarian stimulation. This can result in a hyper-estrogenic state, which in turn can lead to ovarian hyperstimulation syndrome (OHSS) associated with both venous and arterial thromboembolism. This chapter addresses clinically relevant thrombotic and haemostatic aspects of assisted conception, including the diagnosis, treatment and prevention of OHSS-related thromboembolism.

16.1 Introduction

In the UK, 1 in 6 couples have difficulty in conceiving. The use of assisted conception is on the rise worldwide, and over 35,000 procedures are performed annually in the UK alone. It is estimated that 4.2 % of babies in Europe are born as a consequence of these techniques [1].

In vitro fertilization (IVF) treatment involves ovarian stimulation with exogenous hormones.

This can result in a hyper-estrogenic status which in turn can cause ovarian hyperstimulation syndrome (OHSS). OHSS is a systemic disease resulting from the release of vasoactive products from overstimulated ovaries. The syndrome has a broad spectrum of presentation, ranging from mild illness needing only careful observation to severe disease requiring hospitalization and intensive care. OHSS is associated with both venous and arterial thromboembolic complications.

16.2 Incidence of OHSS-Related Thrombosis

The absolute incidence of venous thromboembolism secondary to assisted conception treatment is small and estimated to be 0.08–0.11 % [2], an incidence similar to that of pregnancy-associated venous thromboembolism, whereas

I. Koita-Kazi, MRCOG (✉) • P. Serhal, MRCOG
Centre for Reproductive and Genetic Health (CRGH),
Eastman Dental Hospital, 256 Gray's Inn Road,
London WC1X 8LD, UK
e-mail: irfana.koita-kazi@uclh.nhs.uk;
paul.serhal@uclh.nhs.uk

H. Cohen, P. O'Brien (eds.), *Disorders of Thrombosis and Hemostasis in Pregnancy*,
DOI 10.1007/978-1-4471-4411-3_16, © Springer-Verlag London 2012

the incidence of arterial thromboembolism is reported to be several times lower [3]. The ratio of venous to arterial thrombosis is estimated to be 3:1 [4]. A Danish study of 30,884 women which compared the incidence rates of venous and arterial thromboses with previously published estimates of the risk of thrombosis among young Danish women found no evidence that assisted reproduction increased the risk of thrombosis [5].

16.3 Hemostatic Changes Associated with Assisted Conception

Ovarian stimulation during IVF treatment results in a dramatic increase of as much as 20–50 times baseline estradiol levels [6]. The possibility that elevated estradiol levels may be linked to arterial and venous thrombosis stems from previous studies conducted on oral contraceptive pill use [7] and hormone replacement therapy [8].

A number of studies have reported prothrombotic changes during the IVF process. These include increased levels of factor VIII, von Willebrand factor and fibrinogen, decreased levels of the naturally occurring anticoagulants antithrombin, protein C and S as well as increased levels of the coagulation activation markers prothrombin fragment F1.2 and thrombin-antithrombin complexes. Analysis of whole blood using thromboelastography has suggested changes towards hypercoagulability, although parameters remained within normal limits. Westerlund et al. reported that the endogenous thrombin potential (ETP), a key parameter of the thrombin generation test which provides information about the dynamics of thrombin generation, was increased in women undergoing IVF [9–22]. Platelet function appears to remain unchanged [16].

In women with OHSS, the prothrombotic changes may be more pronounced [23–25]. Excessive coagulation activation reflected by raised D-dimer levels and thrombin-antithrombin complexes seen in women with OHSS who do not fall pregnant despite higher oocyte yield suggests

that prothrombotic mechanisms play a role in implantation [24].

16.4 Mechanism of Venous and Arterial Thrombosis in Assisted Conception

In women undergoing assisted conception, OHSS is the main predisposing factor for both arterial and venous thrombotic events. The pathophysiology of OHSS is characterized by the release of vasoactive substances which result in increased capillary permeability, leading to leakage of fluid from the vascular compartment. This causes third-space fluid accumulation and intravascular dehydration.

Factors that have been suggested in the process leading to OHSS include:
- Increased exudation of protein-rich fluid from the ovaries or peritoneal surfaces [26–29]
- Increased levels of prorenin and renin in follicular fluid [30, 31]
- Angiotensin-mediated changes in capillary permeability [31, 32]
- Vascular endothelial growth factor (VEGF)/ Vascular permeability factor (VPF): expression and production within the ovary appear critical for normal reproductive function [33]

Arterial thrombosis is most likely due to thromboembolic events. Autopsy findings in a patient who died from stroke revealed small brain thrombi with otherwise normal vessels [34]. Similarly, angiography and MRI studies in several reported cases suggest isolated thrombi within affected vessels [35–38].

Women who have an underlying thrombophilia and who fall pregnant as a result of the assisted conception are more likely to develop venous thrombosis. The supraphysiological estrogenic state secondary to ovarian stimulation may add to the hypercoagulability in these patients and result in venous thrombosis. Bauersachs et al. [39] and Salomon et al. [40] put forward two theories for the specific, yet unusual, localisation of DVT in OHSS. Bauersachs et al. hypothesized that ascitic fluid high in estrogen, particularly in women with OHSS, drained into the thoracic duct. This lymphatic fluid then drains into the left subclavian vein resulting in a local area of high estrogen level leading to thrombosis in these neck veins. Salomon et al. hypothesized that the rudimentary brachial cysts in the neck fill with fluid due to OHSS causing mechanical obstruction at the base of the jugular and subclavian veins leading to upper extremity thrombosis.

Apart from OHSS, other risk factors for venous thromboembolism include a previous personal or family history of venous thromboembolism, concurrent medical conditions such as chronic infective or inflammatory disorders, and obesity.

16.5 Diagnosis of OHSS-Related Thrombosis

Women at high risk of developing OHSS include:

- Those with polycystic ovaries
- Those under 30 years of age
- Those with low body weight
- Use of high doses of gonadotrophins for stimulation
- Use of gonadotrophin releasing hormone (GnRH) agonists, luteinizing hormone (LH), or human chorionic gonadotrophin (hCG)
- Development of multiple follicles during treatment
- High absolute or rapidly rising serum estradiol levels
- Increased number of eggs retrieved
- Previous history of OHSS

Women are classified as having mild, moderate, severe or critical OHSS based on the clinical severity at presentation. Those who develop thromboembolism lie in the critical category.

The drugs used for hormonal manipulation include follicle-stimulating hormone (FSH), human menopausal gonadotrophin (hMG), GnRH, GnRH agonist, clomiphene citrate, and hCG. Clomiphene citrate and GnRH are only rarely associated with OHSS [41].

The commonest reported site for both arterial and venous thrombotic events is the head and neck region although an underreporting of lower extremity venous thrombosis cannot be excluded. The predominant sites of involvement of venous thromboembolism are the veins in the neck and upper extremities in 80 % of cases [3]. Arterial events most commonly (two-thirds) present as cerebrovascular accidents or stroke; the remaining third present in extremities or with myocardial infarction. This is in stark contrast to the classical left iliofemoral deep vein thrombosis seen in pregnancy. The sites for OHSS-related thrombosis reported in the literature include the superior sagittal sinus, internal jugular vein, superior vena cava, thromboembolism extending from the right ovarian vein to the inferior vena cava, basilar artery, subclavian vein, central retinal vein, and the internal carotid vein.

Arterial thrombotic events invariably present early, that is within 2 weeks after embryo transfer, and occur along with the development of OHSS. Venous thromboembolic events, however, may present at any time from within a week after embryo transfer to 12 weeks of gestation, well beyond the resolution of clinical OHSS.

Almost all cases of venous thromboembolism occur in women who are pregnant; in contrast, only half of those who develop arterial thrombosis are pregnant.

The causes of death reported in the literature include acute respiratory distress syndrome, cerebral infarction, and hepatorenal failure (reported in a woman with preexisting hepatitis C) [42].

Symptoms and signs suggestive of thromboembolism demand prompt additional diagnostic measures. These include arterial blood gas measurement and appropriate imaging tailored to the individual situation and may include Doppler/Duplex ultrasound of the vasculature of the site involved, CT pulmonary angiography (CTPA), and brain imaging: CT/CT venography and/or MRI.

Thromboembolic events can occur in the absence of other clinical features of OHSS, particularly in patients with severe prothrombotic abnormalities, for example combined heritable thrombophilias or antiphospholipid syndrome. Neck pain and swelling in a pregnant woman, especially one that has undergone IVF, should be taken seriously and investigated with Duplex scanning and/or MR angiography. Unusual neurological symptomatology following ovarian stimulation should raise the possibility of a thrombotic episode in an uncommon location, prompting referral for expert opinion [42] and appropriate investigation.

16.6 Treatment of OHSS-Related Thromboembolism

Women who develop thromboembolism secondary to assisted conception treatment should be promptly admitted to hospital and managed by a multidisciplinary team. If there is also severe OHSS, pulmonary embolus or head/neck thrombosis, intensive care admission may be advisable until the woman's condition is controlled.

The treatment of venous thromboembolism involves the use of therapeutic doses of low molecular weight heparin (LMWH) and thrombolysis if indicated [43]. Anticoagulation should be under the supervision of a hematologist and for an appropriate period depending on the site of thrombosis and presence of pregnancy. Similarly, the management of arterial thrombosis should be tailored to the clinical presentation of the condition, with input by appropriate specialists, such as neurologists.

It is concerning that some studies have demonstrated thrombosis in association with OHSS despite prophylactic [44, 45] and even therapeutic anticoagulation [46]. It has been suggested that this may be due to localized increase in activation of coagulation and raised concentrations of estradiol resulting in impairment of the endothelium's antithrombotic properties [39].

16.6.1 The Role of Heparin in Assisted Conception

Heparin can alter the hemostatic response to controlled ovarian stimulation and modify the risk of thrombosis associated with exogenous gonadotrophin use. Vascular endothelial growth factor

(VEGF), a proangiogenic factor, plays a major role in the pathogenesis of in OHSS, and heparin may have a direct role in OHSS due to its action on VEGF. There is increasing evidence that heparin can influence many of the basic physiological processes that are required for blastocyst apposition, adherence and implantation. In addition, heparin seems to have a role in trophoblast differentiation and invasion. This is likely to have the potential to improve pregnancy rates, perinatal outcome and live birthrates. However, there is little substantive evidence to support its use in assisted conception [1].

16.6.2 Reporting of Adverse Incidents

The Human Fertilisation and Embryology Authority (HFEA) is a licensing body that regulates all the fertility units in the UK. All adverse incidents occurring at the treatment center must be reported to the HFEA by telephone within 12 working hours of the identification of the incident and submission of an incident report form is required within 24 working hours.

In the UK, any death related to OHSS, irrespective of whether the woman was pregnant, must be reported to the Confidential Enquiries into Maternal Deaths.

16.7 Prevention of OHSS

Measures that can prevent OHSS include:
(a) Controlled ovarian stimulation using the lowest effective dose, especially in those women with risk factors for OHSS
(b) Coasting, that is, cessation of ovarian stimulation
(c) Delaying administration of hCG until estradiol levels have fallen significantly or plateau
(d) Cycle cancellation prior to hCG administration
(e) A lower dose of hCG, that is 5,000 IU instead of 10,000 IU, or a single bolus of GnRH agonist to trigger ovulation in a GnRH antagonist-based protocol

(f) Use of progesterone instead of hCG for luteal support

(g) Cryopreservation of all embryos

Thromboprophylaxis should be initiated in all women admitted to hospital with OHSS, but is particularly important in those with a personal or family history of thromboembolic events, thrombophilia, or vascular anomalies. Antiembolism stockings and prophylactic heparin therapy should be used. This should be continued at least until discharge from hospital or resolution of symptoms. The risk of thrombosis appears to persist into the first trimester of pregnancy so, LMWH prophylaxis should be continued until the end of the first trimester and possibly longer, depending on other risk factors and the course of the OHSS [47]. The use of intermittent pneumatic compression devices is useful in patients who are confined to bed.

Routine screening for thrombophilia in all women undergoing assisted conception is not warranted, although testing may be helpful for those with a personal or family history of thrombosis [42]. The British Committee for Standards in Haematology (BCSH) Haemostasis and Thrombosis Task Force states that, as the incidence of severe OHSS is so low, the predictive value of thrombophilia testing would be very low and testing should not be used to influence antithrombotic strategies in women commencing ovarian stimulation [48]. However, in the absence of well-designed trials, a pragmatic approach to the prevention of thromboembolism is needed. Hence, all women undergoing ovarian stimulation should undergo risk assessment for thrombosis. Women with a previous history or additional current risk factors for venous thromboembolism and with known thrombophilia should be closely monitored. Low molecular weight heparin thromboprophylaxis (e.g. 40 mg enoxaparin or 5,000 IU dalteparin daily or 12 hourly) along with graduated compression stockings should be initiated depending on the clinical situation. These measures may well need to be continued throughout pregnancy in high-risk women. Those on long-term oral anticoagulantion should be switched to therapeutic dose LMWH.

16.8 Heritable and Acquired Thrombophilia in Assisted Conception

Adverse perinatal outcome in women with thrombophilia has led to the speculation that these conditions may also play a role in subfertility, especially recurrent implantation failure. Proposed mechanisms include local microthrombosis at the site of implantation which impairs invasion of maternal vessels by syncitiotrophoblast and leads to implantation failure (Alijotas-Reig et al, 2009). However, due to the low and varying prevalence of inherited thrombophilia, the small studies which have been conducted so far have been unable to confirm whether thrombophilia is contributory to subfertility [1].

An increased incidence of Factor V Leiden and prothrombin G20210 heterozygotes was reported in women failing to conceive after three or more IVF–embryo transfer cycles [49]. In a larger study, 90 women who failed to fall pregnant after three embryo transfers were compared with two separate control groups containing women who conceived after their first attempt ($n = 90$) and another group containing women who conceived spontaneously ($n = 100$). The study group was found to have an increased incidence of homozygosity for the MTHFR C677TT polymorphism and combined thrombophilias but not isolated Factor V Leiden [50]. Other studies have replicated the findings of an increased prevalence of heritable thrombophilia in women with recurrent implantation failure [51, 52] compared with those who conceived spontaneously or after their first cycle of IVF treatment.

The role of acquired thrombophilia, namely antiphospholipid syndrome, in subfertility is also debatable. As with heritable thrombophilias, large multicenter trials would be needed in order to reach a consensus on which antibodies should be tested for and what level corresponds to a clinically significant result. Women who do not conceive after three embryo transfers may exhibit an increased prevalence of antiphospholipid antibodies [50, 53, 54]. In women with thrombotic or obstetric antiphospholipid syndrome [55], therapeutic or prophylactic dose LMWH respectively plus low dose aspirin should be started at the time of ovarian stimulation and anticoagulation continued throughout pregnancy and anticoagulation continued for at least six weeks postpartum. Infertile women, and those with recurrent IVF implantation failure, have an increased incidence of antiphospholipid antibodies (22 % and 30 %, respectively) compared with a healthy, fertile population (1–3 %). Despite this increased incidence, antiphospholipid antibodies are not predictive of an adverse outcome from IVF [56], and treatment of these women with antithrombotic therapy remains empirical. Support for the view that prothrombotic changes may impact on the outcome of IVF comes from a randomized placebo-controlled trial which included 83 women with recurrent IVF failure (3 or more unsuccessful IVF cycles) who had at least one inherited or acquired thrombophilic defect (antiphospholipid antibodies). The primary outcomes (implantation, pregnancy and live birth rates) were all significantly higher in patients treated with LMWH during IVF treatment starting on the day of embryo transfer, versus the placebo-treated controls [57].

Learning Points
- OHSS is the main predisposing factor in both arterial and venous thrombotic events associated with assisted conception.
- Venous thromboembolism is the commonest thrombotic complication seen in assisted conception, with thrombosis occurring mainly in the neck and upper extremities. These women are more likely to be pregnant.
- Arterial events present early (within 2 weeks of embryo transfer) compared to venous events and are mainly due to thromboembolism.
- Unusual neurological symptomatology following ovarian stimulation should raise the possibility of a thrombotic episode in an uncommon location, prompting referral for a neurological opinion and appropriate investigation.
- All women undergoing ovarian stimulation should undergo risk assessment for thromboembolism so that timely preventive measures can be taken.

Case Study 1

A case of forearm amputation after ovarian stimulation for IVF–ET (embryo transfer) [58].

A 41-year-old woman affected by primary subfertility had ovarian stimulation for IVF treatment in a university hospital. The patient underwent many cycles of IVF–ET with administration of purified FSH (75 IU 10 times per day, for 12 days). Nine oocytes were obtained and 7 oocytes were inseminated in vitro.

A few days later, the patient showed absolute arterial insufficiency and an ischemic hand. Angiography confirmed thrombi in the subclavian artery. She was treated with thrombolysis and underwent thromboendarterectomy. In summary, this patient developed ovarian hyperstimulation syndrome associated with subclavian artery thrombosis, recurring twice after thromboarterectomy and leading to amputation of her forearm.

Case Study 2

Lower limb DVT followed by internal jugular vein thrombosis as a complication of IVF in a woman heterozygous for the prothrombin 3'UTR and factor V Leiden mutations [59].

A 30-year-old woman heterozygous for both the prothrombin 3'UTR and factor V Leiden mutations underwent IVF treatment. Two embryos were transferred following ovarian stimulation. She presented with lower limb swelling due to proximal deep vein thrombosis which was diagnosed on Doppler ultrasound. Transvaginal ultrasound at 5 weeks' gestation revealed twin gestational sacs, hyperstimulated ovaries, and free fluid in both adnexa. She was started on therapeutic anticoagulant therapy with subcutaneous low molecular weight heparin (enoxaparin 0.75mg/kg b.d.). Despite this, she subsequently developed pain and restricted movements, particularly involving the right side of the neck, due to an internal jugular vein thrombosis extending into the subclavian, axillary and cephalic veins on that side. In view of this patient's history of two DVTs in pregnancy, together with her underlying combined thrombophilia, she remained on therapeutic anticoagulation throughout her pregnancy. She delivered healthy twins by Caesarean section at 38 weeks and had no further thrombotic problems postnatally.

References

1. Nelson SM, Greer IA. The potential role of heparin in assisted conception. Hum Reprod Update. 2008; 14(6):623–45.
2. Mara M, Koryntova D, Rezabek K, et al. Thromboembolic complications in patients undergoing in vitro fertilization: retrospective clinical study. Ceska Gynekol. 2004;69:312–6 [Czech].
3. Chan WS. The 'ART' of thrombosis: a review of arterial and venous thrombosis in assisted reproductive technology. Curr Opin Obstet Gynecol. 2009;21: 207–18.
4. Aboulghar MA, Mansour RT, Serour GI, et al. Moderate Ovarian Hyperstimulation Syndrome complicated by deep cerebrovascular thrombosis. Hum Reprod. 1998;13:2088.
5. Hansen AT, Kesmodel US, Juul S, Hyas AM. No evidence that assisted reproduction increases the risk of thrombosis: a Danish National cohort study. Human Reproduction. 2012;27:1499–1503
6. Whelan JG, Vlahos NF. The ovarian hyperstimulation syndrome. Fertil Steril. 2000;73:83–896.
7. Douketis JD, Ginsberg JS, Holbrook A, et al. A reevaluation of the risk for Venous thromboembolism with the use of oral contraceptives and hormone replacement therapy. Arch Intern Med. 1997;157: 1522–30.
8. Rossouw JE, Anderson GL, Prentice RL, Writing Group for the Women's Health Initiative Investigators, et al. Risks and benefits of estrogen plus progestin in healthy postmenopausal women: principal results from the Women's Health Initiative Randomized Controlled Trial. JAMA. 2002;288:321–33.
9. Biron C, Galtier-Dereure F, Rabesandratana H, et al. Hemostasis parameters during ovarian stimulation for in vitro fertilization: results of a prospective study. Fertil Steril. 1997;67:104–9.
10. Kim HC, Kemmann E, Shelden RM, Saidi P. Response of blood coagulation parameters to elevated endogenous 17 beta-estradiol levels induced by human menopausal gonadotropins. Am J Obstet Gynecol. 1981;140:807–10.
11. Aune B, Hoie KE, Oian P, et al. Does ovarian stimulation for in-vitro fertilization induce a hypercoagulable state? Hum Reprod. 1991;6:925–7.
12. Rice VC, Richard-Davis G, Saleh AA, et al. Fibrinolytic parameters in women undergoing ovulation induction. Am J Obstet Gynecol. 1993;169: 1549–53.
13. Aune B, Oian P, Osterud B. Enhanced sensitivity of the extrinsic coagulation system during ovarian stimulation for in-vitro fertilization. Hum Reprod. 1993;8: 1349–52.
14. Bremme K, Wramsby H, Andersson O, et al. Do lowered factor VII levels at extremely high endogenous oestradiol levels protect against thrombin formation? Blood Coagul Fibrinolysis. 1994;5:205–10.
15. Andersson O, Blomback M, Bremme K, Wramsby H. Prediction of changes in levels of haemostatic variables during natural menstrual cycle and ovarian hyperstimulation. Thromb Haemost. 1997;77: 901–4.
16. Richard-Davis G, Montgomery-Rice V, Mammen EF, et al. In vitro platelet function in controlled ovarian hyperstimulation cycles. Fertil Steril. 1997;67:923–7.
17. Lox C, Canez M, Prien S. The influence of hyperestrogenism during in vitro fertilization on the fibrinolytic mechanism. Int J Fertil Womens Med. 1998;43:34–9.
18. Magnani B, Tsen L, Datta S, Bader A. In vitro fertilization. Do short-term changes in estrogen levels produce increased fibrinolysis? Am J Clin Pathol. 1999; 112:485–91.
19. Curvers J, Nap AW, Thomassen MC, Nienhuis SJ, Hamulyak K, Evers JL, Tans G, Rosing J. Effect of in vitro fertilization treatment and subsequent pregnancy on the protein C pathway. Br J Haematol. 2001; 115:400–7.
20. Harnett MJ, Bhavani-Shankar K, Datta S, Tsen LC. In vitro fertilization-induced alterations in coagulation and fibrinolysis as measured by thromboelastography. Anesth Analg. 2002;95:1063–6.
21. Westerlund E, Henriksson P, Wallén H, Hovatta O, Wallberg KR, Antovic A.Thromb Res. Detection of a procoagulable state during controlled ovarian hyperstimulation for in vitro fertilization with global assays of haemostasis. 2012;130(4):649–53.
22. Bar J, Orvieto R, Lahav J, et al. Effect of urinary versus recombinant follicle stimulating hormone on platelet function and other hemostatic variables in controlled ovarian hyperstimulation. Fertil Steril. 2004;82:1564–9.
23. Phillips LL, Gladstone W, Vande Wiele R, et al. Studies of the coagulation and fibrinolytic systems in hyperstimulation syndrome after administration of human gonadotropins. J Reprod Med. 1975;14: 138–43.

24. Kodama H, Fukuda J, Karube H, et al. Status of the coagulation and fibrinolytic systems in ovarian hyperstimulation syndrome. Fertil Steril. 1996;66:417–24.

25. Rogolino A, Coccia ME, Fedi S, et al. Hypercoagulability, high tissue factor and low tissue factor pathway inhibitor levels in severe ovarian hyperstimulation syndrome: possible association with clinical outcome. Blood Coagul Fibrinolysis. 2002;14:27–282.

26. Bergh PA, Navot D. Ovarian hyperstimulation syndrome: a review of pathophysiology. J Assist Reprod Genet. 1992;9:429–38.

27. Koninckx PR, Heyns W, Verhoeven G, Van Baelen H, Lissens WD, et al. Biochemical characterization of peritoneal fluid in women during the menstrual cycle. J Clin Endocrinol Metab. 1980;51:1239–44.

28. Koninckx PR, Renaer M, Brosens IA. Origin of peritoneal fluid in women: an ovarian exudation product. Br J Obstet Gynaecol. 1980;87:177–83.

29. Donnez J, Langerock S, Thomas K. Peritoneal fluid volume and 17 bestradiol and progesterone concentrations in ovulatory, anovulatory and postmenopausal women. Obstet Gynecol. 1982;59:687–92.

30. Sealey JE, Atlas SA, Glorioso N, Manapat H, Laragh JH. Cyclical secretion of prorenin during the menstrual cycle: synchronization with luteinizing hormone and progesterone. Proc Natl Acad Sci U S A. 1985;82:8705–9.

31. Derkx FH, Alberda AT, Zeilmaker GH, Schalekamp MA. High concentrations of immunoreactive renin, prorenin and enzymatically-active renin in human ovarian follicular fluid. Br J Obstet Gynaecol. 1987; 94:4–9.

32. Lightman A, Tarlatzis BC, Rzasa PJ, Culler MD, Caride VJ, NegroVilar AF, et al. The ovarian renin-angiotensin system: renin-like activity and angiotensin II/III immunoreactivity in gonadotropin-stimulated and unstimulated human follicular fluid. Am J Obstet Gynecol. 1987;156:808–16.

33. Geva E, Jaffe RB. Role of vascular endothelial growth factor in ovarian physiology and pathology. Fertil Steril. 2000;74:429–38.

34. Cluroe AD, Synek BJ. A fatal case of ovarian hyperstimulation syndrome with cerebral infarction. Pathology. 1995;27:344–6.

35. Togay-Isikay C, Celik T, Ustuner I, Yigit A. Ischaemic stroke associated with ovarian hyperstimulation syndrome and factor V Leiden mutation. Aust N Z J Obstet Gynaecol. 2004;44:264–6.

36. Demirol A, Guven S, Gurgan T. Aphasia: an early uncommon complication of ovarian stimulation without ovarian hyperstimulation syndrome. Reprod Biomed Online. 2007;14:29–31.

37. Song TJ, Lee SY, Oh SH, Lee KY. Multiple cerebral infarctions associated with polycystic ovaries and ovarian hyperstimulation syndrome [letter]. Eur Neurol. 2008;59:76–8.

38. Bartkova A, Sanak D, Dostal J, et al. Acute ischaemic stroke in pregnancy: a severe complication of ovarian hyperstimulation syndrome. Neurol Sci. 2008; 29:463–6.

39. Bauersachs RM, Manolopoulos K, Hoppe I, et al. More on: the 'ART' behind the clot – solving the mystery. J Thromb Haemost. 2007;5:438–9.

40. Salomon O, Schiby G, Heiman Z, et al. Combined jugular and subclavian vein thrombosis following assisted reproductive technology: new observation. Fertil Steril. 2009;92(2):620–5.

41. American Society for Reproductive Medicine. Ovarian hyperstimulation syndrome. Fertil Steril. 2008;90:S188–93.

42. Royal College of Obstetricians and Gynaecologists. The management of ovarian hyperstimulation syndrome, green-TOP guideline no 5. London: RCOG Press; 2006.

43. Kearon C, Akl EA, Comerota AJ, Prandoni P, Bounameaux H, Goldhaber SZ, Nelson ME, Wells PS, Gould MK, Dentali F, Crowther M, and Kahn SR. Antithrombotic therapy for VTE Disease. Antithrombotic Therapy and Prevention of Thrombosis, 9th ed: American College of Chest Physicians Evidence-Based Clinical Practice Guidelines. Chest 2012;141(2)(Suppl):e419S–e494S.

44. Arya R, Shehata HA, Patel RK, Sahu S, Rajasingam D, Harrington KF, Nelson-Piercy C, Parsons JH. Internal jugular vein thrombosis after assisted conception therapy. Br J Haematol. 2001;115:153–5.

45. Hignett M, Spence JE, Claman P. Internal jugular vein thrombosis: a late complication of ovarian hyperstimulation syndrome despite mini-dose heparin prophylaxis. Hum Reprod. 1995;10:3121–3.

46. McGowan BM, Kay LA, Perry DJ. Deep vein thrombosis followed by internal jugular vein thrombosis as a complication of in vitro fertilization in a woman heterozygous for the prothrombin 30 UTR and factor V Leiden mutations. Am J Hematol. 2003;73:276–8.

47. Mathur R, Evbuomwan I, Jenkins J. Prevention and management of ovarian hyperstimulation syndrome. Curr Obstet Gynaecol. 2005;15:132–8.

48. Baglin T, Gray E, Greaves M, Hunt BJ, Keeling D, Machin S, Mackie I, Makris M, Nokes T, Perry D, Tait RC, Walker I, Watson H. Clinical guidelines for testing for heritable thrombophilia. British Journal of Haematology. 2010;149:209–20.

49. Grandone E, Colaizzo D, Lo Bue A, Checola MG, Cittadini E, Margaglione M. Inherited thrombophilia and in vitro fertilization implantation failure. Fertil Steril. 2001;76:201–2.

50. Qublan HS, Eid SS, Ababneh HA, Amarin ZO, Smadi AZ, Al-Khafaji FF, Khader YS. Acquired and inherited thrombophilia: implication in recurrent IVF and embryo transfer failure. Hum Reprod. 2006;21: 2694–8.

51. Azem F, Many A, Yovel I, Amit A, Lessing JB, Kupferminc MJ. Increased rates of thrombophilia in women with repeated IVF failures. Hum Reprod. 2004;19:368–70.

52. Coulam CB, Jeyendran RS, Fishel LA, Roussev R. Multiple thrombophilic gene mutations are risk factors for implantation failure. Reprod Biomed Online. 2006;12:322–7.

53. Balasch J, Fabregues F, Creus M, Reverter JC, Carmona F, Tassies D, Font J, Vanrell JA. Pregnancy: antiphospholipid antibodies and human reproductive failure. Hum Reprod. 1996;11:2310–5.

54. Vaquero E, Lazzarin N, Caserta D, Valensise H, Baldi M, Moscarini M, Arduini D. Diagnostic evaluation of women experiencing repeated in vitro fertilization failure. Eur J Obstet Gynecol Reprod Biol. 2006;125:79–84.

55. Miyakis S, Lockshin MD, Atsumi T, Branch DW, Brey RL, Cervera R, Derksen RHWM, De Groot PG, Koike T, Meroni PL, et al. International consensus statement on an update of the classification criteria for definite antiphospholipid syndrome (APS). J Thromb Haemost. 2006;4:295–306.

56. Buckingham KL and Chamley LW. A critical assessment of the role of antiphospholipid antibodies in infertility. J Reprod Immunol 2009;80:132–45

57. Qublan H, Amarin Z, Dabbas M, Farraj AE, Beni-Merei Z, Al-Akash H, Bdoor AN, Nawasreh M, Malkawi S, Diab F, Al-Ahmad N, Balawneh M, Abu-Salim A. Low-molecular weight heparin in the treatment of recurrent IVF-ET failure and thrombophilia: a prospective randomised placebo-controlled trial. Hum Fertil (Camb). 2008;11(4):246–53.

58. Mancini A, Milardi D, Di Pietro ML, Giacchi E, Spagnolo AG, Di Donna V, De Marinis L, Jensen L. A case of forearm amputation after ovarian stimulation for IVF-ET. Fertil Steril. 2001;76(1): 198–200.

59. McGovan B, Kay L, Perry D. DVT followed by internal jugular vein thrombosis as a complication of IVF in a woman heterozygous for the prothrombin 3'UTR and factor V Leiden mutations. Am J Hematol. 2003; 73:276–8.

Index

H. Cohen, P. O'Brien (eds.), *Disorders of Thrombosis and Hemostasis in Pregnancy*,
DOI 10.1007/978-1-4471-4411-3, © Springer-Verlag London 2012

Printed by Printforce, the Netherlands